T0366464

MEDICAL APHORISMS

TREATISES 6-9

◆

## THE MEDICAL WORKS
## OF MOSES MAIMONIDES

Medical Aphorisms: Treatises 1–5

Medical Aphorisms: Treatises 6–9

On Asthma

◆   ◆   ◆

*Forthcoming Titles*

Abridgments of the Works of Galen

Commentary on Hippocrates' Aphorisms

Medical Aphorisms: Treatises 10–15

Medical Aphorisms: Treatises 16–21

Medical Aphorisms: Treatises 22–25

Medical Aphorisms: Indexes and Glossaries

On Asthma, Volume 2

On Coitus

On Hemorrhoids

On Poisons and the Protection against Lethal Drugs

The Regimen of Health

*Maimonides*

# Medical Aphorisms
# Treatises 6–9

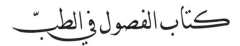

*A parallel Arabic-English edition*
*edited, translated, and annotated by*

## Gerrit Bos

◆ ◆ ◆

PART OF THE MEDICAL WORKS
OF MOSES MAIMONIDES

*Brigham Young University Press* ◆ *Provo, Utah* ◆ *2007*

LIBRARY OF CONGRESS CATALOGUING-IN-PUBLICATION DATA

Maimonides, Moses, 1135–1204.
   [Kitāb al-fuṣūl fī al-ṭibb. Treatises 6–9. English & Arabic]
   Medical aphorisms. Treatises 6–9 : a parallel Arabic-English
edition = Kitāb al-fuṣūl fī al-ṭibb / Maimonides ; edited, translated,
and annotated by Gerrit Bos.
     p.  cm.—(The medical works of Moses Maimonides)
     Includes bibliographical references and index.
     ISBN–13: 978–0–8425–2664–7 (alk. paper)
     ISBN–10: 0–8425–2664–1
     I. Bos, Gerrit, 1948– II. Title. III. Title: Kitāb al-fuṣūl fī al-ṭibb.
IV. Title: Fuṣūl fī al-ṭibb. V. Series.
     R128.3. M62513   2006
     610.92—dc22                            2006101770

PRINTED IN THE UNITED STATES OF AMERICA.

1 2 3 4 5 6 7 8 9    13 12 11 10 09 08 07
*First Edition*

TO JAN BOS

*In Fond Memory*

# Contents

❖   ❖   ❖

## *Kitāb al-fuṣūl fī al-ṭibb* (Medical Aphorisms)

❖   ❖   ❖

Bibliographies *(continued)*

# Sigla and Abbreviations

## Arabic Manuscripts

**A**    Ayasofia 3631, Galen, *Fī al-ḥarakāt al-muᶜtāṣa* (forthcoming edition and translation G. Bos and V. Nutton).

**C**    Cairo, *Dalʾat ṭibb* 550, Arabic translation of Galen, *In Hippocratis De aere aquis locis commentarius*, forthcoming edition by G. Strohmaier.

**G**    Gotha, orient. 1937, fols. 6–273, *K. al-fuṣūl fī l-ṭibb*.

**L**    Leiden 1344, Or. 128,1, fols. 1–140, *K. al-fuṣūl fī l-ṭibb*.

**P**    Paris, Bibliothèque nationale, héb. 1210, fols. 1–130, *K. al-fuṣūl fī l-ṭibb*.

**E**    Escorial, Real Bibliotheca de El Escorial 868, fols. 117–26, *K. al-fuṣūl fī l-ṭibb*.

**Es**    Escorial, Real Bibliotheca de El Escorial 869, fols. 176–1, *K. al-fuṣūl fī l-ṭibb*.

**H**    Paris 2853, *K. fī manāfiᶜ al-aᶜḍāᶜ (De usu partium)*, Arabic translation by Ḥubaysh, revised by Ḥunayn.

**O**    Oxford, Bodleian, Uri 412, Poc. 319, cat. Neubauer 2113, *K. al-fuṣūl fī l-ṭibb*.

**Ox**    Oxford, Bodleian, Hunt. Donat 33, Uri 423, cat. Neubauer 2114, *K. al-fuṣūl fī l-ṭibb*.

**W**    Wellcome Or. 14a, *K. al-mawāḍiᶜ al-ālima (De locis affectis)*, Arabic translation by Ḥunayn.

## Hebrew Translations

**B**    Berlin Or. Qu. 512, *Pirḳe Mosheh bi-refuʾah*, Hebrew translation by Zeraḥyah Ben Isaac Ben Sheʾaltiel Ḥen.

**M**    Munich 111, *Pirḳe Mosheh bi-refuʾah*, Hebrew translation by Zeraḥyah Ben Isaac Ben Sheʾaltiel Ḥen.

**N**      Paris, Bibliothèque nationale, héb. 1173, *Pirḳe Mosheh bi-refu'ah*, Hebrew translation by Nathan ha-Me'ati.

**Oh**     Oxford, Bodleian, Mich. Add. 42, cat. Neubauer 2117, *Pirḳe Mosheh bi-refu'ah*, Hebrew translation by Nathan ha-Me'ati.

**Z**      Both Zeraḥyah translations (**B** & **M**) taken together.

A superscripted 1 after a siglum (e.g. **Es¹**) indicates a note in the margin of that manuscript. A superscripted 2 indicates a note above the line.

## Other

**Bo**     Maimonides, *Aphorismi*, ed. Bologna 1489 (Latin).

**CMG**   Corpus Medicorum Graecorum.

**m**      Maimonides, *Pirḳe Mosheh*, Hebrew translation by Nathan ha-Me'ati, ed. Muntner.

**r**       Maimonides, *Aphorisms*, English translation by Rosner.

◆  ◆  ◆

< >      supplied by editor, in Arabic and Hebrew text

[  ]      supplied by translator, in English text

*add.*     added in

*om.*     omitted in

(!)       corrupt reading

(?)       doubtful reading

## Transliteration and Citation Style

Transliterations from Arabic and Hebrew follow the romanization tables established by the American Library Association and the Library of Congress (*ALA-LC Romanization Tables: Transliteration Schemes for Non-Roman Scripts*. Compiled and edited by Randall K. Barry. Washington, D.C.: Library of Congress, 1997; available on-line at www.loc.gov/catdir/cpso/roman.html).

Passages from the *Aphorisms* are referenced by treatise and section number (e.g., 3.12). Maimonides' introduction is designated as treatise 0.

# Foreword

Brigham Young University and its Middle Eastern Texts Initiative are pleased to sponsor and publish the Medical Works of Moses Maimonides. The texts that appear in this series are among the cultural treasures of the world, representing as they do the medieval efflorescence of Arabic-Islamic civilization—a civilization in which works of impressive intellectual stature were composed not only by Muslims but also by Christians, Jews, and others in a quest for knowledge that transcended religious and ethnic boundaries. Together they not only preserved the best of Greek thought but enhanced it, added to it, and built upon it a corpus of scientific and philosophical understanding that is properly the inheritance of all the peoples of the world.

As an institution of The Church of Jesus Christ of Latter-day Saints, Brigham Young University is honored to collaborate with Gerrit Bos and other members of the academic community in bringing this series to fruition, making these texts available to many for the first time. In doing so, we at the Middle Eastern Texts Initiative hope to serve our fellow human beings of all creeds and cultures. We also follow the admonition of our own religious tradition, to "seek . . . out of the best books words of wisdom," believing, indeed, that "the glory of God is intelligence."

—Daniel C. Peterson
—D. Morgan Davis

# Preface

This edition of Maimonides' *Medical Aphorisms: Treatises 6–9* is the second volume in a series of five volumes which will cover all 25 treatises. It is part of a project initiated at University College London, sponsored by the Wellcome Trust, and now proceeding at the Martin Buber Institute for Jewish Studies at the University of Cologne with the financial support of the Deutsche Forschungsgemeinschaft. The project aims to provide critical editions in the original Arabic together with English translations of Maimonides' medical works that are still in manuscript. Thus, it includes: *Treatise on Asthma* (in print), *Medical Aphorisms: Treatises 1–5* (in print), *Commentary on Hippocrates' Aphorisms, Treatise on Poisons,* and *Abridgments of the Works of Galen.* At a later stage we hope to look closely at those works that have appeared in critical editions in the original Arabic in the past but may now have to be revised in light of new manuscript findings. These works are: *Treatise on Hemorrhoids, Treatise on Coitus, Regimen of Health,* and *On the Elucidation of Some Symptoms and the Response to Them*—all of them edited by Kroner. The series is published by the Middle Eastern Texts Initiative at Brigham Young University's Neal A. Maxwell Institute for Religious Scholarship. On this occasion I thank Professor Daniel C. Peterson, under whose direction this series has been prepared for publication, and his colleague, Dr. D. Morgan Davis, for their enthusiastic support of the project and dedication to it. Thanks are also due to Muḥammad S. Eissa, Angela C. Barrionuevo, and Steve Stay for their diligent editorial work. I thank Professor Vivian Nutton for his help in correctly understanding and translating many Greek passages from the Galenic medical corpus, Professor Lawrence I. Conrad for his careful review of the manuscript, and Dr. Carsten Schliwski for his general assistance in the preparation of this volume.

# Translator's Introduction

In my edition of volume one of the *Medical Aphorisms*, I have said but little concerning the kind of compilation with which we are dealing. It was merely characterized as "a medical work."[1] However, recent research has shown beyond any doubt that it is nothing other than a notebook[2] and thus in a way comparable to the *K. al-ḥāwī fī al-ṭibb* (Liber continens) composed by the Arab physician al-Rāzī (865–932), which consists of the author's personal notes from a wide range of sources together with his clinical observations which he edited in some twenty-five volumes. Therefore, Maimonides' *Medical Aphorisms* cannot be characterized as a medical equivalent of the *Mishneh Torah,* as was noted rightly by Herbert Davidson in his extensive description of the character of this work.[3]

Since the publication of volume one of the *Medical Aphorisms*, I have found further evidence of the interest Maimonides' compendium excited in Jewish circles. For example, it is quoted throughout MS Berlin, Staats-bibliothek, fol. or. 3088, which dates from the fourteenth to fifteenth centuries and is a collection of notes by an anonymous physician based on a large variety of medical works.[4] Further, Jacob Zahalon, the seventeenth-century Jewish physician in Rome, quotes from the Hebrew translation of the *Medical Aphorisms* that he himself prepared from a Latin translation.[5]

This second volume of the *Medical Aphorisms* compiled by Moses Maimonides (1138–1204)[6] covers treatises 6–9. The central subjects of these treatises are prognosis (treatise 6), aetiology (treatise 7), therapy (treatise 8), and pathology (treatise 9). Most of these aphorisms are based on the works of Galen, and some of them go back to works that are no longer available in the original Greek. An example is the following aphorism (9.11):

> If a person is overcome by a torpor, one should grasp the tip of the tongue and press it completely down. Then one should look for a receptacle with a narrow opening, and put some [moist] liquid food into it,

and put it into the mouth on the base [of the tongue], and pour the contents into the esophagus.

This aphorism is a quotation from Galen's *De motibus manifestis et obscuris*.[7] It only survives in Latin translations by Mark of Toledo and Niccolò da Reggio[8] and in an Arabic translation entitled *Fī al-ḥarakāt al-muʿtāṣa*, which has been preserved in MS Ayasofia 3631 and which Vivian Nutton and I are currently editing. Muntner assumed that the Hebrew translation of Galen's *De motibus,* entitled *Ba-Tenuʿot ha-mukhraḥot,* was identical with Galen's *Peri thorakos kai pneumonos kineseos*.[9] This assumption was adopted by Rosner as well.[10]

On other occasions, Maimonides quotes from a Galenic treatise that has been preserved only in an Arabic translation, but the text he adduces is missing from that particular translation. For example, in aphorism 7.51 he quotes from Galen's *De somno et vigilia:*

> If someone wishes to raise his voice, he should become accustomed to opening his mouth wide so that he lets in much air, which widens the larynx. Then the voice is loud. Therefore, those whose larynx is narrow and small have thin, small voices without any substance so that they are broken off quickly. But those whose larynx is wide have a full and powerful voice. Children, women, and eunuchs have thin and weak voices because their larynx is small.

Since Maimonides' quotation is not found in the Arabic translation, Nabielek, the editor and translator of the Arabic, concludes that the original text of this treatise must have been more extensive.[11] But, paradoxically, he also concludes that because of the similarity between Maimonides' text and the relevant passage from Oribasius' *Collectiones medicae,* the latter must have been the source that Maimonides copied from.[12]

In one case Maimonides quotes from a text under a title that, to the best of my knowledge, has not been preserved in bibliographical literature.[13] Maimonides remarks (9.101):

> Much flesh and fat is harmful and detrimental and gives the body an ugly appearance and hinders its activities and movements. Therefore, those suffering from it should travel a lot and do much walking in the sun. Travel over sea is especially good because the sea air dissolves the [superfluous] moistures. One should let them eat foods with little nourishment, such as vegetables, and that which contains heat, such as onions, garlic, and salted fish, and that which strengthens but does not moisten, such as lean roasted meat. One should not let them bathe

in any hot water except that of thermal springs. One should keep them a little thirsty and make their bodies firm in any possible manner. *De extenuatione corporum pinguium.*

Although the Arabic title of this aphorism, *Fī tahzīl al-ajsād al-ᶜabla* (A Slimming [Diet] for Fat Bodies) is reminiscent of Galen's *Fī al-tadbīr al-mulaṭṭif* (On the Thinning Diet), it is unlikely that the former title is just another name for the latter, especially because this quotation does not appear in the text edited by Kalbfleisch.[14] Moreover, the difference in title between the two Galenic treatises is supported by both Hebrew translators. The title *Fī tahzīl al-ajsād al-ᶜabla* is translated by Nathan ha-Meᵓati as *Be-hattakhat ha-geshamim he-ᶜavim we-ha-shemenim* and by Zeraḥyah Ben Isaac Ben Sheᵓaltiel Ḥen as *Be-harazut(!) ha-guf ha-shamen,* while *Fī al-tadbīr al-mulaṭṭif* is translated by both as *Ba-hanhagah ha-medaqdeqet.*

Sometimes Maimonides quotes from treatises ascribed to Galen whose authenticity is doubtful. This is the case for his quotations from *De signis mortis* (On the Signs of Death). An example is aphorism 6.48:

> [If someone has] hiccups accompanied by tumors in the liver, or if someone cannot sleep and suffers from tremors, or if someone suffering from dropsy is affected by cough, he will die. But if someone suffering from hiccups is affected by spontaneous strong sneezing, his hiccups will stop. *De signis mortis.*[15]

The title of this treatise does not appear in the bibliographical literature—neither under the authentic works nor under the spurious ones.[16] The Arabic tradition has preserved a number of texts under this title ascribed to Hippocrates, all in manuscript, whose central subject is the signs of death derived from the efflorences of the skin. Another text under this title, ascribed to the famous philosopher and physician al-Kindī, is actually an adaptation of a part of Hippocrates' *Prognostics.*[17]

On many occasions Maimonides quotes from Pseudo-Galen's commentary on Hippocrates' *De humoribus.* These quotations are a valuable source for reconstructing part of Galen's genuine commentary to this book since the text edited by Kühn is, as Deichgräber showed, a Renaissance forgery.[18] On that occasion Deichgräber also demonstrated that Maimonides' quotations closely parallel those of Oribasius. But at the same time he warned against too much optimism since both Maimonides and Oribasius tend to abbreviate the original Galenic text.[19] Deichgräber's analysis of these quotations also shows the importance of the availability of a critical original text of Maimonides' *Medical Aphorisms.* In one case he uses a corrupt Latin version to conclude that Maimonides' summary of the Galenic text is unique for its brevity insofar as it summarizes fifteen lines of the Greek text into one line.[20]

The importance of a critical edition of Maimonides' *Medical Aphorisms* based on all the available manuscripts can also be demonstrated from Deller's translations of Maimonides' quotations from Galen's *Commentaries on Hippocrates' Epidemics.*[21] His translation is sometimes faulty as it is based on a corrupt version found in the only manuscript consulted for the Arabic edition: MS Leiden 128, 1. An example of such a corruption is provided in aphorism 6.40:

> In some acute diseases bad humors stream to the lungs in such a small quantity that they do not cause any tumors, and they are excreted with the sputum. Someone with no experience will think that the patient suffers from pleurisy or pneumonia, but this is not the case.

Instead of "stream to" *(yataḥallab ilā)* he translates *lösen sich auf in* ("dissolve in"), following the corruption of MS Leiden: *yataḥallal.*[22] And in aphorism 7.66, where Galen speaks about pain with numbness occurring in the legs in the case of kidney diseases, his version for "pain with numbness" is "Schmerz verbunden mit Kälte" (pain associated with cold) since he follows MS **L**, which does not read *al-wajᶜ maᶜa khadr,* but *al-wajᶜ maᶜa bard.*

As I showed in the introduction to the edition of *Medical Aphorisms* 1–5, abbreviation is an important and recurring element in the reformulation process of the Galenic text. A telling example is provided by aphorism 6.37. When speaking about the different symptoms of phrenitis, Galen mentions the following: "Sometimes we observe an irrational forgetfulness, when, for instance, the patients ask for the urinal but do not pass their water, or forget to surrender the urinal after having voided." This text is summarized by Maimonides as "short-term memory loss." It is clear that Maimonides has summarized and abbreviated nonessential parts of this text. Yet it is important to note that Maimonides is not satisfied with merely quoting or reformulating the Galenic text. In several instances Maimonides reflects upon these texts and arrives at certain conclusions regarding their correctness or incorrectness. Thus he remarks in aphorism 7.72 that Galen's statement that one cannot know the cause for laughing when the armpits are tickled or when one sees funny things is correct, because "laughter is a specific characteristic of human beings," and the specific characteristics of any species of animals, plants, and minerals cannot be explained etiologically.

On other occasions Maimonides adds certain elements to the Galenic text, possibly because he feels they are essential. Thus, after recording Galen's statement (9.57) "if someone suffers from indigestion and the like and from a burning in the stomach that is so severe that one imagines that there is an inflamed tumor there, he will benefit from a salve prepared with quince oil," Maimonides adds that it is his practice to heat the oils in a double vessel[23] because their strength is lost if they are heated in any other way. This addition to the Galenic text gives us a glimpse into Maimonides' personal medical practice. It shows that at least occasionally he prepared his own salves and medicaments. As we know from the Cairo Genizah, even famous physicians did this. On the other hand, numerous prescriptions have been preserved in the Genizah that are undoubtedly instructions given to a pharmacist.[24]

In another addition to the Galenic text (6.94), Maimonides deals with a central aspect of the medical art: the role of nature. He remarks that just as the leading faculty in the body, i.e., nature, acts sparingly with regard to the eminent activities in the body and always strives to maintain the more eminent one(s) even at the cost of the less eminent one(s), in the same way it acts sparingly with regard to changes in the complexion of the patient. Maimonides concludes that precise knowledge of the role of nature and its effects can provide the physician with data important for medical prognosis.

In one case Maimonides' personal comment on a Galenic text gives us additional valuable information about his training as a doctor. In aphorism 8.69 Galen remarks that the occurrence of diabetes is very rare and that he personally has only seen it twice. Maimonides observes:

> I too have not seen it in the Maghreb, nor did any one of the elders under whom I studied inform me that he had seen it. However, here in Egypt I have seen more than twenty people affected by this disease in approximately ten years. This is to show you that this disease occurs mostly in hot countries. Perhaps the water of the Nile, because of its sweetness, plays a role in this.

This report provides further evidence for the supposition that Maimonides got some sort of formal medical training, which usually involved studying under other physicians, while residing in the Maghreb.[25] Maimonides' personal note is similar to one found in *On Asthma*, where he remarks, in the context of his account of a notorious medical incident that occurred in the Maghreb, that he studied under a learned physician.[26] Moreover, in the same book he refers to his contacts with physicians from the Maghreb.[27]

Maimonides' additions to the Galenic text may also take the form of critical comments. This is clearly the case when he reviews Galen's discussion of syncope and its causes in aphorism 7.8. Maimonides criticizes him for not being consistent and for being unmethodical in his classification of these causes. Maimonides' criticism is aimed at Galen's discussion in *De methodo medendi:* Galen first mentions a variety of causes for syncope[28] and then remarks that there are four other causes.[29] Maimonides exclaims: "I wish I knew why only some causes were given a specific number but not all of them" (7.8). He adds that what is even worse is that Galen, after naming these four causes, remarks: "And if you want, you can add another one to these four—namely, a bad temperament of the organs" (7.8). Maimonides is once again implicitly critical of Galen when he concludes that since syncope is so serious and since it is often followed by death, a physician should have a comprehensive knowledge of all its causes and should mention all of them. If he has a detailed and exact knowledge of its causes, he knows how to treat the illness when it occurs. And in the name of Abū Marwān b. Zuhr he adds that "when a patient suffers from syncope without the physician knowing about it until it [actually] happens and without his having warned against it, then this physician is undoubtedly responsible for the death of the patient" (7.8). The matter is of such vital importance in Maimonides' eyes that he resorts to a rearrangement and systematization of Galen's discussion in *De methodo medendi.* Thus, Maimonides summarizes in aphorism 7.10:

> Syncope is a quick collapse of the faculties of the body. The existence and permanence of the faculties in their essential nature depends on the balance of the pneumata, humors, and organs in their quantity and quality. The cause for the collapse of the faculties (namely, syncope) can be a quantitative or qualitative change of the pneumata, or a quantitative or qualitative change of the humors, or a quantitative or qualitative change of the organs. The causes of syncope can thus be limited to these three classes, and since each class consists of two subclasses (namely, a quantitative change and a qualitative change) we [actually] have six classes.

On another occasion Maimonides criticizes Galen for making contradictory statements. This is the case in aphorism 7.44, where he quotes the following text from Galen's *De tremore, palpitatione, rigore et convulsione:* "If the cold [only] moves the outer surface [of the body] with a shivering movement and shakes it at the moment of the onset of a fever attack but does not move the whole body, this is called 'shivering.' Shivering is an affliction occurring only to the skin. Its significance for the skin is the same as that of rigor for the whole body." Maimonides then exclaims: "But in *De febribus* 2 he said that shivering is something less severe than rigor but more cold."

In aphorism 9.127 Maimonides criticizes Galen for not mentioning Aristotle's discussion of the topic of spasms occurring to babies in the latter's *De animalibus* 9. In this case Maimonides' critique is unjustified, as Galen dealt with this matter extensively in his commentary on Hippocrates' *Prognostics* 3.34.

These examples show clearly that in spite of the high regard he had for Galen as a physician, Maimonides surely was not blind to his faults. This of course becomes especially clear from his systematic criticism of Galen in treatise 25.

## Manuscripts of the *Kitāb al-fuṣūl fī al-ṭibb* (Medical Aphorisms)

This work is known to be extant in the following manuscripts:

(1) Gotha 1937 (**G**); fols. 6–273 (fol. 7 numbered twice); Naskh script.[30] A considerable section of the text, from treatise 6.10 beginning at *al-mawt* to treatise 7.16 ending at *min amthāl*, is missing.[31] According to the colophon on fol. 273a that appears after aphorism 25.55, the scribe copied the text from a copy of the original redaction of the work by Maimonides' nephew Abū l-Maʾālī (or al-Maʾānī) ibn Yūsuf ibn ʿAbdallāh.[32] The scribe adds that he found a note in the text in which Abū al-Maʾālī remarks that in the case of the first twenty-four *maqālāt*, Maimonides would correct his autograph notes and that he, Abū al-Maʾālī, would then make a fair copy and correct it in Maimonides' presence, but that the text of the twenty-fifth *maqāla* was copied by him in the beginning of the year 602 A.H. (August 1205), after the death of Maimonides, so that the latter had not been able to do the redaction.[33] Although it is generally agreed that this manuscript has preserved the best readings,[34] it should be noted that in some cases the text suffers from a certain carelessness by the scribe, resulting in mistakes and corruptions. Moreover, the language he employs is sometimes extremely vulgar and colloquial. Another characteristic of the text is that the central issue of many aphorisms is indicated in the margin using terminology derived from the text itself.

(2) Leiden 1344, Or. 128, 1 (**L**); 140 fols; Maghribī script.[35] The manuscript ends on fol. 140b with the following colophon:

> This is the end of the treatise—praise be to God—and the completion
> of the *Book of Aphorisms* of the most perfect and unique scholar Mūsā
> ibn Maymūn ibn ʿUbaydallāh, the Israelite, from Cordova—may God
> be pleased with him. The copying [of the text] was completed in the
> month of May of the year 1362 according to the calendar of al-Ṣufr
> in the city of Ṭulayṭula—may God protect it—and it was written by
> Yūsuf ibn Isḥāq ibn Shabbathay, the Israelite.

The calendar of al-Ṣufr was common in Spain, especially among Christians, and started about thirty-eight years before the Christian calendar.[36]
Accordingly the manuscript was written in May 1324 in Toledo. More
than any of the other manuscripts, the language of this manuscript con-
forms to the rules of classical Arabic; the influence of vulgarization is
thus far less pronounced than in the others. Just like **G**, it has many marginal catchwords.

(3) Paris BN, héb. 1210 (**P**); fols. 1–130; Judeo-Arabic; no date.[37] The
manuscript only contains treatises 1–9 (the last one incomplete), part of
treatise 24, and the major part of treatise 25. Missing also is 8.42–59.
According to the inscription on fol. 1v, the manuscript was once in the
possession of R. Meir ha-QNZ(?)Y. The text has been copied carefully,
so that there are only a few mistakes; the top section has been stained to
the degree that the first lines are hard to read.

(4) Escorial, Real Biblioteca de El Escorial 868 (**E**); fols. 117–26
(numbered in reverse order); Maghribī script.[38] According to the colophon
this text was copied in the city of Qalʿa (=Alcalá) by Mūsā b. Sūshān
al-Yahūdī in the year 1380 (read 1389), corresponding to the year 5149
since the creation. The text offers a close parallel to manuscript **L**, both
having many otherwise unique readings in common, including whole
paragraphs not appearing in any other manuscript—as, for instance,
treatise 3.52. Like **L**, it has several marginal catchwords, but not as many
and they use different terminology.

(5) Escorial, Real Biblioteca de El Escorial 869 (**S**); fols. 176–1
(numbered in reverse order); Oriental script; no date.[39] The text, missing an important section between treatises 10.27 and 21.73, finishes at
treatise 25.58. The text of this manuscript is closely related to **G**.

(6) Oxford, Bodleian, Uri 412, Poc. 319, cat. Neubauer 2113 (**B**); fols.
1–123; Judeo-Arabic; Sephardic semicursive script.[40] According to the
colophon, the text was copied by Makhluf ben Rabbi Shmuʾel he-Ḥazan
DMNSY (from Mans?) and completed on the 11th of Elul 5112 (1352
CE).[41] Numerous Hebrew versions derived from the Hebrew translation

prepared by Nathan ha-Meʾati have been added to the text above the lines and in the margins. The text suffers from many omissions and corruptions, but does provide some unique variant readings—as, for instance, treatise 3.22: المركب; a unique, correct version according to Galen's τῆς συνθέτου σαρκὸς.[42]

(7) Oxford, Bodleian, Hunt. Donat 33, Uri 423, cat. Neubauer 2114 (**O**); 78 fols; Sephardic semicursive script; ca. 1300 (?).[43] The text begins with treatise 23, continues with the end of treatise 6 to treatise 24 (incomplete, large sections missing), and ends with 12. The text has a few catchwords, some in Judeo-Arabic and some in Arabic. This manuscript is closely related to manuscripts **E** and **L**, sharing many characteristic readings.

(8) Oxford, Bodleian, Hunt. 356, Uri 426, cat. Neubauer 2115; 107 fols., Oriental semicursive script; late thirteenth century.[44] The text runs from treatise 10 (but not its beginning) to treatise 24 (but not to its end). A later scribe has falsified some of the headings of this manuscript.[45]

(9) Göttingen 99. This manuscript was copied by Antonius Deussingius in the year 1635 in Leiden from **L**.[46]

(10) Istanbul Velieddin 2525.[47]

For this edition of Maimonides' *Medical Aphorisms: Treatises 6–9*, the following manuscripts have been consulted: Gotha 1937 (**G**), Leiden 1344 (**L**), Paris 1210 (**P**), Escorial 868 (**E**) and 869 (**S**), and Oxford 2113 (**B**) and 2114 (**O**). These manuscripts can be divided into two main groups: **S** and **G**; and **E**, **L**, **B**, **O**, and **P**. The edition is based mainly on **G** and **S**.

The edition of the text of Maimonides' *Medical Aphorisms* in Arabic rather than Hebrew characters has been inspired by Maimonides' own practice. According to recent scholarship there is reason to assume that Maimonides composed a first draft of his medical works intended for private use in Arabic written in Hebrew characters, since it was easier for him to write in Hebrew than in Arabic, and that these works were subsequently transcribed in Arabic characters when intended for public use. Thus, Stern remarks that "all of Maimonides' medical works were naturally published in Arabic script, since otherwise they would have been of no use to the non-Jewish public," and adds that Maimonides first drafted the text in Hebrew script, because the Hebrew script was easier for him, and then had it transcribed into the Arabic script.[48] Stern's point of view has been endorsed by Hopkins, who remarks that although we have sporadic autograph examples of his Arabic handwriting, Maimonides always used the Hebrew script when writing privately.[49] Other scholars have expressed (partly) different opinions in this matter. Meyerhof remarks that Maimonides composed all of his medical writings in Arabic, probably using Arabic characters, since he had nothing to hide from the Muslims.[50] Blau suggests that Jewish authors addressing a general public including Muslims and Christians (as in the case of medical writings) might have used Arabic script, but when addressing a Jewish audience might have used Hebrew characters.[51] Langermann remarks that it seems likely that many of Maimonides' medical writings were originally written in Arabic characters and only afterwards transcribed into Hebrew characters.[52]

For editing the Arabic text, which is written in the Middle Arabic typical for this genre, I have adhered to the guidelines formulated by Oliver Kahl. Morphological and syntactical errors and even grievous offences against the grammar of classical Arabic have neither been included in the apparatus nor changed or corrected at all. Nor have peculiarities of orthography been included in the critical apparatus. They have either been spelled in the conventional way or allowed to remain in their original forms, as the need for clarity dictated.[53] In some cases I have corrected Maimonides' Arabic version on the basis of corresponding Arabic translations of the Galenic treatises he quotes.

As with *Medical Aphorisms: Treatises 1–5*, this edition is supplemented by a list of faulty readings and translations selected from Muntner's edition[54] of Nathan ha-Meʾati's Hebrew translation[55] and from Rosner's English translation.[56] Since Muntner's edition is eclectic, lacks a critical apparatus, and is replete with errors and therefore unreliable, his readings have been compared throughout with those of manuscript Paris BN hébr. 1173 (**N**), the manuscript on which he based his edition.[57] The list also provides the versions of these particular readings by Zeraḥyah Ben Isaac Ben Sheʾaltiel Ḥen (**Z**), derived from his translation of the *Medical Aphorisms*.[58] It is my hope that on the basis of this list and ideally on the basis of future critical editions of these translations, it will be possible to provide critical evaluations of the translation activity of these two prominent translators. With this goal in mind, a supplemental volume containing a comparative Arabic-Hebrew-English glossary of technical terms used in the *Medical Aphorisms* is being planned. The Hebrew terms will also be listed alphabetically in a separate index with reference to the comparative glossary. Thus, the glossary and indexes may contribute to our knowledge of medieval Hebrew medical terminology. They may also be used to amplify dictionaries of the Hebrew language, or, ideally, to create a dictionary devoted to this particular area. During the compilation of the glossary it has became increasingly clear that both of the Hebrew translations are based on an Arabic text represented by manuscripts **E** and **L**, since they share several unique readings. As explained in the first volume of *Medical Aphorisms*, Zeraḥyah's translation is characterized by many terms in Latin and Romance, and these will be registered in a separate index.

MEDICAL APHORISMS

TREATISES 6–9

◆

*In the name of God,*
*the Merciful, the Compassionate.*
*O Lord, make [our task] easy*

# The Sixth Treatise

*Containing aphorisms concerning the other prognostic signs*

1. One can predict whether an apoplexy will be severe and necessarily fatal or weak and curable—though it is difficult—from the condition of the respiration. For when the movement of the respiration is totally missing, so that it cannot be noticed, it is the fastest [killing][1] kind of apoplexy there is. When the patient breathes with difficulty[2] and strain, the apoplexy is also severe and deadly, but to a lesser degree than the first. If the patient breathes without strain and difficulty but in an irregular and disordered way, the apoplexy is still severe but less so than the previous [example]. And when his respiration is to some extent orderly— although irregular—and is unstrained, the apoplexy is weak and can be cured if proper procedure is followed. *In Hippocratis Aphorismos commentarius* 2.[3]

2. Cessation of respiration occurs either from the weakness of the power which moves the chest or from a severe cold that overpowers the brain.[4] *In Hippocratis Aphorismos commentarius* 4.[5]

بسم الله الرحمن الرحيم ربّ يسّر

# المقالة السادسة

تشتمل على فصول تتعلّق بسائر الاستدلالات

١ . يستدلّ على السكتة هل هي قوية فتقتل ضرورة أو ضعيفة فيمكن برؤها وإن كان

٥      ذلك عسيرا من حال التنفّس فإن عدم حركة التنفّس بالجملة حتّى لا يدرك كان ذلك أوحى

ما يكون من السكتة وإن كان يتنفّس باستكراه ومجاهدة فهي أيضا قوية ومهلكة وهي دون

الأولى . وإن كان تنفّسه بغير جهد ولا استكراه لكنّه تنفّسا مختلفا غير لازم لنظام فهي

أيضا سكتة قوية إلا أنّها دون التي قبلها . ومتى كان تنفّسه لازما لنظام ما فإن كان مختلفا ولا

جهد فيه فهذه سكتة ضعيفة ويمكن برؤها إن تأتّيت في أمرها . في شرحه لثانية الفصول .

٢ . بطلان التنفّس إمّا من ضعف القوّة المحرّكة للصدر وإمّا من برد مفرط يغلب على

١٠      الدماغ. في رابعة الفصول .

---

١ بسم . . . يسّر] om. ELOP ‖ ٥ أوحى] أقوى O ‖ ٦ يتنفّس] التنفّس O ‖ ٨ فإن]
ولا O ‖ ٩ أمرها] أمره EsG ‖ ١٠ إمّا] إنّا O

3. When mental confusion[6] results from heat but without [superfluous] matter, it is similar to the mental confusion caused by drinking wine. When it results from yellow bile, it is accompanied by worry and fear.[7] When the yellow bile becomes increasingly burnt, the confusion turns into madness. *In Hippocratis Aphorismos commentarius* 6.[8]

4. Sneezing in the case of chronic diseases, except for diseases of the chest and lungs, is a good sign because it indicates coction and great strength of the expulsive faculty of the brain. *In Hippocratis Prognostica commentarius* 2.[9]

5. A special symptom for the kind of overfilling that is commensurate to strength is weight, and [a special symptom] for the kind of overfilling that is commensurate to the vessels is stretching. *De venae sectione.*[10]

6. Sometimes the outer vessels are full and stretched while the inner ones are not, as happens when it is hot and when one takes a bath in hot water. At other times the outer vessels are empty while the inner vessels are full, as happens when it is extremely cold. Fullness of the outer vessels, then, is only an indication of an excess of blood when two conditions are fulfilled: (1) the temperatures of the inside and the outside of the body are equal and (2) no unusual heat such as, for instance, ardent fever pervades the body. *De plenitudine.*[11]

7. Four different types of biting chymes occur in our bodies. The type from which itch develops is only slightly biting. A more biting type is the one that produces shivering. The one that is extremely biting causes rigor, and the one that is [even] more biting causes a sensation of ulceration.[12] *De plenitudine.*[13]

8. Says Moses: Consider how only the [different] degrees of sharpness of the humor are turned by him [Galen] into that which forms the difference between itch, shivering, and rigor. There is another distinction between these diseases that he makes in his treatise *De tremore, palpitatione, rigore et convulsione.*[14] I do not say that what he said here is contrary to what he said there. Rather, both statements are true, and by

٣. ما كان من اختلاط العقل من حرارة فقط من غير مادّة فهو شبيه بالاختلاط الكائن من شرب النبيذ. وما كان منه من مرّة صفراء فيكون معه همّ وحرص وإن تزيّدت الصفراء احتراقا صار الاختلاط إلى طريق الجنون. في سادسة الفصول.

٤. العطاس في الأمراض المزمنة غير أمراض الصدر والرئة علامة جيّدة لأنّه يدلّ على النضج وعلى شدّة القوّة الدافعة التي في الدماغ. في شرحه لثانية تقدمة المعرفة.

٥. الدليل الخاصّ بالصنف من الامتلاء الذي يكون بحسب القوّة الثقل. وأمّا بالصنف من الامتلاء الذي يكون بحسب الأوعية فالتمدّد. في مقالته في الفصد.

٦. قد تكون العروق الظاهرة ممتلئة متمدّدة ولا تكون الداخلة كذلك كما يعرض في الحرّ أو عند الاستحمام بالماء الحارّ. وقد تكون العروق الظاهرة فارغة خالية وتكون الداخلة ممتلئة كما يعرض في البرد الشديد. فليس امتلاء العروق الظاهرة دليل على كثرة الدم حتّى تشترط شرطان: أحدهما استواء حرارة باطن البدن وخارجه والثاني أن لا تعمّ البدن حرارة غريبة كالحمّى المحرقة. في مقالته في الكثرة.

٧. الكيموسات اللذّاعة تحدث فينا على أربعة أصناف فإنّ الذي يحدث منها الحكّة هو الذي يلذع لذعا يسيرا والذي يحدث الاقشعرار هو الذي يحدث لذعا أكثر من ذلك والذي يفرط لذعه يحدث النافض والذي يلذع أشدّ من هذا يحدث حسّ التقريح. في مقالته في الكثرة.

٨. قال موسى: تأمّل كيف جعل الفرق بين الحكّة والقشعريرة والنافض مراتب حدّة الخلط فقط وفي ذلك زيادة تبيين ممّا قاله في مقالته في الرعدة والاختلاج والنافض والتشنّج. ولست أقول إنّ هذا الذي قاله هنا خلاف الذي قاله هناك بل القولين صحيحين وبمجموعهما

---

٢ تزيّدت] تزيد O ‖ ٣ إلى] على O ‖ ٦ بالصنف (1st)] في الصنف Es ‖ الذي يكون] الذي يكون O. om ‖ ٨ متمدّدة] ممتدّة L ‖ كذلك] كذاك O ‖ ٩ أو عند] عند EL ‖ ١٤ يسيرا] شديدا EL ‖ ١٨ تبيين] لك add. OP ‖ ١٩ هذا الذي] ما EL

combining them one obtains a complete picture of what he means—
namely, that the places where the biting [chyme affects the body] vary
according to the strength or weakness of the pungency of the chyme. In
his treatise *De tremore, palpitatione, [rigore et convulsione,]* he explains that
in the case of shivering, the biting humor is confined to the skin alone,
while that which produces rigor is in all the parts beneath the skin, and
this is correct.[15] We should also understand from his statement that itch
occurs in the upper layers of the skin and not in those that are adjacent
to the flesh.

9. When sweet phlegm increases in a man's body, he sleeps much.
When acid phlegm increases, he suffers from hunger. When salty phlegm
becomes dominant, he suffers from thirst. When raw phlegm becomes
dominant, it stops the thirst. *De plenitudine.*[16]

10. Pus is formed when innate heat overwhelms those humors in
order to coct and transform them. At that time an extremely severe
pain arises and sometimes even fever. [When the fever is already there],
it rises. When the pus is expelled, the organ becomes completely healthy
again, as it was before. When the innate heat disappears and becomes
weak and does not want at all to coct those humors [because of its
weakness], no pus originates in the organ and neither pain nor fever
develops. Rather, it becomes putrefied and corrupted to such a degree
that one is often forced to cut the corrupted part off completely. So it
may occur with someone that the fever dies away once fatal signs appear
in him and there is no indication of improvement. *In Hippocratis Epidemiarum* 3.1.[17]

11. Sometimes melancholic delusion[18] and phrenitis[19] occur together.
An indication of this is that at one time [someone suffering from it] talks
continually, for this is a symptom of phrenitis, while at another time
he is continually silent, for this is a symptom of melancholic delusion.
*In Hippocratis Epidemiarum* 3.3.[20]

يكمل المعنى . وذلك أنّ مع اختلاف شدّة اللذع وضعفه تختلف أيضا مواضعه . وذلك أنّه بيّن في مقالته في الرعدة والاختلاج أنّ الخلط اللذّاع في حال الاقشعرار هو في الجلد وحده والفاعل للنافض هـو في الأعضاء كلّها التي تحت الجلد وهذا صحيح . وكذلك ينبغي لنا أيضا أن نفهم من قوله أنّ الحكّة هي في سطح الجلد لا فيما يلي اللحم منه .

٩ . يعرض للناس مع البلغم الحلو اذا كثر كثرة النوم واذا كثر البلغم الحامض عرض لهم الجـوع واذا غلب البلغم المالح عرض لهم العطش واذا غلب البلغم الفجّ أبطل العطش . في مقالته في الكثرة والامتلاء .

١٠ . تولّـد المدّة يكون عند اسـتيلاء الحرارة الغريزية علـى تلك الأخلاط لتنضجها وتحيلها . وأشـدّ ما يكون الألم والوجع حينئذ وقد تحدث الحمّى أو تشـتدّ حينئذ . واذا خرجت المدّة بقي العضو سـليما كما كان . فأمّا اذا ضاعت الحرارة الغريزية وخارت ولم تـرم أصـلا إنضاج تلك الأخلاط لضعفها فإنّ العضو لا يتولّد فيه مدّة ولا وجع يعتّد به ولا حمّى بل يعفن ويفسـد حتّى يضطرّ كثيرا ليقطعه بأسره . وعلى هذا المثال يعرض لمن تقلع عنـه الحمّى بعد أن قد ظهرت فيـه دلائل تدلّ على الموت ولم تظهر دلائل تنذر بحير . في الأولى من شرحه لثالثة ابيذيميا .

١١ . قد يتركّب الوسـواس السوداوي والسرسـام وعلامة ذلك أن يحدث مرّة كلام كثير وهو من علامة السرسـام ومرّة صمت دائم وهو من أعلام الوسواس السوداوي . في الثالثة من شرحه لثالثة ابيذيميا .

٢ مقالتـه ] قولـه O || ٤ أنّ ] فـي EL | هي | أنّها ] E? || ٧ والامتلاء [ om. ELOP || ١٠ ضاعت ] حاعت Es : حـارت Es¹G || ١٢ ليقطعه [ قطعه OP || ٣،١٣– ٢٩،١ المـوت . . . أمثـال [ om. G || ١٤ ابيذيميـا ] افيذيميا EL || ١٥–١٧ قد . . . ابيذيميا [ om. E || ١٦ علامة ] علامات LO | أعلام ] علامات L || ١٧ ابيذيميا ] افيذيميا L

12. A surplus of watery moisture is expelled in one of three ways: through diarrhea, through the urine, or through the sweat. It is expelled by nature in whatever way she prefers, to the exclusion of the other two ways. Therefore, when the feces are retained[21] and the urine is withheld while the crisis [of the disease] is near, the patient is necessarily afflicted by rigor followed by sweating. *In Hippocratis Epidemiarum* 6.1.[22]

13. The secretion that dries up on the eyes from conjunctivitis and the sweat that dries up on the face until it becomes like dust are bad signs. Similarly, darkening of vision in acute diseases indicates that the faculty of vision is perishing. *In Hippocratis Epidemiarum* 6.1.[23]

14. When the signs are very bad[24]—whether symptoms or diseases[25]—but the face is fine, very similar to its natural condition, it is a good sign. When the signs are minor[26]—whether symptoms or diseases—and the face is very different from its natural condition, it is a bad sign. *In Hippocratis Epidemiarum* 6.2.[27]

15. There is no person suffering from melancholy who does not fear something that is not frightening or who does not have an imaginary fear of something that is not frightening. When the affliction is mild, he is only afraid of one thing; but when it is more severe, he is afraid of two or three things. And some are afraid of everything because of the severity of the affliction. *In Hippocratis Epidemiarum* 6.3.[28]

16. In his treatise "That the faculties of the soul follow the temperament of the body," Galen has mentioned that the word "melancholy" means "fear" in the Greek language.[29]

١٢ . استخراج الرطوبة المائية إذا كثرت تكون بأحد ثلاثة أنحاء إمّا باختلاف أو بـول أو بعرق . وأيّ جهة من هذه الثلاث مالت إليها دفعتها الطبيعة منها وحبستها من الجهتين الأخريين ولذلك إذا اعتقل البطن واحتبس البول وكان البحران قريب المجيء وجب ضرورة أن يصيب المريض نافض يتلوه عرق . في الأولى من شرحه لسادسة ابيديميا .

٥          ١٣ . ما يجفّ على العينين من الرمص وعلى الوجه من العرق حتّى يصير ذلك كالغبار دليــل ردىء وكذلك ظلمة البصر في الأمراض الحــادّة دليل على موت القوة الباصرة . في الأولى من شرحه لسادسة ابيديميا .

١٤ . إذا كانت الأمارات شديدة الرداة أعراضا كانت أو أمراضا وكان الوجه حسنا شــبيها جدّا بحاله الطبيعية فذلك دليل محمود . وإذا كانت الأمارات يسيرة سواء كانت
١٠          أمراضــا أو أعراضا وكان الوجه مغايرا جدّا لحاله الطبيعية دلّ ذلك على أمر ردىء . في الثانية من شرحه لسادسة ابيديميا .

١٥ . ليس يخلو أحد من أصحاب المالنخوليا من استهوال شيء غير هائل أو التخيّل في شــيء غير هائل أنّه هائل وإن كانت العلّة خفيفة كان الشيء الهائل عنده شيئًا واحدا وإن كانت العلّة أعظم اسـتهول اثنين أو ثلاثة ومنهم من يهوله كلّ شــيء لعظم علّته . في
١٥          الثالثة من شرحه لسادسة ابيديميا .

١٦ . وقد ذكــر في مقالتــه فـي أنّ قوى النفس تابعة لمــزاج البــدن أنّ معنى المالنخوليا في لغة اليونان التفزّع .

---

٤ ابيديميا ] افيديميا EL ‖ ٦ دليل (2nd) L ‖ ٧ ابيديميا ] افيديميا EL ‖ ٩ بحاله ] بالحال EL ‖ ١٠ مغايرا ] مغادرا Es : مغادرا OP : مجاورا ?E | لحاله ] للحال L ‖ ١١ ابيديميا ] افيديميا EL ‖ ١٢ ليس ] لم O | المالنخوليا ] المالنخونيا EL ‖ ١٣ الهائل ] هو add. O ‖ ١٥ ابيديميا ] افيديميا EL ‖ ١٦–١٧ وقد . . . التفزّع ] E¹ ‖ ١٧ المالنخوليا ] المالنخونيا E¹LO

17. When a nosebleed occurs while one is in a healthy condition, it is a sign of bad blood. In this case one should provide the body with good blood by means of fattening kinds of food that do not fill the vessels, such as starch,[30] Roman wheat,[31] milk, young[32] cheese, meat of piglets, and meat of lambs and kids. Sometimes a nosebleed occurs when one is healthy because of an excess of blood. *In Hippocratis Epidemiarum* 6.3.[33]

18. The eyes give a most correct and certain indication of the strength of the body, when one opens them and looks at them[34] with regard to its state of health.[35] *In Hippocratis Epidemiarum* 6.4.[36]

19. The colors of the tongue indicate the dominating chyme in the region of the stomach. The colors of the urine indicate the dominating chyme in the vessels in the regions of the liver, kidneys, and urinary bladder. A dry tongue—that is, a tongue dominated by severe dryness, indicates that ardent fever has burnt the blood. *In Hippocratis Epidemiarum* 6.5.[37]

20. Fat and sweet foods are only enjoyable to a healthy person. Sick people enjoy the rest of the foods apart from these two, commensurate with their illness. *In Hippocratis Epidemiarum* 6.5.[38]

21. Perspiration on the forehead, neck, and chest area indicates weakness of the animal faculty.[39] Frequent dyspepsias and the consumption of things that are partly putrefied[40] and of coarse bread produce abdominal worms.[41] *In Hippocratis Epidemiarum* 6.7.[42]

١٧ . الرعاف الذي يكون في حال الصحّة يدلّ على رداة الدم فينبغي أن يودع البدن دما محمودا بالأغذية المغلّظة التي لا تملأ العروق مثل النشاستج والخندروس واللبن والجبن الرطب ولحم الخنانيص ولحوم الخرفان والجداء . وقد يحدث الرعاف في حال الصحّة من كثرة الدم . في الثالثة من شرحه لسادسة ابيديميا .

١٨ . العينان يدلّان على قوة البدن أصحّ دلالة وأوكدها إذا كان نظرهما وفتحهما على ٥ حال الصحّة . في الرابعة من شرحه لسادسة ابيديميا .

١٩ . ألوان اللسان تدلّ على الكيموس الغالب في المعدة ونواحيها وألوان البول تدلّ على الكيموس الغالب في العروق التي في نواحي الكبد والكلى والمثانة . واللسان القحل وهو الذي قد غلب عليه اليبس الشـديد يدلّ على حمّـى محرقة قد أحرقت الدم . في الخامسة من شرحه لسادسة ابيديميا . ١٠

٢٠ . ليس يستلذّ الطعام الدسم والطعام الحلو إلا من كان صحيحا فقط . وأمّا المرضى فيستلذّون سائر الطعوم غير هذين بحسب مرضهم . في الخامسة من شرحه لسادسة ابيديميا .

٢١ . عرق الجبهة والرقبـة وناحية الصدر يدلّ على ضعف القوة الحيوانية . وترادف التخم وأكل الأشـياء التي قد شـابهها عفونة والخبز الخشـن يولّد الحيات في البطن . في السابعة من شرحه لسادسة ابيديميا . ١٥

---

٢ المغلّظة] الغليظة Es ‖ ٤ ابيديميا] افديميا EL ‖ ٥–٦ العينـان . . . ابيديميا] افيديميا L ‖ يـدلّان] om. E ‖ أصحّ دلالة وأوكدها] add. LP | دلالة صحيحة] om. LP ‖ ٦ ابيديميا] افيديميا L ‖ ٨ الكيموس] الخلط EL ‖ ١٠ الخامسـة] ثامنة Es ‖ ابيديميا] افيديميا EL ‖ ١١ ليـس] لم O | والطعام الحلو والحلـو EL ‖ ١٢ ابيديميا] افيديميا EL ‖ ١٣ وناحية] وناحي L ‖ ١٥ ابيديميا] افيديميا EL

22. Sometimes physicians are mistaken by thinking that the blood has increased in the body, while [in reality] it has not increased. Rather, because of the heat of the air, or anger, or fever, something happens to it that is similar to the high tide of the sea. Conversely, they sometimes think that the blood has diminished, while [in reality] it has not diminished. Rather, because of the cold that pushes the blood inwards, something happens to it that is similar to the low tide of the sea. *In Hippocratis De humoribus commentarius* 1.[43]

23. Black bile is a very deadly [sign][44] when it appears in the spittle, vomit, urine, or excrements. After it [in danger] comes yellow bile when it appears pure. The other humors are less dangerous when they appear in a pure form in one of these [excretions]. *In Hippocratis De humoribus commentarius* 2.[45]

24. If a growth appears on the tongue similar to the black seed of the castor oil plant,[46] the patient will not survive to the second day. If a black tumor similar to the seed of the bitter vetch[47] appears on the fingers of the hands in combination with any fever and severe pain, the patient will die on the fourth day. *De signis mortis.*[48]

25. Black chymes are often excreted with vomiting or diarrhea, and this can in some cases be a good sign. But when black bile is excreted with vomiting or diarrhea, it indicates death; its development in the body is a fatal sign, since it originates from the burning of the turbid and residual part of the blood. When it originates from the burning of yellow bile, the damage to the organs is [even] worse because it corrodes them. It is the clearest sign of [impending] death. *De atra bile.*[49]

26. If someone has long experience with these two chymes, he will easily understand the reason why the excretion of black bile from the body indicates [impending] death. Someone who is inexperienced will either be amazed, or he will not believe it and say: How can the excretion of something that is extremely harmful have a fatal effect on the body? *De atra bile.*[50]

٢٢ . قد ينخدع بعض الأطبّاء ويظنّ أنّ الدم كثر في البدن وما كثر بل عرض له من حرّ
الهواء أو الغضب أو الحمّى ما يعرض للبحر من المدّ . ويظنّ أنّه قد نقص وما نقص بل يعرض له
من البرد الذي دفعه لداخل البدن ما يعرض للبحر من الجزر . في أولى من شرحه للأخلاط .

٢٣ . المرّة السوداء قتّالة جدّا متى ظهرت في البزاق أو في القيء أو في البول أو في
البراز . ثمّ من بعدها المرّة الصفراء إذا ظهرت صرفة . وسائر الأخلاط أقلّ غائلة إذا ظهرت
صرفة في أحد هذه . في الثانية من شرح الأخلاط .

٢٤ . إن ظهر على اللسان بثر شبه حبّ الخروع أسود لم يعش لليوم الثاني . وإن ظهر
على أصابع اليدين مع أيّ حمّى كانت ورم أسود شبه حبّ الكرسنّة مع وجع شديد مات
في الرابع . في مقالته في علامات الموت .

٢٥ . كثيرا ما يخرج بالقيء أو بالإسهال كيموسات سود وقد يدلّ خروجها على
خير عدّة مرّات . وأمّا المرّة السوداء فمتى خرجت بالقيء أو بالإسهال دلّت على الهلاك
لأنّ تولّدها في البدن هو دليل الهلاك وهي تتولّد من احتراق عكر الدم وثفله . وإن
تولّدت من احتراق الصفراء كانت نكايتها للأعضاء أشدّ وتأكلها أكلا وهي أدلّ على
الهلاك . في مقالته في المرّة السوداء .

٢٦ . من طالت تجربته لأمر هذين الكيموسين فإنّه يسهل عليه معرفة السبب
الذي له صار خروج المرّة السوداء من البدن دالّا على الهلاك . وأمّا غير المجرّب
فيتعجّب أو ينكر ويقول كيف صار خروج الشيء الضارّ المفرط الضرر مهلكا
للبدن . في مقالته في المرّة السوداء .

١ كثـر (1st)] كثيـر EL || ٢ الحمّى] الحمّام Es || ويظنّ] أبضا add. L || ٤ قتّالة] قاتلة
Es | متـى] مـا add. EL | البزاق] البصاق EL | القيء] أو في الأخلاط add. L ||
٥ صرفة] في أحد هذه add. EL || ٧ شبه] شبيه O | لم يعش] لا يعيش O | لليوم الثاني]
اليوم والثاني Es : إلى اليوم الثاني EL || ١٦ دالّا] : دلالة Es²  Es : دالّا

27. When the disease is stronger than the strength of the patient, he will most certainly die. One can take as an indication the observation of increasing signs of the lack of coction day by day. The more one looks closely into the disease, the more fatal signs will appear. *De morborum temporibus.*[51]

28. It is impossible at any time that a sign becomes visible that indicates coction but does not indicate something very good. When the flow of blood from a site in the body, perspiration, and tumors[52] occur at the proper time, the body may benefit from it, but otherwise not. *De crisibus* 1.[53]

29. Signs of coction indicate that the patient will recover and do not necessarily indicate that a crisis will befall him, because the illness will dissolve slowly. *De crisibus* 1.[54]

30. The superfluity in each part of the body indicates its condition. When it is cocted, it indicates that it is healthy; and when it is not cocted, it indicates that it is ill. The urine indicates the coction in the vessels, the excrements indicate the coction in the abdomen, and the sputum indicates the coction in the respiratory organs. *De crisibus* 1.[55]

31. To lie on one's back and to open one's mouth, which are the only ways through which snoring takes place, indicate weakness or drunkenness or relaxation.[56] *De motu musculorum.*[57]

32. The madness occurring from melancholic humor is not as bad as that arising from the burning of bilious humor. Phlegmatic humor does not cause any madness at all. *In Hippocratis Aphorismos commentarius* 6.[58]

٢٧. متى كان المرض أعظم من القوة مات المريض لا محالة وتستدلّ على ذلك بأنّك تـرى علامات عدم النضج متزيّدة يوما بعد يـوم. وكلّ ما أمعن في المرض تظهر العلامات المهلكة. في مقالته في أوقات الأمراض.

٢٨. ليس يمكن في وقت من الأوقات أن تظهر علامة تدلّ على النضج فلا تدلّ على خير عظيم. أمّا الدم الذي يجري من موضع من البدن والعرق والخراجات فإن ظهرت في وقتها فقد ينتفع بها وإن ظهرت في غير وقتها لم ينتفع بها. أولى البحران.

٢٩. علامات النضج تدلّ على أنّ المريض يسلم وليست تدلّ ضرورة على أنّ المريض يأتيه بحران لأنّه قد يتحلّل المرض قليلا قليلا. في الأولى من البحران.

٣٠. فضلة كلّ عضو تدلّ على حاله فإن كانت نضيجة دلّت على صحّته وإن كانت غير نضيجة دلّت على سـقمه. والبول يدلّ على النضج الـذي يكون في العروق والبراز يـدلّ على النضج الـذي يكون في البطن والنفث يدلّ على النضج الذي يكون في آلات التنفّس. في الأولى من البحران.

٣١. الاسـتلقاء على القفاء وفتح الفم الّذان لا يكون الغطيط إلا بهما هما علامتان يدلّان على ضعف أو على سكر أو استرخاء. في الثانية من كتاب حركات العضل.

٣٢. الجنون الكائن من الخلط السوداوي أقلّ رداة من الكائن من احتراق الصفراء. أمّا الخلط البلغمي فلا يحدث عنه جنون بتّة. في شرحه لسادسة الفصول.

٥ موضـع] مواضع L | ظهـرت] تظهر O ‖ ٨ يأتيه بحران] Es² : يهلك Es | لأنّه . . . البحـران] om. O | في الأولـى] Es² : أوّل ثانية Es ‖ ١٣ الـذان] الذي LO : التي E ‖ ١٤ سكر] سكنة Es : سدد O ‖ ١٥ الكائن (1st) . . . الصفراء] الحادث من احتراق الصفرة أقلّ رداة من الكائن من المرّة السوداء O | الصفراء] المرّة السوداء L : والجنون الكائن من احتراق الصفراء أقلّ رداة من الكائن من المرّة السوداء add. E Es P

33. When the substance of the brain is dominated by the humor that results from the burning of yellow bile, delusion and delirium[59] associated with fever[60] arise from it. The delirium that occurs at the climax of ardent fevers is caused by hot vapors arising to the brain. *De locis affectis* 3.[61]

34. If someone is affected by vertigo and dizziness, he blacks out and falls down on minor occasions[62] when he is turned around.[63] If someone is affected by vertigo or dizziness that originates from the cardia of the stomach, it is preceded by palpitation of the heart[64] and nausea. *De locis affectis* 3.[65]

35. Some of those who suffer from migraine feel the sensation of the pain on the outside of the skull, while others feel it deep inside the head. The pain of [those suffering from] migraine ends at the line that separates the two halves of the head. When the pain originates from wind, it comes necessarily with tension; if it originates from bilious superfluities, the patient feels a sharp pain. When it arises from an excess of humors, he has a feeling of heaviness next to the pain. When the [feeling of] heaviness is combined with a red complexion and heat, then those excessive humors are hot; but when it is not accompanied by redness and heat, those excessive humors are not hot. *De locis affectis* 3.[66]

36. The movement of the tongue comes from the seventh pair of cranial nerves. When an affliction occurs to both the right part and the left part of the brain at the origin of this seventh pair, the patient is in danger of suffering a stroke.[67] When one part of it is afflicted, the patient will suffer from paralysis.[68] This paralysis will harm the movement of one half of the tongue and it may also harm other parts of the body beneath the head at different times. *De locis affectis* 4.[69]

٣٣. إذا غلب على جرم الدماغ الخلط الذي يحدث عن احتراق الصفراء فيحدث
عنه الوسواس والاختلاط الذي يكون مع حرارة. فأمّا الاختلاط الذي يحدث في منتهى
الحمّيات المحرقة فحدوثه عن ما يصعد إلى الدماغ من الأبخرة الحارّة. في ثالثة التعرّف.

٣٤. من يصيبه السدر والدوار تظلم أعينهم ويسقطون ويدار بهم من أسباب يسيرة.

٥ ومن يصيبه السدر والدوار من قبل فم المعدة يتقدّم ذلك خفقان وتهوّع. في ثالثة التعرّف.

٣٥. أصحاب الشقيقة بعضهم يجد مسّ الوجع خارجا عن القحف وبعضهم يجده
يبلغ إلى عمق الرأس. والوجع ينتهي في الشقيقة إلى الحدّ الفاصل بين شقّي الرأس. فإن
كان الوجع عن ريح فيكون مع الوجع تمدّد لازم له وإن كان عن فضول مرارية وجد وجعا
لذّاعا فإن كان عن كثرة من الأخلاط فيحسّ معه بثقل فإن اقترن مع الثقل حمرة ولون وحرارة
١٠ فتلك الأخلاط الكثيرة حارّة وما لم تكن معه حمرة ولا حرارة فتلك الأخلاط الكثيرة غير
حارّة. في ثالثة التعرّف.

٣٦. حركة اللسان من الزوج السابع من أزواج عصب الدماغ وإذا اعتلّ الجزء الأيمن
والجزء الأيسر من الدماغ في موضع منشأ هذا الزوج السابع فصاحب العلّة على خطر
من *السكتة. وإن اعتلّ منه شقّ واحد فالأمر يؤول بصاحبه إلى الاسترخاء وهذا
١٥ الاسترخاء يضرّ بحركة اللسان في نصفه وقد يضرّ أعضاء آخر أسفل من الرأس في وقت
دون وقت. رابعة التعرّف.

---

٢ مع] عن Es | حرارة] جذام EL | الاختلاط الذي يحدث] الاختلاطات التي
تحدث EsP | المحرقة] Es² : المفرطة EsP | ٣ المحرقة] Es² | فحدوثه] Es | فحدوثها EsP | ٥ يصيبهم]
Es | ٨ ريح] رياح EL | له] om. L | وجد] يجد L | ١٣ الزوج] الجزء ELP ||
١٤ *السكتة] السبات ELOP : السكات Es || ١٥–١٦ في وقت دون وقت] om. Es

37. The signs of phrenitis are sixteen: sleeplessness or disturbed sleep, delirium manifesting itself gradually, acute fever which never subsides, short-term memory loss,[70] lack of thirst, very aggressive and insolent behavior[71] shown by the patient, deep and intermittent respiration,[72] a small and hard pulse, picking flocks from garments or straw from walls,[73] roughness of the tongue, pain in the back of the head, a dry discharge from the eyes[74] and an acid tear streaming from one eye, drops of blood dripping from the nose, acoustic hallucinations,[75] loss of the sensation of touch throughout the body even [when one is touched] with force,[76] and the patient lies prostrate and is unresponsive to questions. All these symptoms can occur simultaneously, but sometimes only a majority thereof. *De locis affectis* 5.[77]

38. If a nosebleed comes from the side opposite to where the illness is, it is a bad sign. But if it comes from the same side as the illness, it is a good sign. *De crisibus* 3.[78]

39. Just as those animals and plants which grow more rapidly have a shorter life span and those which grow more slowly have a longer life span, so too is the situation regarding fevers and tumors and all other occurrences. That which develops faster is of shorter duration. *In Hippocratis Epidemiarum* 2.1.[79]

40. In some acute diseases bad humors stream[80] to the lungs in such a small quantity that they do not cause any tumors, and they are excreted with the sputum. Someone with no experience will think that the patient suffers from pleurisy or pneumonia, but this is not the case. *In Hippocratis Epidemiarum* 3.1.[81]

41. A malignant cough is one whose cause is either a catarrh which descends from the head, or an ulcer or an abscess[82] in one of the respiratory organs, or matter collecting in the chest. A benign cough originates either from a bad temperament[83] of the respiratory organs or from roughness of the pharynx or trachea. In the case of fevers, when the benign

٣٧ . علامات فرانيطس ستّة عشر علامة وهي السهر أو النوم المضطرب واختلاط العقل ويبدو قليلا بعد قليل والحمّى الحادّة التي لا تلين في وقت من الأوقات والنسيان للأمور الحاضرة وقلّة العطش ويبدو من العليل فضل تهجّم وجرأة، التنفّس العظيم متفاوت، صغر النبض مع صلابة، لقط الزئبر من الثياب أو التبن من الحيطان، خشونة اللسان، وجع مؤخّر الـرأس، يبس العينين وترمّصهما وتدمـع واحدة دمعة حادّة. قطرات دم تقطر من الأنف، السمع الكاذب، بطلان حسّ اللمس من سائر الجسد *وإن يقويه. كون العليل ملقا لا يردّ الجواب إلا بكدّ. وهذه العلامات قد توجد معا وقد يوجد أكثرها. خامسة التعرّف.

٣٨ . الرعاف متـى كان من خلاف الجانب الذي فيه العلّة فليس بمحمود ومتى كان من جانب العلّة فهو محمود. ثالثة البحران.

٣٩ . كما أنّ ما كان من الحيوان والنبات أسـرع نشـء كان أقصر مدّة وما كان أبطأ نشء كان أطول مدّة كذلك الحال في الحمّيات والأورام وسائر ما يعرض. ما كان منها أسرع حركة كان أقصر مدّة. في الأولى من شرحه لثانية ابيديميا.

٤٠ . قـد تتحلّب في بعض الأمراض الحادّة أخـلاط ردئة إلى الرئة ويكون مقدارها يسيرا فلا تحدث ورما وتخرج بالنفث فيظنّ من لا دربة له أنّ بالعليل ذات الجنب أو ذات الرئة وليست به. في الأولى من شرحه لثالثة ابيديميا.

٤١ . السعال الخبيث هو الذي سـببه نزلة تنحدر من الرأس أو قرحة أو خراج في بعض آلات التنفّس أو مادّة تجتمع في الصدر. والسعال السـليم هو الذي يكون من سوء مزاج آلات التنفّس أو من خشـونة الحلق أو من خشـونة قصبة الرئة. والسعال السليم في

---

١ فرانيطس] فرانيس O || ٣ فضل تهجّم وجرأة] قلّة حرارة وتهجّم Es | العظيم متفاوت] عظيم التفاوت Es || ٤ خشونة اللسان] خشونة يسيرة للسان Es || ٥ واحدة دمعة] inv. EL || ٦ السمـع] السرع Es | ٦*وإن يقويه] أويقاربه MSS || ١٢ ابيديميا] افيديميا EL || ١٣ تتحلّب] يتحلّل L || ١٥ ابيديميا] افيديميا EL || ١٧–١٨ أو . . . آلات التنفّس om. O

cough is very strong, it heats the sides of the chest and lungs and increases the strength of the fever and the severity of the thirst. But when [the cough] is weak and occurs only at long intervals,[84] it stimulates the organs to attract a moderate quantity of fine moisture, which diminishes the thirst and the heat of the fever. *In Hippocratis Epidemiarum* 6.2.[85]

42. It has been clarified that bad respiration associated with the movement of all the muscles of the chest and the intercostal muscles has three causes: either a weakness of the power [that moves the muscles of the chest,][86] or a narrowing in the respiratory organs, or heat dominating the heart and the lungs. If the only cause is the domination of heat, the respiration is rapid, strong, and frequent while the air is expelled in puffs of boiling hot air. If the only cause is the weakness of the power [which moves the muscles of the chest], the respiration is neither rapid nor frequent, the air is expelled through the mouth without any puffs whatsoever, and during inhalation one can see the two sides of the nostrils which are called "leaves"[87] contract. This is a strong indication of the weakness of the power. If the only cause is the narrowing in the respiratory organs, one can see the chest expand greatly, and [during] the expansion [the respiration] is rapid and frequent, although the air is expelled freely without puffs. *De locis affectis* 4.[88]

43. When a usual[89] or unusual bad temperament occurs in the lungs, it causes cough. If the regular bad temperament is insignificant, it changes the rhythm of the respiration. But when it is severe and hot, it causes a desire to inhale cold air and to drink something cold. When this lasts for a long time, it causes fever. A cold bad temperament is followed by a desire for hot air and hot drinks as long as it is insignificant. But when it gets worse, the lungs[90] are filled with matter. *De locis affectis* 4.[91]

الحمّيات إن كان شـــديدا قويا أسـخن نواحي الصدر والرئة وزاد في قوة الحمّى وفي شدّة
العطش وإن كان ضعيفا وفي ما بين مدد طويلة حرّك الأعضاء لجذب رطوبة دقيقة معتدلة
الكمّية تنقص من العطش ومن حرارة الحمّى . في الثانية من شرحه لسادسة ابيديميا .

٤٢ . قد تبيّن أنّ ســـوء التنفّس الكائن بتحريـك جميع عضل الصدر وعضل ما بين
الأضــلاع له ثلاثة أسـباب : إمّا ضعف قوة أو ضيـق آلات التنفّس أو حرارة غالبة على
القلب والرئة . فإن كان السـبب اسـتيلاء الحرارة فقط فيكون التنفّس سريعا قويا متواترا
ويكون خروج الهواء بالتنفّس مع نفخة هواء حارّ يغلي . وإن كان السـبب ضعف القوة
فقط فلا يكون التنفّس لا سـريعا ولا متواترا ويخـرج الهواء مطلقا دون نفخة بالفم وترى
المنخرين في دخول الهواء تنقبض طرفاهما المسمّى الورقتين وهذا دليل عظيم على ضعف
القوة . وإن كان السبب ضيق آلات التنفّس وحده فإنّ الصدر تراه ينبسط إلى مسافة كثيرة
ويكون انبساطه سريعا متواترا وخروج الهواء بلا نفخة . رابعة التعرّف .

٤٣ . متى حدث في الرئة سوء مزاج مستوي أو غير مستوي أحدث سعالا وإن كان
سوء المزاج المستوي يسيرا غيّر وزن التنفّس . وإن كان قويا حارّا أحدث شهوة استنشاق
الهواء البارد وشــرب الشيء البارد . وإذا طالت به المدّة أحدث الحمّى . وأمّا سوء المزاج
البارد فيتبعه شهوة الهواء الحارّ وشرب الشيء الحارّ ما دام يسيرا وإذا تزيّد وعظم امتلأت
الرئة موادّا . رابعة التعرّف .

٢ مــدد ] مدّة Es O ‖ ٣ ابيديميا ] افيديميا EL ‖ ٧ نفخة ] وهو add. EL ‖ ٩ طرفاهما ]
أطرافهــا O | الورقتين ] ارنبتــين L(!) ‖ ١٠ كثيــرة ] كبيـرة Es ‖ ١٢ أو غيـر مســتوي ]
وإن ] ومتى EL | om. O

44. The indications of the culmination[92] of pleurisy are that the pain is chronic and that it is not assuaged by the application of warm compresses. Indications of a severe and malignant pleurisy are that the sputum increases in viscosity and that it cannot be expelled because it adheres to the diseased organs and is stuck in them. *In Hippocratis De acutorum morborum [victu et] Galeni commentarius* 1.[93]

45. If someone resembles a person suffering from dropsy in his nature, he is quickly affected by this disease. Similarly, if someone resembles a person suffering from phthisis, soon he will suffer from it, and someone who resembles a person suffering from delusion rapidly develops this disease. This type of analogy can be applied to any disease and to respiratory afflictions, as in the case of someone who moves fast and who [acts like] a fool, for he quickly falls into a delirium. *In Hippocratis Epidemiarum* 6.7.[94]

46. He also said in commentary 3 to *Epidemics* 3: light-witted, troubled,[95] and foolish people become delirious for the slightest reason. But someone with the opposite [nature] only suffers from delirium through a major cause. *In Hippocratis Epidemiarum* 3.3.[96]

47. If someone suffers from a tumor in the liver, his complexion is pale and green. If someone has a tumor in the spleen, his complexion is green and dark. If someone has a tumor in the lungs, his complexion is pale and faded. But this will only be the case if these tumors are not inflamed. *In Hippocratis De humoribus commentarius* 3.[97]

48. [If someone has] hiccups accompanied by tumors in the liver,[98] or if someone cannot sleep and suffers from tremors,[99] or if someone suffering from dropsy is affected by cough, he will die. But if someone suffering from hiccups is affected by spontaneous strong sneezing, his hiccups will stop. *De signis mortis.*[100]

٤٤ . الدلائل التي تدلّ على منتهى ذات الجنب دوام الوجع وأن لا يخفّ منه شـيء بالتكميـد . والدلائل التي تدلّ على عظم ذات الجنـب وخباثتها هي تزيّد البصاق لزوجة وامتناعه من الخروج لالتزاقه ولحوجه في الأعضاء العليلة . في شرحه لأولى الأمراض الحادّة .

٤٥ . من هو بطبيعته يشبه المستسقى فالاستسقاء يسرع إليه وكذلك من هو كالمسلول فالسلّ يسـرع إليه ومن هو كالموسوس فالوسواس يسرع إليه وهو القياس في كلّ علّة وفي أعراض التنفّس كمن هو سـريع الحركة سـفيها فإنّه سـريع الوقوع في اخـتلاط العقل . في سابعة شرحه لسادسة ابيديميا .

٤٦ . وقال أيضا في ثالثة شرحه لثالثة ابيديميا إنّ السخيف من الناس القلق الأخرق يعرض له اضطراب العقل من أدنى سـبب . وأمّا الذي هو على خلاف ذلك فليس يخرج عن عقله إلا بسبب عظيم .

٤٧ . من كبده وارمة يكون لونه أبيض أخضر ولون من طحاله وارم أخضر أسـود . ومـن رئته وارمة يكون لونه أبيض مذبل . وإنّما تكون ألوانهم هكذا إذا كانت أورامهم غير ملتهبة . في شرحه لثالثة الأخلاط .

٤٨ . الفواق مع أورام الكبد ومن كان به سهر فيعرض له كزاز ومن كان به استسقاء فعرض له سعال مات ومن كان به فواق وعرض له عطاس شديد من قبل نفسه انحلّ فواقه . في مقالته في علامات الموت .

١ منـه] معـه O || ٢ وخباثتها] في خباثها Es : وخباثها O | البصـاق] البزاق OP || ٣ لالتزاقـه] لالتصاقه Es || ٦ التنفّس] النفس Es²O || ٧ ابيديميا] افيديميا EL || ٨ في ثالثة شرحه لثالثة] في ثالثة L : في شـرحه لثالثة Es | القلـق الأخرق] الخلق الأخلاق EL || ٩ اضطـراب] اختلاط EL || ١٢ يكون] ترى O : يرى P | مذبـل] مرهل L : مهل E add. EsO ] ردئ ١٤ الكبد]

49. A bad temperament of the heart occurs in one of two ways: either in the moistures specific to the heart or in its solid substance itself. A bad temperament of the moistures is accompanied by palpitation[101] of the entire heart. A bad temperament of the solid heart substance itself is free from palpitation. *De pulsu* 15.[102]

50. Marasmus[103] is mostly caused by [inflamed] tumors[104] in the liver and stomach when not treated properly. *De febribus* 1.[105]

51. An ulcer in the lungs called phthisis causes the nails to become curved as a bow.[106] When the tongue becomes black, it indicates ardent fever. The particular discoloration indicating weakness of the liver is different from the particular discoloration caused by [a disease of] the spleen. *De locis affectis* 1.[107]

52. The indications of hypochondriac melancholia[108] are that the ingestion of food is followed by sour eructations, watery[109] sputum in large quantity, a burning [sensation] in the hypochondria and a gurgling sound[110] not occurring until one hour after the ingestion of food. Despondency[111] and sadness also occur while the mind is affected by something similar to melancholic delusion. Some of these patients develop severe abominal pains, which in a few of them extend to the back. Others vomit their food after some time or the next day. They only find relief through emesis or evacuation of the bowels or a good digestion. *De locis affectis* 3.[112]

53. Contraction[113] of the hypochondria is a special sign of an inflammation of the diaphragm[114] and appears from the very beginning. Similarly, when phrenitis has been established,[115] the hypochondria contracts in the very end. During an inflammation of the diaphragm, respiration is variable; sometimes it is shallow[116] and frequent, and at other times it is deep and similar to groaning.[117] *De locis affectis* 5.[118]

54. The symptoms which always accompany pleurisy are five [in number]: acute fever, goading pain in the side, shallow and frequent respiration, serrated pulse and cough, mostly accompanied by colored sputum. A patient [suffering from this disease] may also cough without sputum. This indicates either imminent death or a prolonged illness. *De locis affectis* 5.[119]

٤٩ . سوء مزاج القلب يكون على ضربين إمّا في الرطوبات التي له خاصّة وإمّا في نفس جرمه الصلب . وسوء المزاج الكائن في رطوباته يكون مع اختلاط من القلب كلّه . وسوء مزاج نفس جرمه الصلب يكون خلوًا من الاختلاط . خامسة عشر النبض .

٥٠ . الذبول أكثر ما يحدث عن أورام الكبد والمعدة إذا لم تعالج بالصواب . في الأولى من الحمّيات .

٥١ . يحدث بسبب القرحة التي تكون في الرئة ويقال لها السلّ تقوّس الأظفار . وإذا اسودّ اللسان فهو دليل على حمّى محرقة . واللون الحائل الدالّ على ضعف الكبد له خصوصية غير خصوصية اللون الحائل الذي سببه الطحال . أولى التعرّف .

٥٢ . علامات المراقّية أن يتبع بعد تناول الطعام جشاء حامض ويزاق رطب كثير المقدار وحرقة في ما دون الشراسيف وقرقرة لا تحدث إلا بعد تناول الطعام بساعة . ويحدث خبث النفس وكآبة ويعرض للعقل مثل أعراض الوسواس السوداوي ويحدث لبعضهم وجع في البطن شديد يبلغ في بعضهم إلى الظهر . وبعضهم يتقيّأ طعامه بعد مدّة أو في اليوم الثاني ولا يجدون راحة إلا بالقيء أو بالبراز أو بجودة الاستمراء . ثالثة التعرّف .

٥٣ . انجذاب الشراسيف إلى فوق علامة خاصّة لورم الحجاب تظهر من أوّل الأمر على المكان . وكذلك إذا استحكم فرانيطس انجذب الشراسيف في آخر الأمر . وفي ورم الحجاب التنفّس مختلف مدّة يصغر ويتواتر ومدّة يعظم ويصير شبيها بالزفرات . خامسة التعرّف .

٥٤ . الأعراض اللازمة لذات الجنب ولا تفارقها خمسة : الحمّى الحادّة والوجع الناخس في الجنب والتنفّس الصغير المتواتر والنبض المنشاري والسعال وهو في الأكثر مع نفث ملوّن . وقد يسعل ولا ينفث وهو يدلّ إمّا على موت عاجل أو على طول من المرض . خامسة التعرّف .

---

٧ وإذا اسودّ] واسوداء EL ‖ ٩ ويزاق] وبصاق L ‖ ١٤ خاصّة] خاصّية EL خاصّة] من] om. O ‖ في EL : om. Es ‖ ١٥ انجذب] انجذبت EL ‖ ١٨ ملوّن]

55. There are eight symptoms of an inflammation in the liver:[120]
burning fever, severe thirst, a total lack of appetite, a tongue which
becomes initially red and then black, vomiting of bile which initially
has the color of egg yolks and then turns verdigris green, a pain in the
right side which extends to the collarbone, especially when the hypochondria is pulled upwards, and occasionally the patient has a mild
cough and a sensation of heaviness inherent to the right side,[121] and he
often complains of [pain in] the ribs of the back if the liver is in its
natural structure attached to those ribs.[122] If the liver itself is not weakened by the inflammation, the patient suffers from constipation.[123] *De
locis affectis* 5.[124]

56. Everyone I observed as suffering from a painful illness of the
esophagus would feel the pain between his shoulders. The reason for
this is that the esophagus stretches along the spinal column. *De locis
affectis* 5.[125]

57. Sometimes an inflammation[126] begins on the convex side of the
liver, whereas at other times it begins on the concave side. When it
begins on the convex side, it causes so much pain and provokes so much
cough that the patient feels as if his collarbone is pulled down. When
the inflammation begins on the concave side of the liver, the lack of
appetite, severe thirst, throwing up of bile, and nausea it causes are
worse than [the problems] caused by an inflammation on the convex
side. *De locis affectis* 5.[127]

58. When the liver becomes ill because of a cold bad temperament,
it often begins without fever at the time when serous, thin blood is
excreted with the excrements. When this lasts for a long time, it is followed by fevers because the blood of the liver is corrupted. Someone
who is neither familiar with this disease nor experienced in it may think
lightly of these fevers or suppose that the patient has no fever at all. *De
locis affectis* 5.[128]

٥٥ . علامـات الأورام الحـارّة في الكبد ثمانية علامات وهي الحمّى المحرقة والعطش
المبرّح وبطلان الشـهوة بالكلّية واحمرار اللسـان أوّلا ثمّ يسـودّ وقيء مـرار محّي أوّلا
وفـي آخـر الأمـر زنجاري ووجع في الجانب الأيمن يمتّد إلى الترقوة وبخاصّة إذا جذبت
ما دون الشراسـيف إلى فوق ويسـعل سعالايسيرا في بعض الأوقات ويجد حسّ الثقل
ويحسّـه معلّقا من الجانب الأيمن ومرارا كثيرة يشتكون ضلوع الخلف إذا كانت الكبد في ٥
خلقتها مضامّة لتلك الأضلاع . وإن لم تكن الكبد في نفسـها ضعيفة مع الورم احتبسـت
طبيعة المريض . خامسة التعرّف .

٥٦ . جميع من رأيته ممّن أصابته في مريئه علّة موجعة كان يجد مسّ الوجع بين كتفيه
والسبب في ذلك كون المريء ممدودا على عظم الصلب . خامسة التعرّف .

٥٧ . قـد يحدث الورم في الجانب المحدّب أوّلا وقد يبتدئ من الجانب المقعّر . والذي ١٠
يكون ابتداؤه من الجانب المحدّب يحدث من الوجع ومن تحريك السعالات أكثر حتّى يحسّ
الترقوة تجذب إلى أسـفل . والذي يبتدئ من مقعّر الكبد يحدث من تعطيل الشهوة وشدّة
العطش وقيء المرار والتهوّع أكثر ممّا يحدثه ورم المحدّب . خامسة التعرّف .

٥٨ . إذا اعتلّت الكبد من سـوء مزاج بارد قد يبتدئ مـرارا كثيرة بلا حمّى في
وقت ما يخرج بالتغوّط صديد دم رقيق . فإذا طالت المدّة تبع ذلك حمّيات لأنّ دم الكبد ١٥
يفسـد . ومن لا دربة له بهذه العلّة ولم يجرّبها يسـتخفّ بهذه الحمّيات أو يظنّ أنّ المريض
ليس بمحموم . خامسة التعرّف .

٢ محّي] يحي O(!) ‖ ٣ وفي آخر] وآخر Es O ‖ ٤ سـعالا يسيرا] سعالات يسيرة Es ‖
٥ ويحسّـه] ونخسـة Es O ‖ خلقتها مضامّة] خلفها مضمّة L ‖ ١٠ الورم] Es² : المرض
Es ‖ ١٢ تجذب] تنجذب EL | من (2nd)] فيه L ‖ ١٥ بالتغوّط] بالتغويط EL | صديد]
ثمّ add. EL ‖ ١٦ دربة] خبرة O

59. The disease which causes headache is sometimes in all the parts [of the head] outside the skull and sometimes in all the parts within the skull. But it may also be in only one of those parts, namely the pulsatile vessels,[129] or the nonpulsatile vessels, or the nerves, or the membranes, or the skin. It may [even] be in the brain substance itself. To determine the exact location of the disease is very difficult and only possible for someone who has personally dealt with it and observed it many times. *Mayāmir* 2.[130]

60. A stabbing pain[131] is that which begins from its root and then rapidly passes to the area surrounding that root. This happens in those pains which are extremely severe and strong, such as one-sided headache[132] and inveterate headache.[133] Nerve pains stretch lengthwise all the way from the origin to the end of the nerve, and the patient feels the pain deep in his body. When the pain is in the membrane that lies under the skin[134] and can be stripped off with it, it causes a tensive numb pain.[135] *De locis affectis* 2.[136]

61. Pains in the membranes surrounding the bones are felt by someone suffering from them deep inside. It seems to him that the pain is in his very bones. Some people call these pains "bone-piercing."[137] These pains result mostly from physical exercise. *De locis affectis* 2.[138]

62. If someone suffers from pain which only occurs in a pulsatile vessel or nonpulsatile vessel, it seems to him that it is a pain of something that is being stretched, such as a string.[139] But pain of the flesh does not extend over a great distance.[140] *De locis affectis* 2.

63. Cold sweat cannot possibly come from sites with high fevers because, had it come from there, it would be hot because of the fever. Rather, it comes from sites that have cooled off because the innate heat has become weak or nearly extinguished. Therefore, it is a sign of [imminent] death or of a prolonged illness. But it only indicates a prolonged illness when a large quantity of cold moistures dominates the body. *In Hippocratis Aphorismos commentarius* 4.[141]

٥٩ . العلّة الموجبة للصداع قد تكون في جميع الأجزاء التي خارج عظم القحف وقد تكون في جميع الأجزاء التي داخله وقد تكون في بعض تلك الأجزاء أعني في جنس العروق الضوارب فقط أو غير الضوارب أو في جنس العصب أو جنس الأغشية أو في جنس الجلد أو تكون العلّة في نفس جرم الدماغ. وتعرّف مواضع العلّة بالحقيقة أمر عسر

٥ شاقّ ليس يقدر عليه إلا من باشره ورآه مرارا كثيرة. ثانية الميامر.

٦٠ . الوجع الذي يعدو عدوانا هو الذي يبتدئ من أصله ثمّ يمرّ بسرعة إلى الموضع الذي حول ذلك الأصل. وذلك يحدث في الأوجاع التي هي في غاية الصعوبة والشدّة كوجع الشقيقة والبيضة. وأوجاع العصب تمتدّ طولا غاية الامتداد إلى مبدأ العصبة ومنتهاها ويحسّ المريض وجع العصب في عمق البدن. وإن كان الوجع في الغشاء

١٠ المستبطن للجلد الذي ينسلخ معه فيحدث عنه وجع امتدادي خدري. ثانية التعرّف.

٦١ . أوجاع الأغشية التي تحيط بالعظام يجد العليل حسّها في عمق ويخيّل إليه أنّ الوجع في نفس عظامه. وقوم يسمّون هذه مثقّبة العظام وأكثر ما يحدث من الرياضة. ثانية التعرّف.

٦٢ . الوجع الخاصّ بالعرق الضارب وغير الضارب يخيّل لصاحبه أنّه وجع جسم ممدود بمنزلة الوتر. ووجع اللحم لا يوجد يمتدّ إلى مسافة كثيرة. ثانية التعرّف.

٦٣ . العرق البارد لا يمكن أن يجيء من المواضع التي فيها الحمّى الشديدة لأنّه لو جاء

١٥ منها سخن بحرارة الحمّى. وإنّما يجيء من مواضع قد بردت لضعف الحرارة الغريزية أو لقربها من الانطفاء. ولذلك يدلّ إمّا على الموت أو على طول المرض وإنّما يدلّ على طول المرض إذا غلبت على البدن رطوبات كثيرة باردة. في شرحه لرابعة الفصول.

---

١ للصداع] للسعال L | عظم] عظام Es | ٢ تلك [om. Es O | في] من Es | ٤ مواضع] موضع L | ٦ عدوانا] كثيرا add. EEs¹L | ١١ تحيط] تحجد : L تحدث E | ١٤ كثيرة] كثيرة : OP بعيدة E | ١٥–١٦ فيها . . . مواضع [om. L | ١٤,١٨–١٥,١ باردة . . . كثيرة [om. L

64. A frequent occurrence of rigor during a fever is a fatal sign because it shakes the body so much that the body's strength dwindles, irrespective of whether evacuation follows thereafter or not. *In Hippocratis Aphorismos commentarius* 4.[142]

65. Sweat tastes salty with healthy people and tastes the same with ill persons. But in the latter case the saltiness undergoes a minor change and tends towards the taste of the dominating humor which caused the disease. *In Hippocratis Epidemiarum* 2.1.[143]

66. The main thing [to do] if one wants to make a diagnosis of the diseased spots of the hypochondria when they are tense is to palpate them so that you will know whether there is an inflamed swelling or a hard swelling or flatulence or pus or much feces. When one has diagnosed the illness in the hypochondria, one should apply oneself to dissolve it. *In Hippocratis Epidemiarum* 2.6.[144]

67. Loss of appetite is sometimes caused by [too much] humor in the cardia of the stomach or by the humor's bad quality or by the loss[145] of strength in the stomach. When the nature of the liver is harmed, the loss of appetite can be so severe that the patient would rather die than taste something. *In Hippocratis Epidemiarum* 3.1.[146]

68. The most benign tumors[147] are those that tend mostly to go outwards; then follow the ones which have a pointed head;[148] then the ones with a [less pointed] head.[149] Also benign are tumors which tend downwards[150] and those that do not have two heads.[151] Those tumors which are the absolute opposite to these are all of the worst kind. The most benign suppurating tumors are those which suppurate evenly[152] and are not very hard.[153] *In Hippocratis Epidemiarum* 6.1.[154]

69. In most chronic diseases the fingers turn cold. But in hectic fevers they stay warm. Because of the small quantity of flesh on the fingers, the heat which is firmly established in the main organs appears in them.[155] *In Hippocratis Prognostica commentaria* 3.[156]

70. If someone suffers from a spasm as a result of a blow or from the ingestion of a purgative, he will die. If someone has a spasm in the front and back [of the body] and then has to laugh, he will die on the spot. *De signis mortis.*[157]

٦٤ . حدوث النافض مرارا كثيرة في الحمّى من علامات الهلاك لزعزعته البدن تخور القوة تبعه استفراغ أو لم يتبعه . في شرحه لرابعة الفصول .

٦٥ . طعـم العرق فـي الأصحّاء مالح وكذلك في المرضى إلا أنّه تغيّر ملوحته قليلا وتميل إلى طعم الخلط الغالب المولد للمرض . في الأولى من شرحه لثانية ابيديميا .

٦٦ . عمـود الأمـر في تعرّف علل ما دون الشراسيـف إذا كانت ممدّدة هو أن تغمز عليها بيدك فتعرف بذلك هل فيها ورم حارّ أو ورم صلب أو نفخة أو مدّة أو رجيع كثير . فإذا علمت العلّة التي فيها حينئذ تقبل على أنّ تحلّها . في سادسة شرحه لثانية ابيديميا .

٦٧ . بطلان الشهوة ربّما كان بسبب خلط في فم المعدة أو كيفية منكرة أو موت القوة التي في المعدة . فإذا عرضت آفة للطبيعة التي في الكبد عرض من بطلان الشهوة أمر فادح حتّى يختار صاحب تلك الحال الموت على أن يطعم شيئًا . في الأولى من شرحه لثالثة ابيديميا .

٦٨ . أحمد الأورام أشدّها ميلا إلى خارج. ثمّ ما كان منها محدّد الرأس. ثمّ ما كان مروّسا .وما كان منها مائلا إلى أسفل فهو أحمد . وما لم يكن منها ذا رأسين فهو أحمد . وما كان منها على غاية المضادّة لهذه فهو أرداها كلّها . وكلّ ما ينضج منها فأحمده ما كان نضجه مستويا ولا يكون حوله صلابة . في الأولى من شرحه لسادسة ابيديميا .

٦٩ . في أكثر الأمراض المزمنة تبرد الأصابع . أمّا في حمّيات الدقّ فإنّها تسخن لقلّة لحم الأصابع تظهر الحرارة التي قد تمكّنت من الأعضاء الأصلية . في شرحه لثالثة تقدمة المعرفة .

٧٠ . من عرض له التشنّج من ضربة أو من شرب دواء مسهل مات . ومن كان به تشنّج من أمام ومن خلف وعرض له الضحك مات من ساعته . في مقالته في علامات الموت .

---

٤ ابيديميا] افيديميا EL || ٥ عمود] عماد ELP | علل] علل ELP | إذا كانت ممدّدة] om. EL | إذا كان ممدّدا] L || ٧ تحلّها] تحلّها Es | ابيديميا] افيديميا EL || ١٠ ابيديميا] افيديميا EL || ١١ محدّد] محدّب L || ١٤ ولا يكون] ولم تكن L | ابيديميا] افيديميا EL || ١٥-١٦ لحم الأصابع] اللحم في الأصابع EL

71. If someone with an intestinal ulcer suffers from severe thirst and gets a black pustule resembling a bitter vetch [kernel] behind the ears, he will die. When chyme streams down to the thighs, it is difficult to cure them. *De signis mortis.*[158]

*5*

72. When one of the intestines develops an ulcer caused by black bile, it cannot be cured. When it develops an ulcer caused by yellow bile, it is difficult to heal. The same holds for the other internal organs. *De atra bile.*[159]

73. When these four signs combine—the stool is soft and cohesive;[160]
*10*      it is discharged neither before nor after its usual time, and its quantity is commensurate with the food intake—it is an indication that the food is well-digested and that the stool is digested and cocted. Occasionally one of these is lacking but the stool is [still] digested and cocted. *De crisibus* 1.[161]

*15*

74. Sometimes something is well-digested and firmly cocted in the stomach, and [yet] the stool is dry because the heat around the stomach or intestines has dried its moistures. Sometimes it is softer[162] than normal because of the weakness of the faculty that transports the food to the organs. Sometimes its evacuation is delayed because its passage
*20*      through the intestines goes very slowly. Sometimes the stool is evacuated before the proper time because of the weakness of the retentive faculty in one of the intestines. If this is accompanied by [a sensation of] biting,[163] it indicates that [some sort of] irritation stimulated the expulsive faculty to evacuate it; this was not because of a deficiency which
*25*      affected its digestion in the stomach. *De crisibus* 1.[164]

75. When a soft, cohesive stool is discharged at the normal time, but in a quantity smaller than appropriate in comparison with the amount of food ingested, it indicates that some of it remains in one of the intestines, and this.is bad in any case. *De crisibus* 1.[165]

*30*

76. A stool that indicates bad digestion is coarse, not ground up, and of a soft consistency, retaining the quality of the food from which it is a residue. *De crisibus* 1.[166]

٧١ . من كانت به قرحة الأمعاء فعرض له عطش شديد وظهر خلف أذنه بثر أسود شبه الكرسنّة مات . والساقان اللّذان ينحدر لهما كيموس بروءهما عسر . في مقالته في علامات الموت .

٧٢ . إذا قرح معاء من الأمعاء من المرّة السوداء لم يكن له بروء . وإذا قرح من الصفراء عسر بروءه وكذلك حال غيرها من الأعضاء الباطنة . في مقالته في المرّة السوداء .

٧٣ . إذا كان البراز لينا متّصلا لا يتقدّم عن وقت عادته ولا يتأخّر وكان مقداره على قياس ما يتناول من الطعام فإنّ اجتماع هذه الأربعة أدلّة دليل على حسن استمراء الطعام وكون البراز منهضما نضيجا . وقد يفقد أحد هذه الأربعة ويكون منهضما نضيجا . أولى البحران .

٧٤ . قد يعرض للشيء الذي انهضم في المعدة هضما جيّدا واستحكم نضجه أن يكون البراز يابسا من أجل حرارة حول المعدة أو الأمعاء نشفت رطوباته . وقد يكون أرقّ ممّا ينبغي لضعف القوة المنفذة بالغذاء للأعضاء . وقد يبطأ عن وقت خروجه لبطء مروره في الأمعاء . وقد يخرج قبل الوقت لضعف القوة الماسكة في أحد الأمعاء . وإن كان ذلك مع لذع دلّ على لذع فيه هيّج القوة الدافعة لدفعه ، لا من أجل نقص لحق هضمه في المعدة . أولى البحران .

٧٥ . البراز اللين المتّصل الذي يخرج في وقت العادة إن كان أقلّ ممّا ينبغي بقياس ما يتناول فذلك يدلّ على أنّه قد بقيت منه بقية في بعض الأمعاء وذلك ردئ على أيّ حال كان . في الأولى من البحران .

٧٦ . البراز الدالّ على فساد الهضم هو أن يكون خشنا غير مسحوق رقيق القوام حافظا لكيفية الطعام الذي هو فضلته . أولى البحران .

---

٢ شبه] شبيه ب- Es || ٦ لا] لم L || ٩ الذي] إذا E || ١٢ في الأمعاء] بالأمعاء L || ١٣ لذع فيه] خلط لذاع L | هيّج] يهيج Es : فيهيج EL | لدفعه] om. EL || ١٨ فساد] صحّة O | هو] om. EL

77. An initially green color [of the stool] may eventually turn black, namely when a malignant disease is accompanied by green sputum or green stool or green urine, each of which will later turn black. *De crisibus* 1.[167]

5  78. If you see a person with a stool containing a discharge of something like water in which freshly slaughtered meat has been washed,[168] let it be a sure indication for you of a decline in the strength of the liver. If the blood that is discharged is thick like wine sediment, it is a sign indicating that the liver is burning the blood. If the blood is thin and serous,[169] it

10  indicates that the liver is too weak to make blood. *De locis affectis* 5.[170]

79. First thin serous blood is discharged in the stool, then after a long time thick[171] blood similar to black bile, and eventually the discharge is pure black bile. *De locis affectis* 5.[172]

80. Sometimes the stool has a variety of discharges with a very bad

15  color and smell, and similarly the urine. This is caused by the strength of the liver and organs, which expelled those bad residues which were retained in them. An inexperienced physician can make a mistake in these matters by supposing that the patient is close to death. These kinds of evacuations simply occur after a prolonged disease and after the mani-

20  festation of signs of coction. *De locis affectis* 5.[173]

81. Just as a discharge of blood through the anus occurs to someone whose hand or foot has been cut off, or to someone who gives up physical exercise, or to someone whose hemorrhoidal or menstrual blood was retained, so a similar discharge occurs to some people through vomiting.

25  The blood of those who eliminate blood either through vomiting or through diarrhea is pure like that of slaughtered animals. If the blood is

٧٧ . اللـون الأخضر إنّما يكون عند ما يبتدئ يكون اللون الأسـود وذلك أنّ المرض الخبيـث إذا ظهر فيه قـيء أخضر أو براز أخضر أو بول أخضر يظهر بعد ذلك كلّ واحد من هذه الثلاثة وهو أسـود . أولى البحران .

٧٨ . متى رأيتم إنسـانا برز منه في الغائط شـيء شبيه بغسالة اللحم القريب العهد بالذبح فليكن ذلك لكم علامة صحيحة تدلّ على ضعف قوة الكبد . وإن كان الدم الذي يبـرز غليظا مثل الدردي فتلك علامة تدلّ على أنّ الكبد تحرق الدم . وإن كان الدم رقيقا صديديا دلّ على أنّ الكبد تضعف عن عمل الدم . خامسة التعرّف .

٧٩ . الـدم الصديـدي الرقيق الذي يخرج أوّلا في التغـوّط إذا طالت المدّة خرج دم *غليظ من جنس المرّة السوداء ، ثمّ يخرج آخر الأمر المرّة السوداء محضة .

٨٠ . قـد يخرج بالبراز ألوان مختلفة رديئة جدّة في ألوانها وروائحها وكذلك بالبول . ويكون علّة ذلك قوة الكبد والأعضاء التي دفعت تلك الفضلات الرديئة المحتقنة التي كانت فيها . ويغلط في هذه الأشـياء من كان من الأطبّـاء لا دربة له فيظنّ أنّ المريض قريب من العطب . وأمثـال هذه الاسـتفراغات إنّما تكون بعـد طول من المرض وبعد ظهور علامات النضج . خامسة التعرّف .

٨١ . كمـا يجـيء خروج الدم لمن قطعت يده أو رجله أو مـن عطّل الرياضة أو من احتبس عنه دم البواسـير أو الطمث من المقعدة كذلك قـد يجيء لبعض الناس بالقيء . وهؤلاء يخرج منهم بالقيء أو بالإسـهال دم محض مثل دم الذبيحة . وأمّا ما يكون سـببه

---

١ يكـون (2nd) L] يتبـيّن : P تكـوّن : P || ٩ *غليظ] عبيط MSS | محضة] المحضة Es ||
١٠ بالبراز] البراز ELO | في] om. EL | بالبول] البول EL | التي (2nd)] P om. ||
١١ التي (2nd)] om. P | ١٦ أو الطمث من المقعدة] من المقعدة EL : من المقعدة أو الطمث O || ١٧ الذبيحة] الذباحة P

eliminated because of ripe abscesses bursting, that blood, whether coming out from above or from below, is turbid like wine sediment. *De locis affectis* 5.[174]

82. Bloody diarrhea[175] due to a liver disease may occur suddenly. But if it comes because of [a disease of] the intestines, it does not happen suddenly, but rather begins as a bilious diarrhea which is extremely acrid; this is followed by shreds[176] of intestinal tissue, and then with the shreds some blood is excreted. *De locis affectis* 6.[177]

83. The blood which is excreted from the liver with the stool is sometimes retained for two or three days. It then becomes worse than what it was the first time but is not accompanied by shreds. These two prognostic signs do not occur in any intestinal ulcer. *De locis affectis* 6.[178]

84. The stool that is deep[179] yellow comes from a large amount of yellow bile that streamed to the abdomen. The stool is green when it is mixed with a large quantity of verdigris green bile. When the stool is black, it indicates that it is mixed with black bile or with blood that was burned there. When it tends to lead gray, it indicates that the cold was so severe in the internal organs that they were close to death. One should know from which food the stool is a residue, because sometimes the color of the stool derives from the nature of the [particular] kind of food. In this case the color is not a prognostic sign. *De crisibus* 1.[180]

85. When the stool is greasy, it is a sign that fat has melted. When it is viscous, it indicates melting of the solid parts, which is worse than the previous case. An excessively putrid stool indicates severe putrefaction. All this is on the condition that it[181] is not due to the nature of the food. *De crisibus* 1.[182]

انفجار أورام قد نضجت فإنّ ذلك الدم الذي يجيء من هذه من فوق أو من أسـفل يكون دما درديا عكرا . خامسة التعرّف .

٨٢ . إسـهال الـدم من عِلّة الكبد قد يحدث دفعة . وأمّا الذي من قِبل الأمعاء فلا يحدث دفعة بل يحدث أوّلا إسهال مِرار يلذع غايـة اللذع ثمّ يتبع ذلك خراطة الأمعاء ثمّ يخرج بعد ذلك مع الخِراطة دم قليل . سادسة التعرّف .

٨٣ . الدم الذي يخرج من الكبد مع الغائط قد يحتبس اليومين والثلاثة ويأتي شـرّ ممّا كان في المرّة الأولى وليس يأتي معه خراطة . وهذان علامتان لا يكونان في شيء من قروح الأمعاء . سادسة التعرّف .

٨٤ . البراز الذي لونه أصفر مشبّع يكون من انصباب شـيء كثير من المرّة الصفراء إلى البطن . وأمّا البراز الأخضر فإذا خالطه مِرار زنجاري . وإذا كان أسود فيدلّ على أنّ خالطه مرّة سـوداء أو دم قد احترق هناك . والـذي يضرب إلى الكمودة الرصاصية يدلّ على برد قوي في الأعضاء الباطنة حتّى كأنّها قد صارت في حدّ الموت . وينبغي أن تعلم الغذاء الذي هذا ثِقله لأنّه قد يكون ذلك اللون من طبيعة نوع الغذاء فلا يسـتدلّ من اللون حينئذ على شيء . أولى البحران .

٨٥ . إذا كان البراز دسـما دلّ على أنّ الشـحم هو ذا يـذوب . فإن كان لزجا دلّ على ذوبان الأعضاء الصلبة وهذا أردأ من الأوّل . والمفرط النتن يدلّ على عفونة شديدة . ويشترط في هذا كلّه أن لا يكون ذلك من أجل طبيعة الطعام . أولى البحران .

١٠

٥

١٥

---

٢ درديـا عكرا] عكرا رديا : ردريا عكـرا L || ٣ الأعماء] المعاء EL || ٤ مِرار . . . EO || خراطـة] O¹ || ١٠ خالطه . . . على أنّ] om. O || ١٢ كأنّها] om. L || ١٣ ثقله] فعله O || ١٤ حينئذ] om. L || ١٥ هو ذا] om. EL

86. A foamy stool indicates one of two things: either extreme heat melting the body, whereby foam results from the boiling of the body moistures which were boiled[183] by the extreme heat, or from an anomalous disturbance[184] resulting from the struggle between thick flatulence and moisture.[185] *De crisibus* 1.[186]

87. A stool with different colors indicates that the body suffers from different diseases. Thus, it announces that the disease will be prolonged and malignant, because when diseases multiply they need more time to coct. Their severity and danger is according to their number. *De crisibus* 1.[187]

88. Sometimes the diseases and symptoms[188] caused by the retentive faculty and the expulsive faculty are mixed with one another. An example of this is hiccups. For in the case of hiccups, the stomach has bad contractions over the food, while at the same time the expulsive faculty is making wrong[189] movements. *De [morborum] causis et symptomatibus* 6.[190]

89. Black stool originates either from the domination of burning, from foul putrefaction, or from the streaming of a melancholic humor. *In Hippocratis Aphorismos commentarius* 4.[191]

90. Sometimes a lack of appetite occurs in the beginning of bloody diarrhea.[192] This is not a bad sign, because choleric humors streaming from the liver to the intestines and abrading them stream from there to the stomach so that appetite diminishes. But if the disease is prolonged and a lack of appetite occurs, it is a bad sign because it indicates death of the powers [of the body]. *In Hippocratis Aphorismos commentarius* 6.[193]

91. When blood congeals and coagulates and turns into thick, clotted blood in the urinary bladder and, similarly, when it congeals in the intestines or stomach or chest—and in this case it is worse than in that of the bladder—it causes syncope, pallor,[194] and a small, weak, and

٨٦ . البراز الذي فيه زبد يدلّ على أحد شيئَين : إمّا على حرارة مفرطة تذيب البدن فيحدث الزبد من قبل الشيء الذي يغلي من رطوبات البدن التي أذابتها الحرارة المفرطة وإمّا على اضطراب مختلف من قبل مقاومة ريح غليظة لرطوبة . أولى البحران .

٨٧ . البــراز المختلف الألوان يدلّ على أنّ في البدن أمراض مختلفة ولذلك ينذر من المرض بطول وخبـث لأنّ الأمراض إذا كثرت احتاجت في نضجها إلى زمان أطول وكان صعوبتها وخطرها على حسب كثرتها . أولى البحران .

٨٨ . أعراض القوة الماسكة وأعراض القوة الدافعة قد تختلط بعضها ببعض من ذلك الفواق . فإنّ المعدة في حال الفواق تنقبض على الطعام انقباض سوء والقوة الدافعة تتحرّك أيضا حينئذ حركة منكرة . سادسة العلل والأعراض .

٨٩ . البراز الأسـود يتولّد إمّا من غلبة الاحتراق وإمّا من قبل عفونة منكرة وإمّا من انصباب خلط سوداوي . في شرحه لرابعة الفصول .

٩٠ . قـد يعرض في أوّل اختلاف الدم ذهاب الشـهوة وليس ذلك بعلامة رديئة لأنّ الأخلاط الصفراوية التي تنصبّ من الكبد للمعى فتسحجه تنصبّ منها إلى المعدة فتسقط الشـهوة . أمّا إذا طالت العلّة فيحدث سـقوط الشهوة فهي علامة رديئة لأنّ ذلك يدلّ على موت القوى . في شرحه لسادسة الفصول .

٩١ . الدم إذا جمد وانعقد وصار علقا في المثانة وكذلك إذا جمد في المعى أو المعدة أو الصدر فإنّه في هذه أشـرّ منه في المثانة عرض بسببه غشي وصفرة لون وصار النبض

---

٤ – ٥ من المرض بطول] بطول من المرض Es || ٥ أطول] طويل EL || ٦ حسب] قدر EL || ١١ الفصول] إذا ظهر البراز الأسود في أوّل المرض دلّ على آفة عظيمة حدثت بالكبد وإذا ظهر بعد انتهاء المرض فكثيرا ما يدلّ على خير إذا كان ظهوره بدفع الطبيعة لتلك الفضول الممرّضة . في شرحه لرابعة الفصول . add. Es O P¹ || ١٤ إذا طالت] Beginning of Ox || ١٧ فإنّه في هذه] فإنّ هذه O

frequent pulse. The patient becomes hot[195] and weak. This makes a
person wonder how it is possible that blood—although it is most dear
to nature[196]—causes these bad and malignant symptoms when it leaves
its vessels. Sometimes this is followed—after what we mentioned—by
putrefaction and death of the organs. *De locis affectis* 6.[197]

92. Stones develop only in the kidneys and the urinary bladder,
though according to some people also in the intestine called "colon." *De
locis affectis* 1.[198]

93. That which in the medical art goes according to supposition and
conjecture[199] is in most cases the diagnosis of diseases. However, once
these diseases are known, their treatment is not arrived at through supposition, guesswork, and conjecture, but through certain knowledge.[200]
*Mayāmir* 2.[201]

94. Says Moses: It is well known that the physicians speak about
psychical faculties, animal faculties, and natural faculties. Now, according to this convention I want to call all the activities of the human body
"corporal activities" and say that the most eminent bodily activity is respiration, followed by the pulse, and after that, sensation. The most eminent
sense is seeing, followed by hearing. After sensation comes craving for
food and drink, then speech, and then distinction[202]—that is, thought
and imagination. Then comes the movement of the other parts of the
body, according to their habit. This gradation in eminence is specifically
according to the requirements for life, or its proper continuation.

Following this introduction, you should know that the term *nature*
is a homonym[203] which has many [different] meanings.[204] One of all
these meanings is the faculty which governs the body of living beings,
for the physicians also call this faculty "nature." This faculty always
spares the most eminent activities of the body and always strives to
maintain the integrity of all [its] activities. If a disease-producing cause

صغيرا ضعيفا متواترا وسخن العليل واسترخى . وهذا يدعو الإنسان للتعجّب كيف صار الدم وهو أحبّ الأشياء للطبيعة إذا خرج عن أوعيته حـدث عنه هذه الأعراض الرديئة الخبيثة . وقد يتبعه مع ما ذكرنا تعفّن الأعضاء وموتها . سادسة التعرّف .

٩٢ . تولّـد الحصى لا يكون إلا في الكليتين والمثانة فقط . ويكون أيضا على ما يقول بعض الناس في المعى المسمّى قولون . في الأولى من التعرّف . ٥

٩٣ . الشيء الذي يكون من صناعة الطبّ على طريق التخمين والإزكان إنّما هو على الأكثـر تعرّف الأمراض . أمّا متى علمت الأمراض ووقف عليها فإنّ علاجها ليس يعرف حينئذ بالتخمين والحدس والإزكان بل بالمعرفة اليقينية . ثانية الميامر .

٩٤ . قال موسـى : قد علمت قول الأطبّاء : قوى نفسـانية وقـوى حيوانية وقوى طبيعية . ولنسـمّ الآن في هذا الاصطلاح جميع أفعال بدن الإنسان الأفعال البدنية . فأقول ١٠ إنّ أشرف الأفعال البدنية التنفّس وبعده النبض وبعده الإحساس وأشرف الحواس البصر ثمّ السمع وبعد الإحسـاس شهوة الطعام والشراب وبعد ذلك الكلام وبعد ذلك التمييز أعني به التخيّل والفكر وبعد ذلك حركة سائر الأعضاء على معتّادها . وهذه الرتبة في الشرف إنّما هي بحسب ضرورية الحياة أو صلاحية استمرارها .

وبعد هذه المقدّمة فلتعلم أنّ الطبيعة اسـم مشـترك يقال على معاني كثيرة . من جملة ١٥ تلك المعاني القوة المدبّرة لبدن الحيوان فإنّ الأطبّاء يسـمّونها أيضا طبيعة . وهذه القوة هي أبدا تشـاحح على أشرف الأفعال البدنية وهي أبدا تروم سلامة الأفعال كلّها . فإن حدث

---

١ وسخن] وسكن Es L : وسخن Es² || ٥ في] تكرر Es² || ٧ ليس] لم O || ٩ قول] أقـوال Ox || الأطبّاء] في add. Ox || ١٠ ولنسـمّ] والنفس O : أنا add. Es O P | ١٠- ١١ فأقول . . . النبض] om. O || ١٢ وبعد الإحساس . . . والشراب] O¹ | أعني] الذي add. Ox || ١٤ استمرارها] استمراها O || ١٦ هي] om. P || ١٧ أبدا (1st)] أيضا Es O

develops, it (i.e., nature) opposes it and expels it. If it finds it difficult
to do so,[205] it casts it to that bodily part that is least important and
gives up the activity that is least important. But if nature has difficulty
doing so, it gives up the [next] most important activity and holds on to
the activity that is more important [than the former one], etc. According to this sequence one can distinguish between fatal and nonfatal
diseases and draw conclusions regarding the degree of severity or weakness of the disease and the degree of strength or weakness of nature. For
cessation or disturbance of respiration is fatal without any doubt, and
similarly [cessation of] the pulse, loss or disturbance of vision, loss of
appetite, loss or weakness of speech, amentia or disturbance of the mind;
all these afflictions are fatal indications, and their degree [of severity]
is according to my arrangement and according to the strength of the
particular affliction.

Therefore, a severe stroke is necessarily fatal and a mild one is difficult to heal, as Hippocrates stated.[206] For during this affliction, namely
a stroke, the eminent activities which nature always spares are either
abolished or disturbed. These activities are respiration, mental activity,[207]
speech, sensation, and pulse. The prerequisite for all that I have mentioned is that the loss or impairment of that activity is due to a weakening of the general faculty that governs the body of living beings, and
not just due to a disease of the particular organ performing that activity.

You know that many of those suffering from madness[208] or melancholy
live for a long time, as they have strong bodies. The loss of their mental
activities is only due to an affliction of the brain, and not due to a weakening of the faculty which governs that which occurs to patients during
their agony. Thus, the weakening of vision due to an affliction in the eye
and the weakening of hearing due to an affliction in the inner earhole
is unlike the weakening of vision or hearing—when one dies—due to the
collapse of the general faculty that governs [the body]. The same conditions apply to loss of speech and the other bodily activities. Similarly,
nature acts sparingly with changes in one's complexion. For when the

سـبب من الأسـباب الممرّضة قاومته ودفعته فإن غلبت عن ذلك ألقته لأخسّ الأعضاء وبذلت أخسّ الأفعال . فإن غلبت عن ذلك ما هو أشـرف وتمسّـكت بالأشـرف فالأشرف . وبحسب هذا الترتيب تعلم المرض المهلك من غير المهلك وتستدلّ على مراتب شـدّة المرض وضعفه وعلى مراتب قوة الطبيعة وضعفهـا . فإنّ تعطّل التنفّس أو اختلاله مهلك بلا شكّ وكذلك النبض وكذلك تعطّل البصر أو اختلاله وتعطّل الشهوة وتعطّل الكلام أو ضعفه أو غيبة الذهن أو اختلاله كلّ هذه الأعراض علامات هلاك ومراتبها بحسب ما رتّبت لك وبحسب قوة ذلك العارض .

ولذلك كانت السـكتة القوية مهلكة ضرورة والضعيفة يعسر بروءها كما نصّ أبقراط لأنّ هذه الآفة أعني السـكتة تعطّلت فيها أو اختلّت الأفعال الشـريفة التي تشاحح عليها الطبيعة دائما وهي التنفّس وغياب الذهن والكلام والإحسـاس والنبض . والشرط في كلّ مـا ذكرته أن يكون بطلان ذلك الفعـل أو اختلاله من قبل ضعف القوة العامّة المدبّرة لبدن الحيوان لا من قبل مرض الآلة وحدها الفاعلة لذلك الفعل .

أنت تعلم أنّ كثيرا من المجانين وأصحاب المالنخوليا يعيشون زمانا طويلا وهم أقوياء الأجسـام لأنّ فسـاد أذهانهم من قبل آفة الدماغ وحده لا من قبل ضعف القوة المدبّرة على ما يعتري للمرضى عند النزاع . كما أنّ ضعف البصر الكائن من قبل آفة في العين وضعف السـمع الكائن من قبل آفة في السـماخ ليس هو مثل ضعف البصر أو السمع الكائن عند الموت من قبل سـقوط القوة العامّة المدبّرة . وهكذا يشـترط في تعطيل الكلام وفي سائر الأفعال البدنية . وهكذا أيضا سـحنة الوجه تشاحح الطبيعة على تغييرها . فمتى كانت

---

٢–١ ألقته . . . أشرف] بذلت ما هو أخسّ L ‖ ٣ فالأشرف] في الأشرف P ‖ ٤ التنفّس] النفس P ‖ . . . البصر] om. O ‖ ٥ مهلك . . . البصر] om. O ‖ ٦ الأعراض] الأمراض O ‖ ٧ رتّبت] بيّنت O ‖ ٨ أبقـراط] بوقراط O ‖ ١٣ المالنخوليا] المالنخونيا ELOx ‖ ١٥–١٦ النزاع . . . مثّل] om. L ‖ ١٦ السماخ] الأذن O : الصماخ L

complexion of a patient is close to that which he has when he is healthy, it indicates that nature is strong, and when his complexion is very far from resembling his normal complexion, it indicates that the general strength is weak.[209] Consider this aphorism carefully, for it contains many things relevant to prognosis.

95. In the medical art we can find many symptoms[210] which, when they appear in healthy people, indicate diseases, and which, when they appear in sick people, indicate health. One of these is sleep which is longer and deeper than usual. When it occurs to healthy people, it indicates illness, and when it occurs to sick people, it indicates health. And when a strong appetite occurs to healthy people, there is reason for suspicion,[211] as it indicates a disease, and when it occurs to sick people, it is a laudable sign. Similarly, sneezing, for when it happens often to someone whose health is beyond reproach, it indicates that an affliction has reached the head. And when it occurs to someone who is in a bad state of disease, it indicates that his condition will change for the better. We can find many things of this nature in the art of medicine. *In Timaeum commentarius* 2.[212]

> *This is the end of the sixth treatise,*
> *by the grace of God, praise be to Him.*

◆

أيضا ســحنة وجه المريض قريبا منها في حــال صحّته فتلك علامة على قوة الطبيعة وإن كانت بعيدا جدًّا عن حال الصحّة فذلك من ضعف القوة العامّة . فتدبّر هذا الفصل بتأمّل جيّد فإنّه يشتمل على أجزاء كثيرة من تقدمة المعرفة .

٩٥ . قـد نجد في صناعة الطبّ أعراضا كثيرة متى ظهرت في الأصحّاء دلّت على الأمــراض ومتى ظهرت في المرضى دلّت على الصحّة . من ذلك النوم الكثير المستغرق بأكـــثر مّما جرت به العادة متى عـرض للأصحّاء دلّ على مرض ومتى عرض للمرضى دلّ على الصحّة . وشهوة الطعام القوية متى عرضت للأصحّاء كانت موضع تهمة ودليلا على مرض ومتى عرضت للمرضى كانت دليلا محمودا . وكذلك العطاس فإنّه متى عرض كثيرا لمــن لا يذمّ من صحّته شــيئًا دلّت على أنّ الرأس قد نالتـه آفة ومتى عرض لمن هو بحال سوء من المرض دلّ على أنّ حاله سيتغيّر إلى ما هو أصلح . وقد نجد في صناعة الطبّ أشــياء كثيرة طبعها هذا الطبع . في المقالة الثانية من شرحه لكتاب طيماوس . تمّت المقالة السادسة ولله الحمد والمنّة .

_____

٤ نجد] يوجد LO || ٦ به] عليه EsO || ١٠ إلى ما] لما ELOx || ١١ طبعها] طبيعتها ELOx | ١١–١٢ تمّت . . . والمنّة] om. O : كملت المقالة السادسة والحمد لله P : تمّت المقالة السادسة والحمد لله وعدد فصولها ثلاثة وتسعون فصلا L : كملت المقالة السادسة والحمد لواهب العقل وعدد فصوله xxx Ox : كملت المقالة السادسة ولله الحمد وعدد فصولها ثلاثة وتسعين فصلا E

*In the name of God,*
*the Merciful, the Compassionate.*
*O Lord, make [our task] easy*

# The Seventh Treatise

*Containing aphorisms concerning*
*the causes [of diseases] which are often not known*
*or which are discussed in a confused way*

1. The things which cause a manifest increase in strength are six: (1) moderate wine consumption, (2) moderate food intake, (3) moderate physical exercise, (4) anything that improves a bad temperament of the heart and pulsatile vessels, whether drink or drug, (5) anger[1] and joy, and (6) the coction of the humors so that they start to dissolve or to be evacuated during the crisis. *De pulsu* 13.[2]

2. The things which weaken and diminish one's strength are eight: (1) fasting, (2) sleeplessness, (3) anxiety, (4) excessive evacuation of any type, (5) severe pain in any spot, (6) abdominal pain, especially that followed by fainting, (7) a very bad temperament of whatever type of the humors of the body, and (8) a very bad temperament of whatever type of the organs of the body. *De pulsu* 13.[3]

بسم الله الرحمن الرحيم ربّ يسّر

# المقالة السابعة

تشتمل على فصول تتعلّق بإعطاء أسباب كثيرا ما تُجهل أو يتشوّش القول فيها

١. الأشـياء التي توجب تزيّد القوة وظهورها ستّة أسباب: أحدها شرب النبيذ

٥   باعتدال. الثاني تناول الطعام باعتدال. الثالث الرياضة المعتدلة. الرابع ما يصلح سوء مزاج
القلب والعروق الضوارب شـرابا كان أو دواء. الخامس الغضب والفرح. السـادس نضج
الأخلاط إمّا لتأخذ في التحلّل أو لتستفرغ في البحران. ثالثة عشر النبض.

٢. الأشـياء التي تحمل القوة وتضعفها أحد ثمانية أسـباب: أحدها الصوم والثاني
السـهر والثالث الغمّ والرابع الاسـتفراغ المفرط بـأيّ نوع كان والخامس الوجع الشـديد

١٠  حيـث كان والسـادس وجع المعدة خاصّة الذي يتبعه الغشـي والسابع إفراط سـوء
مـزاج أخلاط البدن أيّ سـوء مزاج كان والثامن إفراط سـوء مزاج أعضـاء البدن أيّ
سوء مزاج كان. ثالثة عشر النبض.

---

١ بسم ... يسّر [om. ELOP : بسم الله الرحمن الرحيم Ox ‖ ٢ السابعة] الثانية Ox ‖
١١–١٢ أخلاط ... مزاج [om. L

3. People can also faint because of the strength of the affections of the soul. This happens mostly to the elderly and to weak people, whatever the cause of their weakness. Many of them faint when they are affected by anxiety, joy, or anger.[4] Sometimes [this] happens to them because their bodies unnecessarily sweat a little bit. *Ad Glauconem [de methodo medendi]* 1.[5]

4. Constant anxiety dissolves the fat and corrupts the moist flesh, while frequent joy corrupts the blood. Similarly, the blood is corrupted by passionate love, lust for money, political leadership, and fame. The corruption of the blood by any of these comes from bad digestion in the stomach and vessels. The dissolution [of the fat] is caused by sleeplessness and by [constantly] thinking about these things. *In Hippocratis De humoribus commentaria* 3.[6]

5. The reason why the organs on the right side have more strength than the organs on the left side is that the liver lies on the right side while the leaning of the heart towards the left side is very small. When this leaning of the heart is slightly greater, the organs on the left become stronger than those on the right, especially if the liver, in such a case, is weak and small. *In Hippocratis Epidemiarum* 2.6.[7]

6. The causes of pain are a dissolution of continuity[8] or a sudden change that occurs to the organ through coercion and harshness.[9] If the change happens slowly, it cannot hurt. Pain does not occur in senseless organs. *De methodo medendi* 12.[10]

7. Any cause of pain inflicts harm through which the expulsive faculty is activated[11] and exerts itself to expel the harmful element. Because of its intense activity to expel the harmful cause, the expulsive faculty often produces a tumor by attracting blood and air together to the [affected] organ. *De methodo medendi* 13.[12]

٣ . قـد يعـرض أيضا الغشـي لقوم من قوة عـوارض النفس وأكثر مـا يعرض ذلك للمشـائخ والضعفاء من أيّ سبب كان ضعفهم . فإنّ كثيرا من هؤلاء إذا اغتمّوا أو سرّوا أو غضبـوا عرض لهم الغشـي وربّما عرض لهم من أدنى رشـح ترشـح أبدانهم من غير حاجة لذلك الرشح . أولى أغلوقن .

٤ . إدامة الهموم تذيب الشـحم وتفسـد اللحم الطري وتواتر اللذّات يفسـد الدم . وكذلك يفسـد الدم العشق ومحبّة الأموال والرياسـة في المدن ونباهة الذكر . وإفساد كلّ واحد من هذه للدم يكون بسبب رداة الهضم العارض في المعدة والعروق والذوبان العارض بسبب السهر والأفكار في هذه الأشياء . في الثالثة من شرح الأخلاط .

٥ . سـبب فضل قوة الأعضاء اليمنى على اليسرى هو كون الكبد في الجانب الأيمن وميل القلب إلى الجانب الأيسر هو ميل قليل جدّا . فإن كان ميله أكثر قليلا صارت بذلك الأعضاء اليسـرى أقوى من اليمنى سـيّما إن كانت الكبد في هذه الحال ضعيفة صغيرة . في السادسة من شرحه لثانية ابيديميا .

٦ . أسباب الأوجاع إمّا تفرّق اتّصال وإمّا تغيّر ما يكون دفعة ويكون يستكره العضو ويعنف به فإنّ التغيّر إذا كان قليلا قليلا فليس يمكن فيه أن يوجع والأعضاء التي لا حسّ لها لا يحدث فيها وجع . ثانية عشر الحيلة .

٧ . السـبب الفاعل للوجع أيّ سـبب كان يوذي وتتحرّك القوة الدافعة وتجهد نفسها لدفع الشـيء الموذي فتحدث مرارا كثيرة ورما بجلبها للعضو دما وروحا معا عند شـدّة حركتها لدفع السبب الموذي . ثالثة عشر الحيلة .

___

٥ تذيب] تذبل Es² ‖ ٦ المدن] المدون Ox ‖ ٧ بسبب رداة] لرداة Es ‖ ٨ في الثالثة من شرح] ثالثة عشر L ‖ ١٠ إلى] في P ‖ ١٢ ابيديميا] افيديميا ELOx ‖ ١٣ الأوجاع] الوجع L ‖ يستكره] يستكرهه O

8. Says Moses: When Galen speaks about the healing of syncope, he
starts by giving its causes; however, he does not describe[13] them as he
usually does when he classifies the [various] kinds of diseases and their
causes and the [various] kinds of symptoms: according to the method
applied in the [medical] art, as in his classification of fevers in their
[various] classes and species. Rather, he describes the causes of syncope
in an amazing way, namely by saying that it can be caused by this and
by that, but does not classify these causes into specific categories.[14] And
[even] more amazing than this is that when he discusses the subject
in detail, he remarks, "The other causes for syncope are four."[15] I wish
I knew why only some causes were given a specific number but not all
of them. Moreover, after mentioning the four [causes] he remarks, "And
if you want, you can add another one to these four—namely, a bad temperament of the organs." In short, he did not give a systematic discussion
in that place, although everything he said is undoubtedly correct. However, as we said, it is disordered.

And since this affliction, namely syncope, is such a serious[16] one and
is a partner and associate of death, which it [often] precedes, a physician should have a comprehensive knowledge of all the causes of syncope
and should always keep them in mind. If he has a detailed and exact
knowledge of its causes, he knows how to treat it when it occurs, and
how to prevent its occurrence, and how to warn against it when its
occurrence is unavoidable. Abū Marwān b. Zuhr[17] and other physicians
said that when a patient suffers from syncope without the physician knowing about it until it [actually] happens and without his having warned
against it, then this physician is undoubtedly responsible for the death
of the patient.[18]

9. Says Moses: This is correct, for if he knew all the causes of syncope,
his most important and desired goal would be to prevent its occurrence,
and whenever something would appear in the condition of the disease
which could trigger syncope, he would hasten to fight that which would
cause syncope if it were neglected. And if he had to give up his fight
against it, he would warn [the patient] against its occurrence. Therefore,
I thought it a good thing to classify the [various] causes of syncope and
to describe its classes and species so that it will be easy to learn them and
know them by heart. All that I will say in the following five aphorisms is

٨ . قال موسى : لمّا شرع جالينوس أن يتكلّم في طبّ الغشي أخذ أن يعطي أسبابه
فلم يحصر أسبابه على طريــق صناعي كما جرت عادته في تقسيم أجناس الأمراض
وأسبابها وأجناس الأعراض وكما فعل في تقسيم الحمّيات لأجناسها وأصنافها . بل ذكر
أسباب الغشي ذكرا عجيبا وذلك أنّه يقول : قد يحدث من كذا وقد يحدث من كذا ولم
٥ يقسّم الأسباب إلى أنواع محصورة . وأعجب من هذا أنّه لمّا أمعن في القول قال : سائر
أسباب الغشي أربعة . فيا ليت شعري كيف لم يحصر الأسباب كلّها بعدد وحصر بعضها .
ثمّ قال بعد أنّ ذكر الأربعة : وإن شئت زدت مع هذه الأربعة سوء مزاج الأعضاء . وبالجملة
لم ينتظم قوله هناك وإن كان كلّما قاله صحيحا بلا شكّ لكنّه غير مرتّب كما قلنا .

ولمّا أن كان هذا العارض أعني الغشي عارضــا مرهقا جدّا جدّا وهو رفيق الموت
١٠ وقرينه المتقدّم له وجب على الطبيب أن يكون عارفا بجميع أسبــاب الغشــي محيطا بها
ذاكرا لها دائما . فإنّه إذا علم أسبابه بتفصيل وتحديد علم كيف يتدارك الغشي إذا وقع
وكيف يتحفّظ من وقوعه وينذر به قبل وقوعه إن لم يكن بدّ من وقوعه فقد قال أبو مروان
بن زهر وغيره إنّه أيّ مريض غشي عليه ولم يعلم الطبيب ذلك حتّى وقع ولم ينذر به فإنّ
ذلك الطبيب أهلك المريض بلا شكّ .

١٥ ٩ . قال موسـى : وهذا صحيح لأنّه لو علم أسبــاب الغشي كلّها لكان أهمّ أغراضه
وأوكدها التحفّظ من وقوع الغشي وكلّما ظهر له في حال المرض أمر يتوقّع منه الغشي بادر
لمقاومة ذلك الأمر الذي يكون سببا للغشي أن أهمل وإن غلب عن مقاومته أنذر بوقوع
الغشي . فلذلك رأيت أن أرتّب أسباب الغشي وأحصر أجناسها وأنواعها كي يسهل علمها
وحفظها . وكلّما أقوله من ذلك في هذه الفصول الخمسة الذي أتي بها بعد هذا هو إمّا نصّ

٣ لأجناسها ] om. L ‖ ٥ أنّه لمّا ] لمّا أنّه Es ‖ ٧ مع ] من Ox ‖ فإنّه : O أنّه ] ٩ مرهقا ] موثقا
Es² ‖ ١٥ أهمّ ] أعمّ Es : أتمّ Es¹O ‖ ١٦ منه ] معه EsO ‖ ١٨ أجناسها ] أجناسه EsP

either a literal quotation from Galen or the intent of his words. But I will express this intent partly in his words and partly in my own words.[19] All this is gleaned from what Galen taught us in *De methodo medendi* 12. This is the right moment to start with those five aphorisms which I promised.[20]

10. Syncope is a quick collapse[21] of the faculties of the body. The existence and permanence of the faculties in their essential nature depends on the balance of the pneumata, humors, and organs in their quantity and quality. The cause for the collapse of the faculties (namely, syncope) can be a quantitative or qualitative change of the pneumata, or a quantitative or qualitative change of the humors, or a quantitative or qualitative change of the organs.[22] The causes of syncope can thus be limited to these three classes, and since each class consists of two subclasses (namely, a quantitative change and a qualitative change) we [actually] have six classes.[23]

11. A change in the main organs that causes syncope is [due either to] a dissolution in their substance—and this is a decrease in quantity—or to their bad temperament because of an excess in one of the four qualities. The substance of the organs is dissolved either because of prolonged chronic diseases or because of acute diseases or because of wasting fevers.[24]

12. A change in the pneumata that causes syncope occurs either because the pneuma dissolves, and this is a quantitative loss, or because the substance of the pneuma is corrupted, and this is a qualitative loss. The corruption of the substance of the pneuma is due to a corruption of the air, or to lethal drugs, or to animal poisons. A dissolution of the pneuma is either due to the movements of the soul[25] such as intense joy, which is called "exultation,"[26] or intense pleasure or intense fear, and similarly, anxiety and anger. As part of all these movements, Galen [also] mentioned pain and sleeplessness.[27] But I say that these two should

كلام جالينوس بعينه أو معانيه لكنّ أعبّر عنه بعبارة بعض تلك العبارة من كلامه وبعضها
من كلامي . وكلّ ذلك ملقوط ممّا علّمنا جالينوس في ثانية عشر الحيلة . وهذا حين أبتدئ
بتلك الفصول الخمسة التي وعدنا بها .

١٠ . الغشــي ســقوط يعرض للقوى بحدّة وسرعة وقوام جوهر القوى وثباته هو
باعتــدال الأرواح والأخلاط والأعضاء في كمّيتها وكيفيتها . فقد يكون ســبب ســقوط
القوى أعني سقوط الغشي من أجل تغيّر الأرواح في كمّيتها أو في كيفيتها وقد يكون سبب ذلك
من أجل تغيّر الأخلاط في كيفيتها أو كمّيتها وقد يكون سبب ذلك من أجل تغيّر الأعضاء
في كيفيتها أو في كمّيتها . فقد انحصرت إذا أسـباب الغشي في هذه الثلاثة أجناس وفي
كلّ الجنس جنسان تغيّر الكمّية وتغيّر الكيفية فهذه ستّة أجناس .

١١ . تغيّر الأعضاء الأصلية الموجب للغشــي هو أن يتحلّل جوهرها وذلك نقصان
كمّية أو بســوء مزاجها بإفراط في أحد الكيفيــات الأربعة . وجوهر الأعضاء يتحلّل إمّا
بطول أمراض مزمنة أو بحدّة أمراض حادّة أو بحمّيات ذوبانية .

١٢ . تغيّر الأرواح الموجب للغشــي إمّا بأن يتحلّل الروح وذلــك نقصان كمّيتها أو
يفســد جوهر الروح وذلك فساد كيفيتها . وفساد جوهر الروح يكون من قبل فساد الهواء
أو من قبل أدوية قتّالة أو من قبل ســموم حيوان . وتحلّل الروح يكون إمّا من قبل حركات
نفسانية كاللذّة الشديدة التي تسمّى فرحا أو السرور الشديد أو الفزع الشديد وكذلك الغمّ
والغضب . ومن جملة هذه الحركات قال جالينوس الوجع والأرق لكنّي أقول إنّه ينبغي أن

---

١ معانيه] معانـاه O || ٤ بحدّة] بغتـة Es | وقوام] يقاوم L | وثباتـه] وثباتها L || ٦-
٧ وقد . . . أو كمّيتها] om. L || ٢٦،٩ - ٢٧،١١ om. E || ١٠ تغيّر] فهذه . . . الكمّية
تغيير L || ١٢ ذوبانية] ذوابنية Ox || ١٣ كمّيتها] كمّيته L

be counted separately because there is nothing stronger for the dissolution of the pneuma than pain, and after that, sleeplessness. Similarly,
the pneuma is dissolved when it becomes excessively thin and fine or
because its vessels become too thin and porous. The pneuma can also be
5      dissolved because of a lack of food or because of severe diarrhea. These
two causes also effect a change in the organs and the humors, but Galen
linked them to the pneuma.[28]

13. A change in the humors that causes syncope occurs either in
their quality [or in their quantity. Their quality changes] when the
10     humors become very thin and fine and dissolve rapidly. Therefore, if one
does not take care to properly nourish these [humors,] syncope occurs
rapidly. Similarly, if the quality of the humors becomes so thick and
viscous that they become crude and raw, they cause syncope for [the fol-
lowing] reasons: (1) the body does not receive enough nutrition, (2) the
15     innate heat is suppressed, (3) the balance of the temperament is changed
and corrupted, and (4) these humors oppress the strength [of the body]
through their abundance—when they neither oppress nor obstruct it,
they cause fainting,[29] not syncope. It is clear to you that a surplus of
humors that causes oppression or obstruction of the strength [of the
20     body] also causes syncope, and this is a change in quantity.

14. It is clear from the foregoing that the causes of syncope comprise
six classes and twenty-one kinds. The first class—namely, a quantitative
change of the organs—consists of three kinds: a chronic disease, an acute
disease, or a wasting fever. The second class—namely, a qualitative change
25     of the organs—consists of four kinds: they become excessively hot or cold
or dry or moist. The third class—namely, a qualitative change of the
pneuma—consists of three kinds, which are corruption of the air, ingestion of a poisonous substance, or the bite of a venomous animal. The fourth
class—namely, a quantitative change of the pneuma, meaning that the
30     pneuma dissolves and disappears or greatly diminishes—consists of seven
kinds: thinness and fineness of the pneumata, or thinness and porousness

تعدّ هذين بانفراد إذ ليس ثمّ سيء أبلغ في تحليل الروح من الوجع وبعده السهر . وكذلك يتحلّل الروح إذا رقّ ولطف بإفراط أو من قبل أنّ أوعيته تسخف وتتخلخل وكذلك يتحلّل الروح من عدم الغذاء ومن إفراط الإسهال . وهذان السببان أيضا يغيّران الأعضاء والأخلاط لكنّ جالينوس للروح نسبها .

١٣ . تغيّر الأخلاط الموجب للغشي إمّا في كيفيتها فبأن ترقّ الأخلاط وتلطف جدّا فهي تتحلّل بسرعة ولذلك إن لم يعتنى بتغذية هؤلاء كما يجب أسرع الغشي . وكذلك إن تغيّرت كيفية الأخلاط إلى الغلظ واللزوجة حتّى صارت نيئة خامة فهي تحدث الغشي لأسباب . أحدها أنّ البدن يقلّ غذاءه والثاني أنّ الحرارة الغريزية تختنق والثالث أنّ اعتدال المزاج يتغيّر ويفسد والرابع أنّها تثقل القوة بكثرتها ومتى لم تثقل ولا سدّدت أحدثت خمولا لا غشيا . فقد تبيّن لك أنّ كثرة الأخلاط أيضا الموجب لإثقال القوة أو للسدد يوجب غشيا وهذا تغيّر في الكمّية .

١٤ . قد تبيّن من كلّ ما قدمناه أنّ أسباب الغشي الجنسية ستّة وأنواعها أحد وعسرون . الجنس الأوّل وهو تغيّر الأعضاء في كمّها أنواعه ثلاثة وهي إمّا مرض مزمن أو مرض حادّ أو حمّى ذوبانية . الجنس الثاني وهو تغيّر الأعضاء في كيفيتها أنواعه أربعة وهي أن تسخن أو تبرد أو تجفّ أو ترطب كلّ ذلك بإفراط . الجنس الثالث وهو تغيّر الروح في كيفيتها وأنواعه ثلاثة وهي فساد الهواء أو تناول شيء من السموم أو نهش حيوان سمّي . الجنس الرابع وهو تغيّر الروح في كمّيتها وهو أن تتحلّل الروح وتذهب أو تنتقص بإفراط أنواعه سبعة : رقّة الأرواح ولطافتها أو سخافة العروق وتخلخلها أو الحركات

of the vessels, or the movements of the soul, or pain, or sleeplessness, or
lack of food, or diarrhea, or other similar evacuations. The fifth class—
namely, a qualitative change of the humors—consists of two kinds, which
are thinness and fineness of the humors or thickness and crudeness
thereof. The sixth class—namely, a quantitative change of the humors—
consists of two kinds: a surplus that oppresses the strength [of the body,]
or a surplus that causes an obstruction. These are all the [various] classes
of the causes of syncope as explained from the words of Galen, and they
number twenty-one causes.

15. Says Moses: The most important way to prevent the occurrence
of syncope is to devote all one's attention during any disease to the
three major organs and the cardia of the stomach because of the close
interaction[30] between the latter and the major organs. One should take
care of the faculties of these organs—namely, through balancing their
temperament by means of that with which one supplies the body and by
means of that which one applies to the organ externally. Having con-
cerned oneself with these organs, one should seek to balance the temperament of the other organs. Similarly, one should give priority to
balancing the pneumata of these three organs. As for the psychical
pneuma, this should be done through the sniffing of aromatic substances. As for the animal pneuma, it should be done through balancing
the outside air, and through opening the pores of the skin, and through
cleansing the respiratory organs from the thick and viscous [humors,]
and through opening the obstruction caused by them, and through the
consumption of that which, in combination with drugs, has the property
to purify the blood of the heart and to remove the turbidity from its air.[31]
As for the natural pneuma, this should be done by the consumption of
food and drink that should be of the best and most balanced quality and
the least detrimental.[32] One should be extremely careful not to let a
patient take any food or drink that is mixed with the slightest [amount
of] putrefaction because these kinds of food produce poisonous humors,
as mentioned by Galen.[33] Similarly, one should be careful not to give a
patient any food that corrupts quickly, such as milk, or those foods
that produce a poisonous humor when they corrupt, such as melon,[34]
cucumber,[35] and gourd.[36] One should be careful that the patient does not

النفسـانية أو الوجع أو الأرق أو عدم الغذاء أو الإسهال ونحوه من الاستفراغات . الجنس الخامس وهو تغيّر الأخلاط في كيفيتها له نوعان وهما رقّة الأخلاط ولطافتها أو غلظها ونيوءتها . الجنس السـادس وهو تغيّر الأخلاط فـي كمّيتها له نوعان : إمّا كثرة تثقل القوة أو كثرة تحدث سددا . فهذا جملة أسباب الغشي النوعية على ما تبيّن من كلام جالينوس وذلك أحد وعشرون سببا .

٥. قال موسـى : آكد الوجوه في التحفّظ من وقوع الغشي هو أن تعنى كلّ العناية في كلّ مرض بالثلاثة الأعضاء الرئيسـة وفم المعدة لعظم المشاركة التي بينه وبين الأعضاء الرئيسة . وتحرز على هذه الأعضاء قواها وذلك بتعديل مزاجها بما تورده البدن وبما تجعل على العضو من خارج وبعد اعتناك بهذه الأعضاء تروم تعديل مزاج سائر الأعضاء وكذلك تقدم العناية بتعديل أرواح هذه الأعضاء الثلاثة . أمّا الروح النفسـانية فبالمشـمومات وأمّا الـروح الحيوانية فبتعديل الهواء الخارج وتفتيح مسـامّ الجلد وتنقية آلات التنفّس من الغلظ واللزوجات وتفتيح سددها وإيراد مع الأدوية ما شأنه أن يروّق دم القلب ويزيل الكدر عن روحه . وأمّا الروح الطبيعية فبما يؤكل ويشـرب وهو أن يكون أفضل غذاء وأعدله وأبعده عن الفسـاد . وتتحفّظ غاية التحفّظ من مناولة المرضى شيئًا من الأطعمة والأشربة التي يشـوبها أيسـر عفونة فإنّ هذه الأغذية تولّد أخلاطا سـمّية كما ذكر جالينوس . وكذلك تتحفّظ من إعطاء المرضى أحد الأغذية التي يسـرع فسـادها كاللبن والأغذية التي يتولّد عنها خلط سـمّي إن فسدت كالبطّيخ والخيار والقرع فإنّ الأخـذ بالاحتياط أن لا ينال

٣ ونيوءتهـا ] ونيبوتها Es P : ونهوتها O : ولزوجتها EL : ليونتها Ox ǁ ٦ آكد ] أوكد EL : اخذ Ox | الوجوه ] الأشياء E : الوجه Ox | كلّ ] غاية O ǁ ٧ لعظم ] لعظيم LOOxP ǁ ٨ تورده ] توربده Ox : داخل add. O ǁ ١٢ مع الأدوية ] om. ELOx | يروّق ] يرقق Ox ǁ ١٣ روحه ] مع الأدوية add. ELOx | وأبعده ] وأعسره L¹ ǁ ١٥ أيسر ] أكثر O

eat any ingredients such as these because we fear that they corrupt or that they are slow to descend[37] and thus cause severe damage. Similarly, one should constantly strengthen the stomach and beware of bad digestion. If one makes these things one's aim, one prevents the occurrence of syncope to the majority of patients under one's care.[38]

16. Emaciation of the body originating from an enlarged spleen has two causes. First, the food is not adequately digested in the liver so that the organs do not receive sufficient food (since the food that is most proper to them in this case is that which is slightly bad). The second cause is that the blood is turbid, and most of it is attracted by the spleen, thus not allowing the body to be nourished by it. *In Hippocratis De aeris [aquis locis] commentarius* 2.[39]

17. If black [bile] dominates someone's body, he is very fond of sexual intercourse because many thick inflating winds collect in his body in the hypochondria. *In Hippocratis Epidemiarum* 6.3.[40]

18. Emaciation of the body occurs either because of weakness of the powers of the flesh or because the pulsatile vessels and nonpulsatile vessels are filled with bad blood. Obesity of the body occurs through the opposite of these two causes—the flesh attracts most of the blood to it, leaving only a small quantity [of it] in the vessels. *In Hippocratis Epidemiarum* 6.3.[41]

19. Humors cause pain in one of six ways: either through their overabundance, their thickness, their viscosity, their heat, their coolness, or through their biting and corrosion[42] of an organ. *In Hippocratis De humoribus commentarius* 1.[43]

20. Just as the humors influence one's character, so one's character influences the humors: if someone is dominated by bile, he is irascible, and when someone is very angry, bilious humors originate in him. *In Hippocratis De humoribus commentarius* 3.[44]

المريض شيئًا من أمثال هذه خشّينا أن تفسد أو يبطأ انحدارها فتؤذي أذية عظيمة . وكذلك تقوّي المعدة دائمًا وتتحفّظ من سـوء الاسـتمراء . فإنّـك إن جعلت هذه الأمور قصدك أمنت حدوث الغشي في معظم من تعانيه .

١٦ . لهزال البدن عن عظم الطحال سببان أحدهما أنّ الغذاء لا ينهضم في الكبد على ما ينبغي فيقلّ غذاء الأعضاء إذ الجيّد الموافق لها في ذلك الرديئ قليلا . والسبب الثاني أنّ الدم يكون عكرا فيجتذب أكثره الطحال فلا يدع البدن يغتذي به . في شرحه للثانية من الأهوية .

١٧ . من يغلب على بدنه السوداء مغرى بالجماع من قبل أن يجتمع في بدنه في ما دون الشراسيف رياح غليظة نافخة كثيرة . في المقالة الثالثة من شرحه لسادسة ابيديميا .

١٨ . هـزال البدن إمّا لضعف قوى اللحم أو لكون العروق الضوارب وغير الضوارب مملوءة دما رديئا . خصب البدن يكون بأضداد هذين السببين حتّى يجذب اللحم معظم الدم فيقلّ ما في العروق . في الثالثة من شرحه لسادسة ابيديميا .

١٩ . الأخلاط تحدث الوجع بأحد ستّة أوجه إمّا بكثرتها أو بغلظها أو بلزوجتها أو بسخونتها أو ببرودتها أو بتلذيعها وأكلها للعضو . في شرحه للأولى من الأخلاط .

٢٠ . كمــا أنّ الأخلاط توثّر فـي الأخلاق كذلك الأخلاق توثّـر في الأخلاط فإنّ مــن غلب عليه المـرار يكون غضوبـا وكلّ من اشـتدّ غضبه يتولّد فيـه أخلاط مرّة . في الثالثة من شرح الأخلاط .

---

٣ أمنت [ من ] ELOx add. ‖ ٤–٦ لهـزال . . . يغتذي به ] وإذا اغتذى جذب الطحال أكثر الغذاء إليه فلا يدع البدن أن يغتذى فيهزل اضطرارا فلهذا قال إنّ اللحم ينحلّ في الطحال وإنّ الطحال هو علّة هزال البدن ليس لهذه العلّة فقط يهزل الطحال البدن كلّه بل لقربه من الكبد فيفسد ويضعف القوّة الهاضمة فيها فإذا ما لم ينهضم الكبد الغذاء على ما ينبغي نحف البدن وانحلّ . . . C, fol. 46v6–10 ‖ عظم ] om. EOx : ضعـف L ‖ ٥ الجيّد ] الغـذاء ELP¹ ‖ ٧ في ما ] سـيما O ‖ ٨ ابيديميا ] افيديميا ELOxP ‖ ٩ هزال ] سـبب هزال E ‖ ١١ ابيديميا ] افيديميا ELOxP

21. Pruritus[45] occurs because of sharp, biting humors that irritate a part of the body and produce a kind of movement that is similar to that which occurs when moving the fingers in the region of the armpit. *In Hippocratis De alimento commentaria* 3.[46]

22. Says Moses: When the biting humor is of a thin consistency and passes through a sensitive organ, one of the four [different] symptoms that he mentioned in his treatise *De plenitudine* is caused in that organ.[47] We have mentioned that particular text in one of the aphorisms [when we discussed] these symptoms.[48] When the biting humor is of a thick consistency or the organ is [only] a little sensitive, it causes the pruritus that he mentioned.

23. Sometimes a vitreous phlegmatic humor collects in the body but does not putrefy and thus causes rigor lasting for many successive days. As long as a person is at rest and does not move at all, the rigor is also at rest. But if he moves, his motion is immediately followed by rigor proportional to the extent of the motion. The stronger and faster the motion, the stronger the rigor. I have seen this affliction and treated it with drugs that heat and dissolve the thick humors, such as the [various] kinds of pepper and mint.[49] *De tremore, [palpitatione, rigore et convulsione].*[50]

24. There are three causes of thickness of blood and its blackness and coagulation so that the vessels are filled with melancholic humor. These causes can occur either together or separately. One of these is that the liver is prepared to produce that superfluity. The second [cause] is that the regimen of food and drink and the like has the property to produce thick blood. The third [cause] is that the condition of the spleen is so weak that it cannot attract all of the superfluity that is produced in the liver. *Ad Glauconem [de medendi methodo]* 2.[51]

25. When sharp humors or sharp drugs that make the organs rough are excessively strong, they produce ulcers in the fleshy parts of the body and caries[52] in the bones. *De [morborum] causis et symptomatibus* 2.[53]

26. Sometimes dementia[54] and forgetfulness occur from extreme old age and senility. This is an indication that the dementia and forgetfulness originate especially from coldness. But all deliria are the result of hot

٢١. الدغدغة تحدث من قبل أخلاط حرّيفة لذّاعة تلذع العضو فيحدث فيه شـبه الحركة التي تحدث من التحريك بالأصابع تحت الإبط ونحوه. في شرحه لثالثة الغذاء.

٢٢. قال موسـى الخلط اللذّاع إن كان رقيق القوام ومرّ بعضو حسّـاس أحدث فيه أحـد الأربعة الأصناف التي ذكرها فـي مقالته في الكثرة. وقـد ذكرنا ذلك الفصل في الاستدلالات من هذه الفصول. أمّا إن كان الخلط اللذّاع غليظ القوام أو يكون العضو قليل الحسّ فيحدث الذعدغة التي ذكر هو. هكذا يبدو إليّ في ذلك.

٢٣. قـد يجتمـع فـي البدن خلط بلغمـي زجاجي ولا يعفن ويحدث نافضا أيّاما كثيرة متوالية. وما دام الإنسـان سـاكنا لا يتحرّك أصلا فيسكن النافض. فإن تحرّك تبع حركته النافض من سـاعته وكان ذلك بحسـب مقادير الحركة. كلّما تحرّك حركة أقوى وأسرع حدث عنها نافض أشدّ. ورأيت هذا العارض وداويته بالأدوية التي تسخن وتقطع الأخلاط الغليظة كالفلافلي والفوذنج. في مقالته في الرعدة.

٢٤. أسباب غلظ الدم وسـواده وخثورته حتّى تمتلئ العروق من الخلط السوداوي ثلاثة إمّا كلّها وإمّا بعضها. أحدها أن تكون الكبد مستعدّة لتوليد ذلك الفضل. والثاني أن يكون التدبير بالأطعمة والأشربة وغير ذلك ممّا شأنه توليد دم غليظ. والثالث أن يكون الطحـال بحـال مـن الضعف يعجز بها عن أن يجتذب إليه كلّمـا يتولّد في الكبد من ذلك الفضل. في ثانية أغلوقا.

٢٥. الأخلاط الحادّة أو الأدوية الحادّة التي تخشّن الأعضاء متى كان معها فضل قوة أحدثت في الأعضاء اللحمية قروحا وفي العظام نخزا. ثانية العلل والأعراض.

٢٦. قد يحدث تخبّل العقل والنسـيان من الشيخوخة القصوى والهرم الشديد وهذا دليل على أنّ تخبّل العقل والنسـيان إنّما يحدثان من قبل البرودة. وجميع الاختلاطات إنّما

٧ أيّامـا] أيّام G ‖ ٩ حركه] حركة O ‖ ١١ والفوذنج] والفوذنجي EEsLP ‖ ١٢ الدم] الورم L ‖ ٣٠،١٧–٤١،٨ أو الأدوية . . . من خواصّ] om. Ox ‖ ١٨ نخزا] om. L

biting humors, particularly yellow bile. Sometimes they occur because of
a hot, bad temperament. Not one of these is caused by a cold humor, except
for the delirium that is called "melancholic delusion." The delirium that
occurs in the last stages of acute fevers is caused by hot biting vapors
5   that rise to the head. *De [morborum] causis et symptomatibus* 5.[55]

27. Pain in membranes is dissimilar because their sensitivity is dissimilar. Some spots are very sensitive while others are hardly sensitive.[56]
But pain in membranes can [also] be dissimilar for a different reason—
namely, that when during [the membrane's] stretching it touches the
10  bone. *De locis affectis* 2.[57]

28. The reason some inflamed tumors are accompanied by pulsation
and others are not is the presence of a sizable pulsatile vessel in the spot
of the [inflamed] tumor. Whenever the [inflamed] tumor expands, it compresses [this vessel] and pulsation occurs. *De locis affectis* 2.[58]

15  29. Just as a thick phlegmatic humor can produce epilepsy, so a
melancholic humor can produce epilepsy when it is retained in the channels of the ventricles of the brain. But when it increases and becomes
dominant[59] in the very substance of the brain, it causes melancholic
delusion. *De locis affectis* 3.[60]

20  30. The cause for the hardening of a [pulsatile] vessel[61] is one of three
things: either dryness, or congealment due to the cold, or stretching.
Dryness occurs in the case of ardent fevers (when they last for a long
time and are bad and malignant) and in the case of melancholy and some
quartan fevers. Congealment originates from anything that produces a
25  vitreous humor in the body. Stretching occurs in the case of diseases that
are of the same type as spasms and in the case of large [inflamed] tumors
and in the case of hardness and rigidity occurring in the substance of
the liver or spleen. *De pulsu* 13.[62]

31. Tapeworms[63] eat anything by which a human being feeds him-
30  self and therefore make the body lean. *De theriaca ad pisonem.*[64]

تتبع الأخلاط الحارّة اللذّاعة بمنزلة المرّة الصفراء خاصّة . وقد يحدث بسبب سوء مزاج حارّ وليس منها شيء يكون السبب فيه خلطا باردا إلا الأختلاط الذي يقال له الوسواس السوداوي . وأمّا يحدث من الاختلاط في أواخر الحمّيات الحادّة فسببه أبخرة حارّة لذّاعة ترتقي إلى الرأس . خامسة العلل والأعراض .

٢٧ . الوجع الذي يكون في الأغشية غير مستوي لأنّ الغشاء حسّه مختلف منه موضع كثير الحسّ وموضع قليل الحسّ . ويختلف وجع الأغشية من وجه آخر لأنّه قد يلقى عند تمدّده عظما . ثانية التعرّف .

٢٨ . السبب في كون بعض الأورام الحارّة يوجد معها ضربان وبعضها دون ضربان هو وجود عرق ضارب ذا قدر في موضع الورم. فكلّما انبسط ضغط الورم وحدث الضربان. ثانية التعرّف .

٢٩ . كما أنّ خلط البلغم الغليظ قد يحدث عنه الصرع كذلك الخلط السوداوي قد يحدث عنه الصرع إذا احتبس في منافذ بطون الدماغ. أمّا متى غلب وكثر في نفس جرم الدماغ فإنّ الذي يحدث عنه الوسواس السوداوي .

٣٠ . الأسباب التي تجعل العرق صلبا أحد ثلاثة أشياء . إمّا يبس وإمّا جمود من قبل البرد وإمّا تمدّد . واليبس يحدث في الحمّيات المحرقة إذا طالت مع رداة وخبث وفي المالنخوليا وبعض حمّيات الربع . والجمود يحدث من كلّ شيء يولّد في البدن خلطا زجاجيا . والتمدّد يحدث في العلل التي من جنس التشنّج وفي الأورام العظيمة وفي الصلابة والجساوة تحدث في جرم الكبد أو الطحال . ثالثة عشر النبض .

٣١ . حبّ القرع يأكل كلّما يغتذي به الإنسان ولذلك يهزل البدن . في مقالة الترياق لقيصر .

---

٨  في كون بعض] الـذي يكون فـي بعـض L  ||  ١١–١٢  كذلك . . . الصرع] G¹O¹  ||
١٦  المالنخوليا] المالنخونيا ELO  |  يحدث] om. EL  ||  ١٩  الترياق] الدرياق EsG

32. Sometimes sneezing is an accidental remedy and cure for moistures that are collected in the lungs, in the stomach, and in the cardia
of the stomach and from which hiccups originate. It removes and expels
them from those places. This is why sneezing [also] cures hiccups—by
5    cleansing all the superfluities that are above the stomach. *De [morborum]*
*causis et symptomatibus* 5.[65]

33. The reason the pain following the extraction of a painful tooth
is necessarily alleviated is that, at that moment, the nerve that was connected to the root of the tooth relaxes because it is severed from the bone
10   that caused its [initial] stretching. And space is formed in the tooth
through which dissolved liquids that have gathered there can emerge.
*Mayāmir* 5.[66]

34. The reason for the breaking and corrosion of teeth lies in their
softness. Therefore, it is necessary to harden and strengthen them with
15   astringent drugs. In the same way their color turns livid[67] and the like
because of bad moistures streaming towards them. Therefore, they
should be treated with drugs that moderately dry—not as some physicians think, that the stronger the drying effect, the more beneficial the
drug. *Mayāmir* 5.[68]

20   35. If an inflamed tumor occurs in a sinewy part of the body, it is
followed by delirium[69] more quickly [than in any other part,] either
because the heat alone ascends to the head through parts connected to
that nerve or because it ascends with a vaporous or smoky gas.[70] *De locis*
*affectis* 3.[71]

25   36. A tremor occurs because of a weakness of the faculty that sup-
ports and moves the body and also because of the natural heaviness of a
part of the body. For when someone [suffering from such a weakness] wants
to move a part of the body, it falls downward due to the weakness of the
force, and because he cannot [support this part of the body,] trembling
30   occurs. But if he did not have any desire at all to move it, he would not
tremble. Similarly, if the motive faculty were totally abolished, no trembling would occur, but relaxation. That impossibility [to move] may be
clarified for you by [thinking of] someone who has a heavy burden upon

٣٢ . العطاس يكون في بعض الأوقات دواء وشفاء بطريق العرض للرطوبات المجتمعة

في الرئة وللرطوبات المجتمعة في المعدة وفي فمها التي يكون عنها الفواق فينفضها ويخرجها

من تلك المواضع . وهذا السبب يكون العطاس شفاء للفواق بتنقيته الفضول كلّها التي فوق

المعدة . خامسة العلل والأعراض .

٣٣ . السبب الموجب لسكون الوجع عند قلع السنّ الألمة أنّ العصبة حينئذ التي تتّصل ٥

بأصل السنّ يذهب تمدّدها من أجل أنّها قد استرخت من الاتّصال والرباط بالعظم الذي بسببه

كانت تتمدّد . وصار لها موضع ينفذ منه ما يتحلّل ممّا كان مجتمع فيها . خامسة الميامر .

٣٤ . سبب تكسير الأسنان وتقتّها من قبل لينها . ومن أجل هذا ينبغي أن نصلّبها

ونقوّيها بالأدوية القابضة . وكذلك تغيّر لونها إلى الخضرة وغيرها من قبل رطوبات رديئة

تتحلّب إليها . ولذلك ينبغي أن تعالج بالأدوية تجفّف تجفيفا معتدلا لا كما يظنّ بعض ١٠

الأطبّاء أنّ كلّما كان أشدّ تجفيفا فهو أنفع . خامسة الميامر .

٣٥ . متى تورّم عضو عصباني ورما حارّا كان اتّباع الاختلاط له أسرع إمّا لأنّ

الحرارة وحدها تصعد إلى الرأس صعودا متّصلا في ذلك العصب أو ترقى مع ريح

بخارية أو دخانية . ثالثة التعرّف .

٣٦ . الرعدة تكون بسبب ضعف القوة الحاملة والمحرّكة للبدن وبسبب ثقل العضو ١٥

الطبيعـي . فـإذا رام تحريك العضو فلأجل ضعف القوة يهوي العضو إلى أسـفل فيحدث

التمانـع فيرتعـد . ولو لم يرم تحريكه أصلا لم يرتعش . وكذلك لو بطلت القوة المحرّكة أصلا

لـم يحدث ارتعاش بل اسـترخاء . ويبيّن لك هذا التمانع فيمـن عليه حمل ثقيل وهو يروم

---

٣ الفضول كلّها التي ] الفضل كلّه الذي ELO || ٤ والأعراض ] om. G || ٥ حينئذ ] G¹ || ٨ تكسير ]
تكثّر OP || ١١ فهو ] كان G || ١٢ الاختلاط ] الأخلاط EEsGOP || ١٣ وحدها ] قصدها
O || ١٣ ترقى ] ترقّى EsO || ١٥ العضو ] EsG || الخلط : Es¹G¹ || ١٧ تحريكه ] تحريك G

himself and wants to lift his feet in order to go [but cannot do so] because his legs tremble. Similarly, if he wants to lift something heavy, his arms tremble. In the same way, when someone is frightened or alarmed and then wants to go or to lift [something heavy], his arms and legs tremble.

5 Alarm and fear undermine one's strength. For this reason, trembling occurs to the elderly and to someone whose body is weakened and emaciated because of a disease. *De tremore, [palpitatione, rigore et convulsione].*[72]

37. Spasms occur because of overfilling or because of emptying. When it occurs because of sleeplessness, exertion, worry, anxiety, or dry ardent

10 fever, the cause of that [kind of] spasm is the dryness and emptying. If someone who is given to rest and ease and to constantly filling [his stomach] and to permanent leisure and idleness is stricken by a spasm, we should suspect that it is caused by overfilling. Similarly, epilepsy is a spasm due to overfilling, possibly occurring when the origin of each

15 nerve is moistened by that thick and viscous moisture.[73] However, this spasm is not continuous as is that which is from the front or back or from both sides together. *De locis affectis* 3.[74]

38. The cause of palpitation is something of the nature and substance of the air that streams to the organs. In its essence there is a

20 thick type of vapor. The cause of a spasm in the case of inflammatory diseases is overfilling and in the case of very ardent and dry fevers is emptying. *De [morborum] causis et symptomatibus* 5.[75]

39. A spasm is caused by a stretching of nerves either because of moisture or because of dryness. The muscles at the origins of nerves

25 also stretch and contract involuntarily, thus causing a spasm. *De tremore, [palpitatione, rigore et convulsione].*[76]

40. The cause of palpitation is a thick wind[77] that is confined to a narrow spot from which it cannot escape. This wind cannot dissolve because of its thickness, and it cannot escape because of the density of the surround-

30 ing bodies. Since it constantly tries to escape, it causes the mentioned palpitation.[78] And since the cause of palpitation is of one kind, its treatment is also of one kind—namely everything that thins and heats. When applied internally or externally, castoreum[79] is especially [good] for this

شــيل رجليه ويمشي فإنّه ترعد رجلاه وكذلك إن شــال شيئًا ثقيلا ارتعدت يداه . وعلى
هذا المثال متى ذعر الإنسان أو فزع ثمّ رام مشيا أو شيلا ارتعدت يداه ورجلاه . فإنّ الفزع
والخوف يهدّان القوّة ولهذا يعرض الارتعاش للشيوخ ولمن قد ضعف ونحل بدنه من المرض .
في مقالته في الرعدة والاختلاج .

٣٧ . التشنّج يكون عن الامتلاء ويكون عن الاستفراغ . فمتى كان حدوث التشنّج من
قبل السهر أو التعب أو الهمّ والغمّ والحمّى اليابسة المحرقة فالسبب في ذلك التشنّج اليبس
والاستفراغ . فأمّا إن كان إنسان صاحب سكون ودعة وتملّؤ في كلّ وقت وإدمان الراحة
والبطالة وأصابه التشنّج فينبغي أن نتوهّم أنّ ذلك من الامتلاء . وكذلك الصرع هو تشنّج
من امتلاء عسى أن يكون منشأ كلّ واحد من الأعصاب يبتلّ بتلك الرطوبة الغليظة اللزجة
إلّا أنّه ليس بدائم كالتشنّج الذي من قدام أو من خلف أو من الوجهين جميعا . ثالثة التعرّف .

٣٨ . ســبب الاختلاج شــيء من طبيعة الهواء وجوهره ينصبّ إلى الأعضاء . وفي
جوهره غلظ من جنس البخار . والســبب الفاعل للتشنّج في العلل الأورامية هو الامتلاء
والفاعل له في الحمّيات المحرقة جدّا اليابسة هو الاستفراغ . خامسة العلل والأعراض .

٣٩ . التشنّج هو تمدّد العصب إمّا من رطوبة أو من يبس . ويتمدّد العضل أيضا
نحو مبادئه ويتقلّص بغير إرادة فيحدث التشنّج . في مقالته في الرعدة .

٤٠ . الاختلاج ســببه ريح غليظة منحصرة في موضع متكاثف لا تجد منه مخلصا
ولا تقدر تتحلّل لغلظها ولا تجد مخلصا لكثافة الأجسام الحاوية لها ولا تزال تطلب الخروج
فتحرّك ما هي فيه تلك الحركة . ومن أجل كون سبب الاختلاج واحدا صار علاجه جنسا
واحدا وهو جميع ما يلطّف ويسخّن . والجندبادستر دواء خاصّ بهذه العلّة إذا شرب وإذا

١ ارتعــدت يداه] ارتعد فـي يديه ورجلاه EL | ٢-١ يــداه ورجلاه . . . وعلى ] om. EL ||
٢ فإنّ] لأنّ EL : P¹ || ٣ يعرض] يحدث L || ٨ أنّ] om. G || ٩ الغليظة] om. EL ||
١٤ هو] و G || ١٥ مبادئه] مواديها O

affliction because it is a drug that is heating, thinning, and extremely drying. According to this reasoning palpitation is especially caused by something cold. *De tremore, [palpitatione, rigore et convulsione].*[80]

41. When someone's body has a bad humor and becomes hot through exertion or something else, he suffers from shivering even when no fever arises. *In Hippocratis Epidemiarum* 6.3.[81]

42. A weakness of the force that is the cause of a tremor does not have one cause but many causes. Sometimes it is caused by malnutrition, as happens in the case of cholera, severe diarrhea, and the frequent loss of blood, and in the case of someone fasting. Sometimes it is caused by the dissolution of the animal faculty,[82] as happens in the case of syncope.[83] Sometimes it is caused by severe cold, which compresses the pores of the nerves so that only weak impulses of that motive faculty get through. Sometimes it is caused by overfilling, which oppresses the force so that it is too weak for motion. Therefore, the remedies that cure tremors are not of one kind. *De tremore, [palpitatione, rigore et convulsione].*[84]

43. A rigor is a severe and suddenly concentrated cold whereby the body goes from a natural to an unnatural condition. That it is a cold affliction is obvious and clear. As for its cause—I mean the cause of a rigor—it is a cold humor that moves and passes through the sensitive organs. Sometimes it is a sharp humor that moves and streams through the sensitive organs. In both cases the innate heat is put to flight by the biting substance and returns to its original site so that the outer parts of the body become cold. Then, when on its return it finds the pores constricted and contracted and its passages obstructed, it stops in its course and returns to its original site and then leaves this site once again. This continues either until it gains the upper hand and heats the outer parts of the body or until it is overpowered and extinguished and the patient dies. During that phase of going back and forth and being hindered [from passing through,] trembling associated with rigor occurs.[85] The difference between a tremor and rigor is that a tremor results from the hindrance between the voluntary strength [of the body] and its natural weight. If

وضع من خارج لأجل أنّه دواء يسخن ويلطّف ويجفّف تجفيفا مستقصى . والاختلاج على هذا القياس إنّما يحدث عن سبب بارد . في مقالته في الرعدة والاختلاج .

٤١ . إذا كان في البدن خلط رديئ فيسخن بتعب أو بغيره يقشعرّ الشخص وإن لم يحدث حمّى . في الثالثة من شرحه لسادسة ابيديميا .

٥ ٤٢ . هذا هو ضعف القوة الذي هو سبب الرعشة ليس سببه واحدا بل أسبابه كثيرة . قد يكون ذلك بسبب عوز الغذاء كما يحدث في الهيضة والاستطلاق الشديد وتواتر خروج الدم ولمن يمسك عن الطعام . وقد يكون بسبب انحلال القوة الحيوانية كما يحدث في الغشي . وقد يكون بسبب برودة شديدة تلزّز مسامّ العصب ولا تنفذ من تلك القوة المحرّكة إلا شيئًا ضعيفا . وقد يكون بسبب امتلاء يثقل القوة فتضعف عن الحركة . ولذلك صارت

١٠ الأشياء التي تداوي الرعشة ليست نوعا واحدا . في مقالته في الرعدة والاختلاج .

٤٣ . النافض برودة مجتمعة في دفعة واحدة عنيفة يصير بها البدن من الحال الطبيعية إلى حال خارجة عن الطبيعة . فأمّا أنّ هذه الآفة باردة فذلك أمر ظاهر مكشوف . وأمّا سببها أعني سبب النافض فقد يكون خلطا باردا عند حركته ومروره بالأعضاء الحسّاسة . وقد يكون خلطا حادّا عند حركته وجريانه على الأعضاء الحسّاسة . وفي

١٥ الحالين جميعا ينهزم الحارّ الغريزي هاربا من الشيء اللذّاع راجعا إلى مبدئه فتبرد ظواهر البدن . ثمّ يكرّ راجعا فيجد المسامّ منقبضا مجتمعا ويسدّ طرقه ويقف في وجهه فيعود راجعا لمبدئه . ثمّ يكرّ خارجا . ولا يزال هذا حتّى يغلب فيسخن ظاهر الجسد أو ينقهر فيطفأ فيموت الشخص . وفي حال تلك المراجعة والممانعة تقع رعدة النافض . والفرق بين الرعدة والنافض هو أنّ الرعدة من الممانعة الواقعة بين القوة الإرادية والثقل الطبيعي . فإن

١ لأجل أنّه] لأنّه P || ٢ بارد] بادي EL || ٣ البدن] المعدة O || ٤ ابيديميا] افيديميا ELP || ١٠ الرعدة] الرعشة EsGP || ١٤ حركته] أيضا add. ELOP || ١٦ ويسدّ] ويستدّ Es || ١٧ الجسد] البدن EL

someone wants to abolish the voluntary strength and does not want [it to perform] any motion, the tremor ceases. But the cessation of a rigor does not depend on one's will—it results from the hindrance between a natural motion (namely that of the innate heat) and that which obstructs
5    its course and its passages and channels. *De tremore, [palpitatione, rigore et convulsione]*.[86]

44. If the cold [only] moves the outer surface [of the body] with a shivering movement and shakes it at the moment of the onset of a fever attack but does not move the whole body, this is called "shivering."
10   Shivering is an affliction occurring only to the skin. Its significance for the skin is the same as that of rigor for the whole body. *De tremore, [palpitatione, rigore et convulsione]*.[87] But in *De febribus* 2 he said that shivering is something less severe than rigor but more cold.[88]

45. For the occurrence of a rigor, it is necessary that the body con-
15   tain a biting substance and that this humor is moved violently, no matter whether the cause of the rigor is a cold or a hot one. Therefore, a rigor starts simultaneously with the attack of tertian or quartan fevers when that humor moves to be expelled. Sometimes a similar thing happens to someone who suffers from indigestion or to someone whose body
20   is full of bad humors and who then exposes himself to the sun or enters the bathhouse or does physical exercise. For if someone does this, he is immediately affected by shivering or sometimes by rigor. *De tremore, [palpitatione, rigore et convulsione]*.[89]

46. Many of those who are affected by rigor are thirsty during that
25   time because the heat remains deep inside the body while the sensation of cold is at that moment in the outer parts of the body, not in the inner ones. *De [morborum] causis et symptomatibus* 5.[90]

47. The causes for bad respiration that force the patient to move all the muscles of the upper chest together with the intercostal ones are
30   one of the following three: either weakened strength, or narrowness and

أراد الإنسـان إبطال القـوة الإرادية ولم يرم حركة بطلت الرعدة. وليس سـكون النافض
بإرادتنا لأنّها ممانعة بين حركة طبيعية وهي حركة الحارّ الغريزي وبين السادّ في وجهه وطرقه
ومجاريه. في مقالته في الرعدة والاختلاج.

٤٤. إن كان البرد يحرّك السطح الظاهر حركة مضطربة وتهزّه عند دخول نوبة الحمّى
ولايحرّك البدن كلّه معا سـمّي قشعريرة. فيكون القشـعريرة إنّما هي عرض يعرض للجلد
وحده ومقامه عند الجلد مقام النافض عند جميع البدن. في مقالته في الرعدة. وفي ثانية
الحمّيات قال القشعريرة شيء أقلّ من النافض وأكثر من البرد.

٤٥. يحتـاج في حدوث النافض إلى أن يكون في البدن شيء لذّاع ويكون ذلك الخلط
يتحرّك حركة شـديدة سواء كان سـبب النافض سببا باردا أو سببا حارّا. ولذلك صار
النافض يبتدئ مع نوبة الحمّى معا في الحميات الغبّ والربع عند حركة ذلك الخلط للخروج.
وقد يعرض شيء شبيه بهذا لمن عرضت له تخمة أو من كان بدنه ممتلئا من الأخلاط الردئة
فتعرّض للشـمس أو دخل الحمّام أو اسـتعمل الرياضة فإنّ من فعل ذلك يجد من ساعته
قشعريرة ومنهم من يصيبه النافض. في مقالته في الرعدة.

٤٦. كثيـر ممـن يعرض له النافض يعطـش في ذلك الوقت لأنّ الحـرارة تكون باقية
فـي باطن البدن وحسّ البـرودة إنّما يكون في ذلك الوقت في الأعضـاء الظاهرة لا في
الباطنة. خامسة العلل والأعراض.

٤٧. أسـباب رداة التنفّـس الموجبة لتحرّك المريـض جميـع عضل صدره الأعلى مع
العضـل الذي بين الأضـلاع أحد ثلاثة أسـباب: إمّا قوّة ضعيفة وإمّا ضيق وضغط في

١ ولم يرم] ولا يروم EL | الرعدة] الرعشة EEsGL: الرعدة L¹ || ٢ وجهه وطرقه] وجه
طرقه Es || ٤ دخول] دخوله L | معا] L || ٥ معه] ELP || ٧-٦ وفي . . . البرد] P¹ ||
٨ شـيء] سـبب ELO || ١٣-١٢ الرياضـة . . . ومنهـم] G¹ | ١٣ من] om. G ||
١٤ لأنّ] فإنّ EsG | ١٥ الأعضاء] G¹

pressure[91] in the respiratory passages,[92] or burning heat in the heart or lungs. When all these three [causes] occur together, the patient dies immediately. When two of them occur together, it is difficult for him to escape, but if only one of them occurs, he will eventually either die or escape. *De locis affectis* 4.[93]

48. Sometimes respiration comes at intervals[94] [and] in great gasps[95] because of harm [that has occurred] to the mind. This illness consists therein that the patient is, as it were, so unmindful and forgetful of his deeds that he does not know when he stops nor when he begins. *In Hippocratis Epidemiarum* 2.1.[96]

Because of the connection between the organs of the chest and the reproductive organs, sometimes a chronic cough stops because of a swelling of the testicles. *In Hippocratis Epidemiarum* 2.1.[97]

49. Thinness and interruption of the voice are only caused by humors that are either abundant or thick or viscous and that obstruct the vessels in the lung. *In Hippocratis Epidemiarum* 2.4.[98]

50. There are two reasons why a patient brings up a small amount of sputum in spite of much coughing: either the humors are so thick and viscous that they get stuck and their expectoration is difficult, or the humors are too thin. For when they are lifted by the air, they are dispersed and sink again. *De locis affectis* 4.[99]

51. If someone wishes to raise his voice, he should become accustomed to opening his mouth wide so that he lets in much air, which widens the larynx. Then the voice is loud. Therefore, those whose larynx is narrow

طريق الهواء ومخترقه وإمّا حرارة كثيرة في القلب أو في الرئة . فإن اجتمعت ثلاثتها مات المريض على المكان . ومتى اجتمع منها اثنتان فعسير ما يتخلّص ومتى كان منها واحد فقط فالمريض يؤول به الأمر إمّا إلى الهلاك وإمّا إلى الخلاص . رابعة التعرّف .

٤٨ . قد يصير التنفّس متفاوتا عظيما لسبب فساد الذهن وعلّة ذلك أنّ المريض كأنّه
يسهو عن أفعاله وينساها حتّى لا يدري متى يمسك عنها ومتى يأخذ فيها . في الثالثة من شرحه للأولى من ابيديميا .

السعال المزمن قد يسكن بورم يحدث في الأثيين من قبل المشاركة التي بين آلات الصدر وآلات التناسل . في الأولى من شرحه لثانية ابيديميا .

٤٩ . رقّة الصوت وانقطاعه إنّما يكون لسبب أخلاط كثيرة أو غليظة أو لزجة تسدّد
العروق التي في الرئة . في الرابعة من شرحه لثانية ابيديميا .

٥٠ . العليل ينفث نفثا يسيرا بسعال كثير على ضربين إمّا بسبب غلظ الأخلاط ولزوجتها فتلجج وتتشبّث ويعسر تخلّصها وإمّا بسبب رقّة الأخلاط . فإذا ارتفعت بالريح التي تصعدها عادت وتفرّقت ورسبت إلى أسفل . رابعة التعرّف .

٥١ . إذا أراد الإنسان أن يرفع صوته فينبغي أن يعوّد نفسه بأن يفتح فمه كثيرا حتّى
يدخل هواء كثيرا يوسع الحلقوم فيكون الصوت جهيرا . ولذلك صار الذين حلوقهم ضيّقة

٣ يؤول] يطول O ‖ ٤ التنفّس] النفس EsG ‖ ٦ للأولى] الأولى EsG | ابيديميا] افيديميا EsG | الأولى من] om. L ‖ ٨ لثانية] الثانية EsG | ابيديميا] افيديميا LP ‖ ٩ لسبب] بسبب ELO ‖ ١٠ لثانية] الثانية G | ابيديميا] افيديميا ELP ‖ ١١ نفثا] شيئا LP ‖ ١٣ ورسبت] وسبحت G¹ : ورسخت Es²GO

and small have thin, small voices without any substance so that they are broken off quickly. But those whose larynx is wide have a full and powerful voice. Children, women, and eunuchs have thin and weak voices because their larynx is small. *De somno et vigilia.*[100]

52. The digestive activity only takes place in the parts that are beneath the cardia of the stomach. Therefore, this part of the stomach causes indigestion when it is indisposed, provided that the indigestion is not caused by foods.[101] *De locis affectis* 5.[102]

53. The cause of a gassy[103] disease [in the stomach] is heat that exceeds the [normal] balance and takes possession of the vessels that receive the food from the stomach so that the blood becomes thick there. An indication that the disturbance lies there is that the food remains undigested in the stomach because of the obstruction of those channels, and those suffering from it vomit their [undigested] food. An indication for the domination of heat in that spot is that they obtain relief by cold things and also that they suffer from burning [fever]. Some people say that the cause of this disease lies in the fact that the opening of the stomach that leads to[104] the intestines is swollen due to an inflamed bloody tumor. This blood is extremely thick and is very much like black bile. *De locis affectis* 3.[105]

54. When there is a large or hard inflamed tumor in the liver, the patient feels the pain in the right collarbone. This results from the stretching of the vessel known as [vena] cava and not from the stretching of the [pleural] membranes. In the case of pleurisy, the pain in the collarbone is the result of the stretching of the [pleural] membranes. *De locis affectis* 2.[106]

55. If you take food without suffering from intestinal rumblings[107] or inflation or palpitation or hiccups, but you do have an unusual feeling of discomfort[108] in your stomach—the food weighs heavily on it—and you do wish that it would descend from it or that eructation would occur to it, and sometimes you also suffer from difficulty of breathing, there is no doubt that the stomach has contracted over the food in a trembling way.[109] *De [morborum] causis et symptomatibus* 3.[110]

صغيرة أصواتهم دقيقة ضعيفة ليس لها مادّة فينقطعون سريعا . فأمّا الذين حلوقهم واسعة فأصواتهم كثيرة قوية . وأمّا الصبيان والنساء والخصيان فأصواتهم دقيقة ضعيفة بحال ضيق حلوقهم . في مقالته في النوم واليقظة .

٥٢ . فعـل الاسـتمراء والهضم إنّما يكون في الأجزاء التي هي أسـفل من فم المعدة ولذلك يكون هذا الجزء من المعدة سببا للتخمة إذا ساءت حاله متى لم يكن سبب التخمة من قبل الأغذية . خامسة التعرّف .

٥٣ . سـبب العلّة النافخة حرارة مجاوزة للاعتدال مستولية على العروق التي تقبل الغذاء من المعدة فيغلظ الدم هناك . والدليل على أنّ العلّة هناك كون الغذاء يبقى في المعدة غير منهضم لانسداد تلك المجاري وكونهم يتقيّؤون طعامهم . والدليل على استيلاء الحرارة هناك كونهم يسـتريحون إلى الأشـياء الباردة وأيضا تلك الحرقة التي تعرض لهم . وبعض الناس يقول إنّ السـبب فـي هذه العلّة كون منفذ المعدة الـلازق بالمعاء وارما ورما حارّا دمويا . وذلك الدم أشدّ غلظا وأقرب إلى السوداوية . ثالثة التعرّف .

٥٤ . إذا كان فـي الكبـد ورم حارّ عظيم أو صلب فيجـد العليل الوجع في الترقوة اليمنى وذلك تابع لتمدّد العرق المعروف بالأجوف لا لتمدّد الأغشية . وأمّا في ذات الجنب فوجع الترقوة تابع لتمدّد الأغشية . ثانية التعرّف .

٥٥ . متى تناولت طعاما ولم يعرض لك معه قرقرة ولا نفخة ولا اختلاج ولا فوائق لكنّك يصيبك في معدتك كرب لا عهد لك بمثله ويثقل عليها ذلك الطعام وتشتاق إلى أن ينحدر عنها أو إلى أن يحدث لها جشاء ووجدت مع ذلك في بعض الأوقات ضيق نفس فلا شكّ عند ذلك أنّ المعدة قد انقبضت على الطعام على جهة الارتعاش . ثالثة العلل والأعراض .

---

١ أصواتهـم] أصواتهـن G | ٢-١ ليـس . . . ضعيفـة] om. L | ٤ الأجـزاء] G¹ ||
٩ طعامهـم] غير منهضم add. EL | ١١ منفـذ] المنفذ G | ١٤ الجنـب] الجانب P ||
١٦ لكنّك] لكنّ EEsLOP | ١٨ جشاء] حامض add. EsG

56. When whiteness dominates in someone['s complexion,] his liver is weak and does not produce much blood. If red spots dominate, his spleen is weak; these red spots are caused by the mixture of melancholic humor with the blood. *In Hippocratis Epidemiarum* 2.1.[111]

57. The first cause of a severe thirst without diabetes[112] is a hot or dry bad temperament, or both, occurring in the stomach and especially in the cardia of the stomach; and after the stomach, the second cause is that this bad temperament affects the liver and especially its concave part. A similar cause is the occurrence of this bad temperament in the esophagus or in the lungs, for it is then transferred to the stomach so that thirst becomes severe. *De locis affectis* 6.[113]

58. Sleep moistens under all circumstances, while sleeplessness dries under all circumstances. Sleep has not the property to heat or to cool, but when it occurs to a body with cold humors, it[114] digests them and cocts them and produces blood from them so that the body is heated. And when sleep occurs [to a body] that suffers from fever caused by the putrefaction of cold humors, it cools the body by extinguishing the heat of the fever and by increasing the innate heat. When the humors are bilious, it[115] selects them and expels them from the body so that it cools off. *In Hippocratis Epidemiarum* 6.4.[116]

59. When evident causes[117] [of an affliction] strike a body that is free of superfluities, the harm inflicted on it can be easily repaired[118] and quickly eliminated. But when they strike the body while it has a surplus of humors or bad [humors,] their effect can be compared to that of a fiery spark on the wood of fatty pine nuts[119] or that of a [burning] wick on sulfur. *In Hippocratis Epidemiarum* 6.8.[120]

٥٦ . مـن كان البيـاض غالبـا عليه فكبده ضعيفـة لا تولّد دمـا كثيـرا . ومن كان النمش غالبا عليه وطحاله ضعيف وسـبب النمش مخالطة الخلط السـوداوي للدم . في الأولى من شرحه لثانية ابيديميا .

٥٧ . العطش الشـديد الذي يكون خلوا من اسـتطلاق البول سببه الأوّل سوء مزاج حارّ أو يابس أو كلاهما معا يحدث في المعدة وخاصّة فمها وسببه الثاني بعد المعدة حدوث هذا السـوء المزاج الكبد وبخاصّة مقعّرها . وكذلك أيضا يكون سببه حدوث هذا السوء مزاج في المريء أو في الرئة فيتأدّى ذلك إلى المعدة فيشتـدّ العطش . سادسـة التعرّف .

٥٨ . النـوم يرطّب في جميع الأحوال والسـهر يجفّف في جميع الأحوال وليس من شـأن النوم أن يسخن أو يبرّد . لكّه إن صادف البدن وفيه أخلاط باردة هضمها وأنضجها وولّد منها دما فيسخن البدن . فإن صادف ⟨البدن و⟩ به حمّى من عفونة أخلاط باردة برّد البـدن بتطفيته لحرارة الحمّى وإنمائه للحرارة الغريزية . وإن كانت الأخلاط من جنس المرار ميّزها ونفضها عن البدن فيبرد . في الرابعة من شرحه لسادسة ابيديميا .

٥٩ . متـى صادفت الأسـباب البادية البدن نقيا من الفضـول كان ما ينال البدن من ضررها سـهل التلافي سـريع الزوال . ومتى صادفته وفيها كثرة من الأخلاط أو رداة فإنّ فعلها هيه فعل شـرارة النار في حطب الصنوبر الدسـم أو فعل الفتيلة في الكبريت . في الثامنة من شرحه لسادسة ابيديميا .

---

٢ الخلط] الدم ELP ‖ ٣ ابيديميا] افيديميا ELP ‖ ٤ البول] البطن EEsOP : البدن L ‖ ٥ يحدث] يوجد L : تجّد E ‖ ٦ الكبد] بالكبد EEsLP ‖ ١١ بتطفيته] بتطفيته G¹ : بتعطيه G : بتعطيته P : بترطيبه EsO ‖ ١٢ ابيديميا] افيديميا ELP ‖ ١٥ فعل (2nd)] بفعل EL

60. Corrosion is caused by biting humors; biting humors are those humors that are sharp, sour, and salty. *In Hippocratis Epidemiarum* 6.8.[121]

61. It is not surprising that one who indulges frequently in sexual intercourse is weak because his whole body is free from [seminal] fluid and pneuma because of their evacuation[122] from it. And besides, there is an accession of pleasure that by itself is enough to weaken and extinguish[123] the animal faculty.[124] Some people who had a sudden intense pleasure died [as a result]. *De semine* 2.[125]

62. The reason for a frequent discharge of feces is one of three: either because of a weakness of the organs due to a bad temperament, as is well known, or because of biting humors that irritate the organ and prompt it to expel [the excrements], or because of excessive sensitivity that is either natural or caused by an ulcer. *De [morborum] causis et symptomatibus* 6.[126]

63. The causes of biting superfluities that necessarily lead to a frequent discharge of feces are four: either the strength of a medication that is received by the body together with the food or without it, or the corruption of food, or biting superfluities that descend from the body into [various] places in the abdomen, or biting superfluities that originate in the stomach or abdomen. *De [morborum] causis et symptomatibus* 6.[127]

64. The cold of the outer parts of the body always hardens the belly, while the cold of the inner parts always softens the belly and sometimes causes diarrhea. *In Hippocratis Epidemiarum* 6.5.[128]

65. When [the part of] the intestine called "colon" becomes full, bad afflictions occur and the stomach feels its pain. The reason for this is that when this [part of the] intestine becomes full, it distends and the pain ascends to the membrane that surrounds the stomach and the intestines. Thus, the stomach feels the pain from there. There is also a muscle that covers both the stomach and the intestines, and when this [part of the] intestine distends, the stomach feels [the pain from] that. *De clysteribus.*[129]

٦٠ . التـأكّل يحدث عن أخلاط لذّاعـة والأخلاط اللذّاعة هـي الحرّيفة الحامضة والمالحة . في السادسة من شرحه لسادسة ابيديميا .

٦١ . ليس بعجب أن يكون من يكثر الجماع يضعف لأنّ البدن كلّه يخلو لما يستفرغ منـه من الروح والرطوبة . ويزيد مـع هذا اللذّة التي هي وحدها علـى الانقراض تبلغ من إخمادهـا للقوة الحيوانيـة وإضعافها إيّاهـا . إنّ قوما فاجأتهم لذّة قوية شـديدة فماتوا . في الثانية من كتابه في المني .

٦٢ . أسباب تواتر خروج البراز أحد ثلاثة أسباب : إمّا لضعف الآلات بسبب سوء مزاج كما علم وإمّا بسبب أخلاط لذّاعة تلذع الآلة فتحثّها على الدفع وإمّا بسبب فضل حسّ إمّا بالطبع وإمّا من أجل قرحة . سادسة العلل والأعراض .

٦٣ . أسـباب الفضول اللاذعة الموجبة لتواتر خروج البراز أربعة : إمّا قوة دوائية ترد على البدن مع الأغذية أو وحدها وإمّا فساد أغذية وإمّا فضول لذّاعة تنحدر من البدن إلى مواضع البطن وإمّا فضول لذّاعة تتولّد في المعدة والبطن . سادسة العلل والأعراض .

٦٤ . برد الأعضاء الظاهرة يشـدّ البطن دائما وبرد الأعضاء الباطنة يلين البطن دائما وربّما أحدث الذرب . في الخامسة من شرحه لسادسة ابيديميا .

٦٥ . أذا امتـلأ المعاء المسـمّى قولـون عرض من ذلك أعراض رديئة وتحسّ المعدة بوجعه . وسبب ذلك أنّ هذا المعاء إذا امتلأ امتدّ فتراقى الوجع إلى الصفاق المحيط بالمعدة والأمعاء فتتألّم المعدة لذلك . وكذلك عضلة منتشرة على المعدة والأمعاء جميعا وإذا امتدّ هذا المعاء أحسّت المعدة بذلك . في مقالته في الحقن .

١–٢ التـأكّل . . . والمالحة ] G¹ || ٢ ابيديميا ] افيديميا ELP || ٤ ويزيد مع ] وأزيد من L || ١٠ اللاذعة ] اللذّاعة ELOP || ١٤ ابيديميا ] افيديميا ELP

66. Pain with numbness[130] occurs in the legs in the case of kidney diseases because of the connection between the kidneys and the legs through the two vessels that descend along the spinal column. These are the vessels known as the [vena] cava and the aorta. *In Hippocratis*
5      *Epidemiarum* 6.1.[131]

67. There are three reasons why a smooth organ becomes rough: either acrid humors pour into it and peel and strip[132] it, or acrid medications have a similar effect on it, or foreign substances adhere to it, such as smoke and dust. The reason why a rough [organ] becomes smooth
10     is that it is soaked and moistened by a fat, soft, or viscous liquid. *De [morborum] causis et symptomatibus* 2.[133]

68. It often happens that symptoms follow each other in a row.[134] The first symptom comes from the disease [itself], the second comes from the first, the third comes from the second, and the fourth from the
15     third. *De [morborum] causis et symptomatibus* 3.[135]

69. If the albuminoid humor is larger or smaller [in quantity] than necessary, it harms vision. When this humor becomes thick, clarity of vision is diminished so that distant objects cannot be seen [at all] and close objects cannot be seen clearly. When it becomes extremely thick, as
20     happens in the case of a cataract, it makes vision impossible. When a part of the eye near the pupil becomes covered [by the thick humor] while another part remains [clear], one clearly sees any one object through the [clear] part, but one cannot see many objects at the same time. When [only] a small amount of thick humor is in the middle of the pupil while
25     the surrounding area remains clear, one sees everything as if one were looking through a window. When the thick substances are spread out and scattered in that spot, it seems to the affected persons as if they see gnats flying outside. Such images often appear to them when they wake up from sleep, and they occur mostly with children and those whose
30     heads are filled with wine or with something else. *De [morborum] causis et symptomatibus* 4.[136]

٦٦ . الوجــع مع خدر في الرجلين في أمراض الكلى يكون لأجل المشـاركة التى بين الكلى وبين الرجلين بالعرقين المنحدرين على الصلب وهما العرق المعروف بالأجوف والعرق الضارب العظيم . في الأولى من شرحه لسادسة ابيديميا .

٦٧ . أسـباب خشونة العضو الأملس ثلاثة : إمّا أخلاط حادّة تنصبّ إليه فتجرده وتقشره وإمّا أدوية حادّة تفعل ذلك فيه أو أجسـام غريبة تلصق به كالدخان والغبار . والسبب في ملاسة الخشن هو أن تستنقع وتبتلّ برطوبة دسمة لدنة أو لزجة . ثانية العلل والأعراض .

٦٨ . قد يتّفق مرارا كثيرة أن تكون أعراض يتلو بعضها بعضا في صنف واحد ويكون العـرض الأوّل منها حادثا عن المرض والثاني حادثا عـن الأوّل والثالث حادثا عن الثاني والرابع حادثا عن الثالث . ثالثة العلل والأعراض .

٦٩ . الرطوبــة البيضيــة إن كانت أكثر أو أقلّ ممّا ينبغـي أضرّت بالبصر وإن غلظت نقصت خلوص البصر حتّى لا يبصر الأشـياء البعيدة ولا يتبيّن القريبة . فإن غلظت غاية الغلـظ بمنزلــة ما يعرض لها في نزول الماء عاقت البصـر . وإن تغطّى بعض ما يلي الحدقة وبقـي بعض أبصر بذلك البعض كلّ شـيء على حدّته ولا يبصر أشـياء كثيرة معا . فإن كانت في وسـط الحدقة رطوبة يسيرة غليظة وما حول ذلك باقيا على صفائه فيبصر في كلّ شـيء يراه شبيها بالكوة . وإن كانت الأشـياء الغليظة متفرّقة متبدّدة في هذا الموضع خيّـل لمن به ذلك أنّـه يرى بقّا يطير من خارج. وكثيرا ما يتخيّلـون عند الانتباه من النوم شـبيها بالصور وأكثر ما يعرض للصبيان ولمن قد امتلأ رأسـه شـرابا أو ضربا آخر من الامتلاء . رابعة العلل والأعراض .

١ خـدر] برد L | لأجـل] من أجل ELOP || ٣ ابيديميا] افيديميا ELP || ٦ ثانية] ثامنة G || ٨ العرض] العارض L || ١١ نقصت] من add. L

70. Just as someone who suffers from a cataract in the eye imagines that the things that are inside the eye are outside, so it happens with the tongue: the faculty of taste turns the quality that lies in the tongue itself into a necessary attribute of the things that are outside [it]. The reason for this is that the foods[137] that one tastes activate the matter residing in the tongue[138] so that one' thinks that the foods themselves contain [the quality of] saltiness and sourness. *De [morborum] causis et symptomatibus* 4.[139]

71. As for laughter occurring through tickling the armpits [on the outside] and the footsoles, as well as laughter which occurs when seeing or hearing comical things, it is absolutely impossible to find out its cause. *De motibus [manifestis et] obscuris.*[140]

72. Says Moses: This statement is correct because laughter is a specific characteristic of human beings. It is well known that each specific property belongs to the generic form,[141] regardless of whether it belongs to the species of animals or plants or minerals. There is no way to give a reason for this. Therefore, one should not look for it in any way, neither regarding laughter nor any other specific property.[142]

73. If someone looks into these things, he will find that nature has [certain] steps: the first is that wherein it departs a short distance from plants, resulting in an animal that has one sense, namely that of touch. The second step is that in which it adds to touch the sense of taste. The third step is that in which one finds an animal who has, next to these two, the sense of smell. The fourth step is that in which it adds to these three the sense of hearing, and the fifth step is that in which is added to these [four the sense of] vision.[143] And sometimes nature molds the eyes[144] and sketches them in a hidden way and forms them without completing their strength, as with the mole.[145] *De semine* 2.

*This is the end of the seventh treatise,*
*by the grace of God, praise be to Him.*

◆

٧٠ . كما أنّ الذي ينزل في عينه الماء يتخيّل الأشياء التي في جوف عينه أنّها من خارج كذلك يعتري في اللسـان أنّ القوة التي يكون بها المذاق توجب الكيفية الموجودة في نفس اللسـان للأشياء التي من خارج. والسبب في ذلك تحريك الشيء الذي يذاق لتلك المادّة المستكنّة في اللسان فيتخيّل أنّ في الأطعمة ملوحة أو حموضة. رابعة العلل والأعراض .

٧١ . أمّا الضحك الذي يكون عند لمس ظاهر الإبطين وأسفل القدمين وكذلك الضحك الذي يصيبنا عند رؤية الأشياء المضحكة أو سماعها فليس إلى معرفة السبب في ذلك سبيلا أصلا . في مقالته في الحركات المعتاصة .

٧٢ . قال موسى : هذا القول صحيح لأنّ الضحك من خواصّ الانسان ومعلوم أنّ كلّ خاصّـة فهي تابعة للصورة النوعية كانت تلك الخاصّية لأيّ نوع كانت من أنواع الحيوان أو النبات أو المعادن فلا وجه لإعطاء السبب في ذلك فليس إذن ممّا يطلب بوجه لا في الضحك ولا في غير ذلك من الخواصّ.

٧٣ . مـن يتفقّد هذه الأمور يجد للطبيعـة درجات : أوّلها الدرجة التي يبعد بها عن النبات قليلا فيكون حيوانا له حاسّة واحدة وهي حاسّة اللمس والدرجة الثانية التي تزيد فيها مع اللمس حاسّـة المذاق والدرجة الثالثة التي توجد له مع هاتين حاسّة الشمّ والدرجة الرابعة التي تزيد مع هذه الثلاثة حاسّـة السمع والخامسة التي يزاد فيها مع هذه البصر . وقد تمّثل البصر وترسمه رسما خفيا وقد تصوّره ولم تكمل قوّته كالخلد . في الثانية من المنّي . تمّت المقالة السابعة ولله الحمد والمنّة .

١ عينه [(1st) عينيه | عينه (2nd) EEsLOP || عينيه ELOP | ٢ في om. EsG

٥–٧ أمّـا . . . أصلا] (1st) | وأمّـا الضحك الذي يكون عند لمس ظاهر مواضع الإبطين وأسـفل القدمين فليس يدخل في هذا الباب ولا أرى إلى معرفة السـبب الذي صارت هذه المواضع إذا لمست هذا اللمس تحرّك الحركة التي تكون عند رؤية الشـيء المضحك أو سـماعه سبيل أصلا

خاصّة (1st) | ٩ خاصّية EL || ١٣ حاسّة Galen, Fī al-ḥarakāt fol. 106r

١٤ توجد] تجد E || ١٦ ولم] ولا ELOOxP | الثانية] الثالثة EsG L

*In the name of God,*
*the Merciful, the Compassionate.*
*O Lord, make [our task] easy*

# The Eighth Treatise

5     *Containing aphorisms concerning the [correct] regimen*
*for the healing of diseases in general*

1. If someone has bad, thin humors in his body, it requires more nutrition, and if he has humors with the opposite quality, it indicates the opposite.[1] If it is impossible to find out the required amount [of food], it

10  is more prudent to change to the consumption of less food rather than more food because one can increase [the consumption of food] when one's strength dwindles but one cannot decrease the [amount of] food that has already gone to the stomach. *De acutorum morborum [victu et] Galeni commentarius* 2.[2]

15  2. The things that help to coct the humors are all those that heat moderately; some of these are foods, some are beverages, some are poultices, and some are fomentations. Moderate massage and moderate bathing equally belong to this category. *In Hippocratis Epidemiarum* 1.2.[3]

بسم الله الرحمن الرحيم ربّ يسّر

# المقالة الثامنة

## يشتمل على فصول تتعلّق بتدبير شفاء الأمراض على العموم

١ . مـن كان فـي بدنه أخلاط ردئـة رقيقة أوجب ذلك تغذيتـه أكثر . ومن كانت

٥ أخلاطه بخلاف ذلك دلّت على الضدّ والانتقال إلى النقصان إذا فاتت معرفة المقدار الذي
ينبغي أحوط من الانتقال إلى الزيادة لأنّك تقدر أن تزيد إن خارت القوّة ولا تقدر أن تنقص
من الطعام الذي قد ورد المعدة . في شرحه لثانية الأمراض الحادّة .

٢ . الأشـياء التي تعين على نضج الأخلاط هي جميع الأشياء التي تسخن باعتدال
وبعضها أطعمة وبعضها أشربة وبعضها أضمدة وبعضها نطولات والدلك المعتدل والاستحمام

١٠ المعتدل من هذا الجنس . في الثانية من شرحه للأولى من ابيديميا .

---

١ بسم . . . يسّر [om. ELOP] || ٤ رقيقة [om. G] || ٦ الزيادة [الزداة G] الرداة G] || ١٠ ابيديميا [
افيديميا ELOxP

3. Raw humors are of two kinds: the first of these is thin and watery, and such [humors] should be evacuated immediately before they become sharp through the heat of the fever and become biting and corrosive. The other kind is thick and viscous and settled in the organs; these [humors] should be cocted first so that they stream easily. *In Hippocratis De humoribus commentarius* 1.[4]

4. Sometimes a patient suffers from three diseases [at the same time]: One of these has already declined, the second is just beginning, and the third is reaching its climax.[5] A patient dies not as a result of the disease that has declined or that is beginning, but because of the disease that is dramatically getting worse. *De totius morbi temporibus.*[6]

5. The first and most difficult thing we should examine is the condition of the three organs from which the faculties [of the body] originate— I mean the heart, the brain, and the liver—next to the condition of the parts that branch out from them—I mean the pulsatile vessels, nerves, and veins. Then we should examine the other parts of the body and look into everything as it is. *De totius morbi temporibus.*[7]

6. All diseases are weaker in their beginning and end and are stronger during their culmination. Between these two stages their condition is intermediate between weakness and strength. During the culmination the dominant treatment should consist of things that alleviate, and in the beginning and end it should consist of things that fight the disease. In the intermediate stages the treatment should be commensurate with [that given during] the two extremes. *De totius morbi temporibus.*[8]

7. When a disease is difficult to coct, the benefit of the therapy becomes apparent only after a long time and after the [same] medica- tion has been taken repeatedly. *In Hippocratis Aphorismos commentarius* 2.[9]

8. One should be anxious and careful not to aggravate the disease and not to destroy the strength of the patient, who is likely to be afflicted for some time,[10] although it is very difficult to achieve both things. For

٣ . الأخلاط النيئة ضربان : أحدهما أن تكون رقيقة مائية وهذه ينبغي أن تستفرغ على المكان من قبل أن تحتدّ بحرارة الحمّى فتصير لذّاعة أكّالة والآخر أن تكون غليظة لزجة متمكّنة في الأعضاء وهذه ينبغي أن تنضج أوّلا حتّى تجري بسهولة . في شرحه للأولى من الأخلاط .

٤ . قـد يمكن أن يكون بالمريض ثلاثة أمراض : أحدها قد انحطّ والثاني في الابتداء والثالث في آخر تزيّده . ويموت المريض لا بـسـبـب المرض الذي انحطّ أو الذي ابتدأ بل من أجل الذي يزيد تزيّدا عظيما . في مقالته في أوقات الأمراض .

٥ . أولى ما ينبغي أن نبحث عنه وأشدّه حال الثلاثة مبادئ التي للقوى أعني القلب والدماغ والكبد وحال الأعضاء المتفرّعة منها أعني العروق الضوارب والأعصاب والأوردة . وبعد ذلك نبحث عن سائر الأعضاء ونعنى بكلّ شيء بحسبه . في مقالته في أوقات الأمراض .

٦ . الأمراض كلّها في أوّلها وآخرها أضعف وفي المنتهى أقوى وفي ما بين هذين الوقتين حالها متوسّطة فيما بين الضعف والقوة . والذي ينبغي أن يكون الغالب في العلاج في وقت المنتهى الأشيـاء المسكّنة وأمّـا في الابتداء والانقضاء فالأشياء المقاومة للمرض وبقياس الطرفين يكون ما يستعمل في الأوقات المتوسّطة . في مقالته في أوقات الأمراض .

٧ . المرض الذي يعسـر نضجه ليس يظهر لما يعالج بـه منفعة بتّة إلّا بعد زمان طويل وتكرار الدواء مرّات كثيرة . في شرحه لثانية الفصول .

٨ . ينبغـي أن تصرّف همّتك وعنايتك أن لا تزيـد في المرض ولا تهدّ قوة المريض مع ما هي مسـتـأنفة من طول معاناة المرض وإن ضبط الأمر من الوجهين جميعا لشـاقّ عسير

٥ آخـر] G¹ || ٧ أولى] أوّل EEsLOOx | أن] om. G || ٩ في مقالته . . . الأمراض] om. G : Es¹ || ١١ متوسّطة] متوسّط EsG | فيمـا] فيما EsG || ١٤ لما] في ما EsG | يعالج] يعالجه Es G | O

to the extent that abstinence is good for rapidly cocting the disease, to that extent it is harmful for the strength [of the patient,] and sometimes it is [even] more [harmful]. And to the extent that food aggravates a disease and delays its coction, to that extent it strengthens [the patient]. Therefore, one should always turn to that [aspect] which is most in need of support. *Ad Glauconem de methodo medendi* 1.[11]

9. One should [try to] determine exactly the proximity and distance of a disease from its culmination. For if one does not know this, one may potentially inflict great harm upon the patient. Similarly, one may sometimes [prescribe] a bad regimen if one does not know when the disease culminates. *De crisibus* 1.[12]

10. If a corruption of the humors occurs together with a weakness of [bodily] strength, there is absolutely no cure for that illness. And if there is something by which it might be healed, it can only be done after a long time, through exertion and strain and the presence of an expert physician. What should be done in this case is that the patient should not be treated with drugs that heal his disease, but one should feed him and revive his strength until his nature[13] is strengthened so much that evacuation does not harm it [at all] or only slightly so. Then one should turn to treating the disease with drugs. *De methodo medendi* 9.[14]

11. One should be extremely careful not to overheat any cold, thick, and viscous humor with blazing hot substances because when these humors dissolve, vapors arise from them that one can neither dissolve nor disperse. The most harmful [situation] is when these humors are between the two membranes of the intestines. These humors can be treated, however, with cutting, thinning remedies that do not overheat. *De methodo medendi* 12.[15]

12. A complete evacuation of the body is [effected] through blood-letting or laxatives or emetics or frequent massage or any kind of exercise, or through bathing in the bathhouse, especially when it has a dissolving effect, or through sharp remedies when they are rubbed on the body, or through abstention from food. Evacuate the body of a patient through that which is most appropriate for him. *De methodo medendi* 14.[16]

من قبل أنّ الحمية بحسب مبلغ نفعها في سرعة نضج المرض تكون أضرارها بالقوة بل ربّما كان أكثر . والغذاء بحسب مبلغ زيادته في قوة المرض وإبطائه بالنضج يكون مبلغ تقويته . فتنحو أبدا نحو أحوجهما إلى المعونة . الأولى من اغلوقن .

٩ . إنّما يقدّر جميع التقدير على حسب قرب منتهى المرض وبعده . وإن جهلت ذلك فليـس تخلو من أن تضرّ المريض مضرّة عظيمة ولا تخلو في وقت من الأوقات من سـوء التدبير متى لم تعلم متى يكون منتهى المرض . أولى البحران .

١٠ . متى عرض فسـاد الأخلاط مع قوة ضعيفة فذلك قوة المرض لا دواء له بتّة . وإن كان لـه ما يداوى به ففي مـدّة طويلة وبجهد وكدّ إن وقع له طبيب حاذق . والذي يجب أن يفعل حينئذ هو أن لا يداوى المريض بشيء ممّا يشفي مرضه بل اغذه وانعش قوته حتّى تقوى الطبيعة حتّى لا يضرّها الاسـتفراغ أو أن يكون أضراره يسـيرة وحينئذ اقبل على مداواة المرض . تاسعة الحيلة .

١١ . كلّ خلط بارد غليظ لزج فاحذر كلّ الحذر أن تسـخنه إسـخانا قويا بأشياء نارية لأنّ تلك الأخلاط إذا ذابت تولّدت منها رياح أن تسـتطيع أن تحلّلها وتفشّها . وأضرّ مـا يكون ذلك إذا كانت تلك الأخلاط بين طبقتي ألأمعاء . وإنّما تداوى هذه الأخلاط بما يقطع ويلطّف من غير أن يسخن إسخانا قويا . ثانية عشر الحيلة .

١٢ . استفراغ البدن كلّه يكون بإخراج الدم أو بالأدوية المطلقة للبطن أو بالادوية المقيّئة أو بالدلك الكثير وبكلّ حركة أيضا أو بالاسـتحمام في الحمّام وخاصّة ما كان منه يحلّل وبالأدوية الحادّة إذا طليت على البدن أو بالإمساك عن الطعام . فاستفرغ بدن المريض بأوفق هذه الأشياء له . آخر الحيلة .

---

٤ على حسـب ] بحسب P ELOOx ‖ ٥ فليـس ] فلن P ELOOx ‖ ٩ المريض ] ELOOx .om ‖ ١٠ الطبيعة ] القوة ELOP ‖ ١١ الحيلة ] من حيلة البر Ox ‖ ١٤ تلك ] om. Es²G ‖ ١٥ الحيلة ] من حيلة البر Ox ‖ ١٩ الأشياء ] كلّها add. EOx | الحيلة ] حيلة البر Ox

One should hasten to evacuate the irritating[17] humor either before it weakens the strength [of the body], or before it increases the heat of the fever, or before such a humor reaches a major organ.[18] *In Hippocratis Aphorismos commentarius* 4.[19]

13. Strong bodies can endure evacuation in one stroke, but in the case of weak bodies, one should evacuate the superfluity many times, for as long as the strength [of the body] can endure it. When the strength [of the body] dwindles, one should stop the evacuation even if there is still some superfluity left [in the body]. *In Hippocratis Aphorismos commentaria* 1.[20]

14. The coction of diseases only takes place through a change of the humors from an unnatural into a natural condition and only when the main organs in which those humors are present are healthy. But when these organs are ill, then the illness has taken possession of the very substance of the body, and the danger is great, and the patient cannot be cured unless the specific strength of these main organs returns to them. *In Hippocratis Epidemiarum* 1.2.[21]

15. When a humor should be evacuated and you see that it tends to be evacuated with the urine, but the kidneys and urinary bladder are sick or weak, direct it to the belly. Similarly, if it tends to the belly but the intestines are ill, direct it to the region of the kidneys and bladder or to the region of the uterus. And what is impossible for you [to direct,] let it [stream] to the region it tends to. *In Hippocratis Epidemiarum* 6.2.[22]

16. When the humors tend [to stream] to the inside, one should attract them to the outside; when they tend [to stream] to the outside, one should attract them to the inside; when they tend [to stream] to the rear, one should attract them to the front; and when they tend [to stream to] one side, one should attract them to the opposite side. *In Hippocratis De humoribus commentarius* 1.[23]

ينبغي أن تبادر باستفراغ الخلط الهائج إمّا من قبل أن تضعف القوة وإمّا من قبل أن تزيد حرارة الحمّى وإمّا من قبل أن تصير تلك الأخلاط إلى عضو شريف . في شرحه لرابعة الفصول .

١٣ . الأبدان القوية تحتمل أن تستفرغ في دفعة واحدة والضعيفة ينبغي أن يخرج منها الفضل في دفعات كثيرة ما دامت القوة تحتمل . وإن خارت القوة فاقطع الاستفراغ وإن كان قد بقي من الفضل بقية . في شرحه للأولى من الفصول .

١٤ . نضج الأمراض إنّما يكون بتغيّر الأخلاط عن الحال الخارجة عن الطبيعة إلى الحال الطبيعية . وإنّما يكون ذلك بالأعضاء الأصلية التي فيها تلك الأخلاط إذا كانت صحيحة . وأمّا متى كانت تلك الأعضاء سقيمة فالمرض متمكّن من نفس جوهر البدن والخطر فيه عظيم وليس يمكن أن يبرأ المريض دون أن تعود إلى تلك الأعضاء الأصلية قوّتها الخصيصة بها . في الثانية من شرحه للأولى من ابيديميا .

١٥ . إذا كان خلط يحتاج أن تستفرغه ورأيته قد مال إلى أن يستفرغ بالبول وكانت الكلى أو المثانة عليلة أو ضعيفة فأمل ذلك الخلط للبطن . وكذلك إن مال إلى البطن وكانت الأمعاء عليلة فأمله إلى ناحية الكلى والمثانة أو إلى ناحية الرحم وما تعاصى عليك فكله إلى ناحية ميله . في الثانية من شرحه للسادسة من ابيديميا .

١٦ . متى مالت الأخلاط إلى داخل فينبغي أن تجذب إلى خارج وإن مالت إلى خارج فينبغي أن تجذب إلى داخل وإن مالت إلى خلف فتجذب إلى قدام وإن مالت إلى قدام فتجذب إلى خلف وإن مالت إلى جانب فتجذب إلى الجانب الآخر . في شرحه للأولى من الأخلاط .

٦-٧ إلى الحال الطبيعية] G¹ || ٩ المريض] المرض E | الأصلية] G¹ || ١٠ ابيديميا] افيديميا ELOxP || ١١-١٤ إذا . . . ابيديميا] om. O || ١٢ فأمل]فاحمل E || ١٣ فأمله]فاحمله E | عليك] G¹ | فكله]فخله E Es²LP || ١٤ ابيديميا] افيديميا ELOxP || ١٥ مالت] سالت ELOx

17. One of the things that attracts in the opposite direction is the binding of the hands and feet when the humor tends to the chest. Similarly, sharp medicines put on hands and feet attract the superfluities towards the head or viscera. *In Hippocratis De humoribus commentarius* 1.[24]

18. One should evacuate the [malignant] humor either at the time that the disease attacks—namely, from above through a nosebleed or through emesis and the like—or at the time that the disease abates— namely, from below through the urine or excrements and the like. *In Hippocratis De humoribus commentarius* 2.[25]

19. Chronic diseases have to be treated by means of a thinning regimen. Indeed, for many of these diseases, this treatment alone is sufficient for their cure. I have seen how many patients who suffered from pains in the joints[26] and asthma and a minor form of epilepsy were completely cured by this regimen. But someone who suffers from chronic epilepsy also derives no small benefit from this thinning regimen. This regimen consists of the continuous [consumption of] foods from which the thinning chyme originates, and of goal-oriented exercise, and of avoidance of any food containing thickness. *De victu attenuante.*[27]

20. If one fixes the time [of consumption] of the food and its quantity and quality, it is sufficient for nature to heal diseases. *In Hippocratis Epidemiarum* 6.5.[28]

21. I know many patients whose strength failed and whom I cured from this affliction by ordering them to abstain from food for a long time while I administered liquid drugs. I know others who suffered from syncope after loss of strength. These I treated by ordering abstention from food and frequent massage of arms and legs. I also ordered massage of the whole spine. These patients regained their strength and recovered fully. With other patients I did the opposite; I prevented them from keeping a restricted diet and administered food. *De optimo medico cognoscendo.*[29]

22. In the case of many people I behaved daringly [in my treatment]. With confidence and certainty, I gave some of them cold water all the time they were ill, and I gave it to others from time to time, although other physicians refrained from letting their patients drink cold water.

١٧. ممّا يجذب على المقابلة شدّ اليدين والرجلين إذا مال الخلط إلى الصدر. وكذلك الأدوية الحرّيفة إذا أدنيت من اليدين والرجلين تجذب الفضول نحو الرأس أو نحو الأحشاء. في شرحه للأولى من الأخلاط.

١٨. ينبغـي لك أن تستفرغ الخلـط إمّا في أوقات النوائب فمـن فوق بالرعاف أو بالقيء ونحو ذلك، وإمّا في أوقات الراحة فمن أسـفل بالبول أو بالبراز وما أشـبه ذلك. في الثانية من شرح الأخلاط.

١٩. الأمراض المزمنة تحتاج إلى التدبير الملطّف حتّى أنّ كثيرا منها يستغني في بروءه بهذا التدبير وحده. وقد رأيت عددا كثيرا ممّن به من أوجاع المفاصل والربو ومن كان به صرع يسيـر برأ بهذا التدبير بروءا تامّا. ومن كان به صرع مزمن فإنّه ينتفع بهذا التدبير الملطّف منفعة ليسـت باليسـيرة. وهذا التدبير هو إدامة الأغذية التي يتولّد عنها كيموس ملطّف والرياضة بالقصد والحذر من كلّ غذاء فيه غلظ. في مقالة في التدبير الملطّف.

٢٠. إذا قدّرت الغذاء في وقته وكمّيته وكيفيته اكتفت به الطبيعة في شفاء الأمراض. في الخامسة من شرحه لسادسة ابيديميا.

٢١. إنّـي لأعرف عدّة من المرضى نقصت قوّتهم فأبرأتهم من هذا العارض بالمنع من الطعام مدّة طويلة مع شرب دواء. وأعرف آخرين ممّن كان قد عرض لهم الغشي فضلا عن نقصـان القوة داويتهم بالمنع من الطعام ودلك اليديـن والرجلين دلكا كثيرا وأمرت مع ذلك بدلك الفقار كلّها فرجعت قوة أولئك المرضى فبروا بروءا تامّا. وآخرين فعلت بهم خلاف ذلك ومنعتهم من الاقتصار وناولتهم الغذاء. في مقالته في محنة الطبيب الفاضل.

٢٢. قد كت أقدم على بشر كثير بعضهم أسقيه الماء البارد بثقة ويقين في وقت مرضه كلّه وفي بعضهم في وقت دون وقت على أنّ غير من الأطبّاء كانوا يجتنبون عن إسقائهم إيّاه.

٢ تجـذب] EL || ٩ بـروءا . . . بهـذا التدبيـر] om. EL || ١١ والرياضـة] G¹ || ١٣ ابيديميا افيديميا [ELOxP || ١٥ كان قد] G¹

With utmost confidence and trust, I let someone who suffered from pure ardent fever (but had no tumor in any part of his viscera) drink cold water. Likewise, in the case of someone else where I was not so sure and confident, I administered [cold water] after I had told his relatives, "If he does not drink cold water, he will most certainly die, but if he drinks it, I hope that he will recover." And I swear by God, all those who drank cold water and whom I had hoped would recover [actually] recovered and regained their health. *De usis.*[30]

23. The diet of convalescents should hold the middle between that of healthy and ill people. Sleeplessness is the most harmful for them. To abandon one's habit is very dangerous not only in the case of the diet of convalescents and their like but also in the treatment of sick people. *De methodo medendi* 7.[31]

24. The quantity of cold water that a fever patient should drink when he suffers from severe thirst should be as much as that which he can swallow without breathing. Cold substances prevent coction, except for oxymel, which does not because of its dissolving strength. *In Hippocratis De acutorum morborum [victu et] Galeni commentarius* 1.[32]

25. Barley groats[33] have the combined beneficial effects of invigorating one's strength and cleansing the respiratory organs of bad humors through cutting and moistening. These beneficial effects cannot be found together in any other substance. If a patient dislikes barley groats, the next best food is rockfish with water, leek,[34] aneth,[35] salt, and a moderate amount[36] of olive oil. If rockfish is unavailable, one should give him a fish that comes close to its temperament, but one should first of all give him some oxymel, except in the case that the nerves[37] are affected. *In Hippocratis De acutorum morborum [victu et] Galeni commentarius* 1.[38]

26. The ingestion of oxymel should precede that of barley broth[39] by two hours so that it can purify, open, and pave the way [for the excretions]. When both are taken at the same time, disturbance[40] occurs to the stomach because they are unequal [in strength]. *In Hippocratis De acutorum morborum [victu et] Galeni commentarius* 3.[41]

أمّا من كانت حمّاه محرقة خالصة ولم يكن في شيء من أحشائه ورم فكنت أسقيه الماء
البارد بغاية الثقة والاتّكال، وكنت أسقي إنسانا آخر وأنا ليس في غاية الثقة والاتّكال بعد
أن أقول لأهله : إن لم يشرب ماء باردا مات لا محالة وإن شربه رجوت له أن يسلم . والله
إنّ كلّ من شرب الماء البارد ممّن رجوت له أن يسلم سلم وعوفي . في مقالته في العادات .

٢٣ . تدبير الناقهين وسـط فيما بين تدبير الأصحّاء وتدبير المرضى . والسـهر أضرّ
شيء بهم وترك العادة خطر عظيم ليس في تدبير الناقهين وأشباههم فقط لكنّ في مداواة
المرضى أيضا . سابعة الحيلة .

٢٤ . مقدار الماء البارد الذي يشربه المحموم عند شدّة العطش ينبغي أن يكون بقدر
ما يمكن المريض أن يتجرّعه من غير أن يستنشق الهواء . والأشياء الباردة تمنع النضج خلا
السكنجبين لأنّ فيه قوة مقطّعة . في شرحه لأولى الأمراض الحادّة .

٢٥ . قـد اجتمع في منافع كشـك الشـعير أنّه يقوّي القوة وينقّـي آلات التنفّس من
الأخــلاط الرديئة بالتقطيع والترطيـب وليس تجتمع هذه المنافع في غيره . ومتى كره المريض
كشـك الشـعير فأصلح الأغذية بعده السمك الصخور بماء وكرّاث وشبثّ وملح وزيت
معتدل . وإن لم يوجد سـمك الصخور فما قارب مزاجه من الأسـماك وينبغي أن يتقّدم
فيعطيه قبل ذلك شـيئًا من السـكنجبين إلا أن يكون يعض الأعضاء العصبية عليلا . في
شرحه لأولى الأمراض الحادّة .

٢٦ . أخذ السـكنجبين قبل أخذ حسـاء الشـعير بمقدار سـاعتين ليجلو ويفتح
ويطرّق . وإن أخـذ في وقـت واحد عرض للمعدة اضطراب لأنّهما غير متشـابهين .
في شرحه لثالثة الأمراض الحادّة .

---

٣ لأهله] هـذا .add E Es²LOOxP ‖ ٤ وعوفي] وعفى L ‖ ٦ شيء] الأشياء
ELOx ‖ ٨ البارد] .om ELOx ‖ ١٠ لأولى] للأولى : .om E EsG ‖ ١٧ حسـاء]
الحسو ELOx ‖ ١٨ لثالثة] الثالثة G

27. Constipation helps the illness to increase and to become more powerful than nature, and sometimes it causes death. Sometimes it also causes various kinds of fevers and various kinds of external and internal tumors. Constipation stirs up every [kind of] pain coming from thick humors; it weakens the powers of nature and corrupts the psychical activities. Sometimes it causes a heavy torpor and loss of reason. *De clysteribus.*[42]

28. When someone after the meal exerts himself and does physical exercise so much that he becomes [very] tired and drinks abundantly,[43] a bilious superfluity collects in his body because of the exertion and a raw uncocted superfluity collects because of the physical exercise performed at an improper time. Diseases become most severe when a large quantity of these two humors collects in the body. *In Hippocratis Epidemiarum* 1.2.[44]

29. Sleep is one of the most harmful things for very cold humors. Similarly,[45] it is harmful in the beginning of fever attacks; it harms the viscera that have a tumor[46] because the heat sinks and the blood sinks with it to the inner [parts of the] body. But if someone's humors are crude or small in quantity or if his strength is weak, sleep is beneficial for him. *In Hippocratis De humoribus commentarius* 1.[47]

30. Sleep in the beginning of [inflamed] tumors[48] that cause fever increases the tumors and the fever. *In Hippocratis Epidemiarum* 6.5.[49]

31. Anxieties are painful affections for the soul.[50] Thoughts and considerations are exercise for the soul. All movements of the soul produce bile. Rest of the soul produces cold phlegmatic humors. [In the case of] cold humors, do not restrict yourself to movements of the body but add to that the movements of the soul [to arouse the innate heat].[51] For the arousal of anger, it is necessary that one recover one's [normal] complexion and that one's humors flow [from the inner parts to the outer parts] of the body.[52] Anger is aroused in someone when the heat of his heart that was weak [is increased]. *In Hippocratis De humoribus commentarius* 1.[53]

٢٧ . احتبـاس الطبـع عونا للمرض في زيادته وقوته على الطبيعة وربّما كان سـببا
للهلاك . وقد يعرض منه أيضا حمّيات على اختلاف أنواعها والأورام الظاهرة والباطنة على
اختلافهـا . واحتباس الطبع يهيج كلّ وجع يكون من الأخلاط الغليظة ويوهن قوى الطبيعة
ويفسد الأفعال النفسانية . وقد يعرض منه السبات الثقيل وذهاب العقل . في مقالته في الحقن .

٢٨ . إذا كان إنسان يتعب تعبا شديدا حتّى يبلغ الإعياء ويشرب شرابا كثيرا ويرتاض
بعد الطعام اجتمع في بدنه فضل مرار من قبل التعب وفضل نيء غير نضيج من قبل رياضة
في غير وقتها . وأصعب ما تكون الأمراض إذا اجتمع من هذين الخلطين في البدن شـيء
كثير . في ثالثة شرحه للأولى من ابيديميا .

٢٩ . النوم من أضرّ الأشـياء للأخلاط الباردة جدّا . وكذلك يضرّ في ابتداء أدوار
الحمّى ويضرّ الأحشاء المتورّمة لأنّ الحرارة تغور ويغور معها الدم إلى داخل البدن . ومن كانت
أخلاطه نيئة أو ناقصة أو كانت قوّته ضعيفة فالنوم ينفعه . في شـرحه للأولى الأخلاط .

٣٠ . النوم في ابتداء الأورام التي تحدث عنها الحمّى تزيد في الورم وتزيد الحمّى . في
الرابعة من شرحه لسادسة ابيديميا .

٣١ . الغمـوم آلام للنفس والأفكار والهموم رياضة النفس . وجميع حركات النفس
تولـد المـرار . وراحتها تولد أخلاطا باردة بلغمية . ولا تقتصـر في الأخلاط الباردة على
حـركات البدن حتّى تضيف لذلك حركات النفس . وتحتاج في تهيّج الغيظ لاسـترداد
اللـون وانصبـاب الأخلاط إلى داخل . ويهيـج الغضب لمن كانت حـرارة قلبه ضعيفة .
في شرحه للأولى من الأخلاط .

---

٧ شيء] فضل ELOOxP ‖ ٨ ابيديميا] افيديميا ELOxP ‖ ٩ الباردة] الحارّة E ‖ وكذلك]
ولذلك EsLOOxP ‖ ١١ للأولى الأخلاط] للأولى من الأخلاط G ‖ ١٣ ابيديميا] افيديميا
ELOxP ‖ ١٦ وتحتاج] وتحتال ELOx

32. Joyful thoughts and expectations[54] rejoice[55] and stimulate the soul, so that the innate heat expands [by it]. Conversely, sad thoughts and expectations distress[56] the soul and cause the innate heat to contract. *In Hippocratis De humoribus commentarius* 2.[57]

5        33. Sleep is of evident benefit in the decline of diseases. It is good against the dryness of the belly, for while the air [entering the body] with the inhalation dries the belly[58] by means of its heat, sleep moistens it. *De somno et vigilia.*[59]

34. Any feebleness[60] caused by a copious evacuation all at once can
10      be cured by wine mixed with cold water, especially when the evacuation is of moistures[61] that stream to the stomach and what is around it. This applies only if there is no inflamed tumor in one of the viscera, no severe headache, no illness that causes a derangement of the mind,[62] no ardent fever, and[63] no illness that has not been cocted yet. In all these cases,
15      drinking wine is so harmful [for the patient] that it almost cannot be cured. *Ad Glauconem [de medendi methodo]* 1.[64]

35. To alleviate the severe pain of inflamed tumors on the outer parts of the body, it is enough to take concentrated grape juice[65] and rose oil mixed with a little melted wax. With this one should moisten a
20      greasy piece of wool and put it on [these tumors]. Make it cold in the summer and lukewarm in the winter. In the same way one should apply poultices. *Ad Glauconem [de medendi methodo]* 2.[66]

36. One should examine the individual characteristics of the natures [of people], because I know some who, having been busy at the begin-
25      ning of the night, missed their [normal] sleeping time and consequently could not sleep for the rest of the night. There are others who, when they taste barley groats, immediately feel sick, and yet others who suffer from heartburn when they take it. *De methodo medendi* 7.[67]

37. Pain arising especially from vaporous wind[68] should be treated
30      with a large cupping glass [applied] with strong heating.[69] You might think that this is a kind of magical treatment regardless of whether the illness is in the intestines or in any other organ of the body, because the very moment that the cupping glass is applied, the pain disappears and the patient

٣٢ . توهّم الأشياء السارّة وترجّيها يبسط النفس وينشطها فتبسط بها الحرارة الغريزية وكذلك توهّم ما يحزن وتوقّعه تنقبض به النفس ويحدث للحرارة الغريزية انقباض . في الثانية من تشريح الأخلاط .

٣٣ . النـوم ظاهر المنفعة في انحطاط الأمراض والنوم ينفع من يبس البطن فإنّ الهواء الذي يكون بالنسيم يبّس البطن بحرارته والنوم يرطّبه . في مقالته في النوم واليقظة .

٣٤ . قد يسكن كلّ غشي يكون من استفراغ كثير دفعة الشراب المزوج بالماء البارد ولا سـيّما متى كان الاستـفراغ من أشياء تنصبّ إلى المعدة وما يليها ، إن لم يمنع من ذلك ورم حارّ في بعض الأحشاء أو صداع شـديد أو علّة غيّرت الذهن أو حمّى محرقة أو مرض لم ينضج بعد . فإنّه يلحق من شرب النبيذ في جميع هذه الأحوال ضرر عظيم يكاد أن لا يكون له بروء . أولى أغلوقن .

٣٥ . ينبغي أن تقتصر في تسكين شـدّة الوجع في أورام ظاهر البدن الحارّة على ما تّتخذ من عقيد العنب ودهن الورد ويسـير من شـمع مذاب فيها وتبلّ فيه صوفة دسـمة وتضعه في الصيف وهو بارد وفي الشتاء وهو فاتر . وكذلك تفعل بالأضمدة . ثانية أغلوقن .

٣٦ . ينبغي أن تنظر في خواصّ الطبائع فإنّي أعرف قوما إن اشـتغلوا في أوّل الليل وفاتهم وقت النوم لم يقدروا أن يناموا بقية ليلتهم . وفي الناس قوم إذا ذاقوا كشك الشعير غثت أنفسهم على المكان وقوم إذا شربوه حمض في معدهم . سابعة الحيلة .

٣٧ . الوجع الحادث من ريح بخارية يداوى خاصّة دون غيره بمحجمة كبيرة تعلق مع نار كثيرة . وأنت تظنّ هذا الضرب من المداواة أنّه ضرب من السحر كانت العلّة في الأمعاء أو في سائر أعضاء البدن وذلك أنّه ساعة تعلق المحجمة يذهب وجعه ويرجع إلى صحّته .

---

١ الأشياء السارّة] G¹ ‖ ٥ البطن]البدن L ‖ ١٤ إن] G¹ ‖ ١٥ لم]لا P : ولا] ولا | ليلتهم] يليهم LOOxP ‖ ١٦ سابعة]G¹ : رابعة] G ‖ ١٧ من]عن ELOOxP ‖ ١٨ وأنت]فإنّك G

regains his health. But if the humor that activated the vapor is [still] there, the pain will necessarily return. Therefore, apply the cupping glass once again until the pain subsides and then evacuate that humor. *De methodo medendi* 12.[70]

38. [Compound] remedies that alleviate pain—namely, those remedies that are mixed with narcotics[71] and soporifics—should only be taken in cases where the pain is strong and severe, such as severe colic, stones, and severe sleeplessness,[72] which dissolve the strength, or if one wants to quiet a severe cough that is difficult [to bear] and detrimental for the patient, such as someone who coughs up blood or who suffers from a very severe catarrh descending from his head. As for cases that are less dangerous than the ones I mentioned, it is sufficient to apply remedies that are not narcotic. *Mayāmir* 8.[73]

39. When one compounds remedies with narcotics to alleviate pain, one should consider three things: first, that [by means of them] one should numb the sensation [of pain]; second, that their application should not be followed by a lasting harm in the [affected] organ; and third, that the affected organ should receive great benefit from them either through dissolving, cutting, or refining the humors that caused the disease or through changing and improving the nature of those humors. I think that Philon composed the remedy named after him[74] only after he had looked into these three [necessary] properties, and it is one of the oldest and most famous remedies. *Mayāmir* 9.[75]

40. If a symptom is accompanied by severe harm that damages the strength of the body, then in order to save the patient from death, the physician is obliged to abandon [the treatment of] the disease [itself] and eliminate the symptom or mitigate its harm, even if this aggravates the disease. Then he turns to the treatment of the harm that occurred because of the treatment of that symptom[76] [and the ensuing neglect of the disease]. Sometimes that harm is completely eliminated, but in other cases it leaves a permanent weakness in or the loss of one of his [bodily] functions, and the patient lives for a long time with that chronic illness. This is the most appropriate [course of action]. *De methodo [medendi]* 12.[77]

وإن كان هنـاك الخلط الفاعل لذلك البخار فإنّ الوجع يعاود ضرورة. فلذلك ترجع وتعلق المحجمة حتّى يسكن الوجع، ثمّ تستفرغ ذلك الخلط. ثانية عشر الحيلة.

٣٨. الأدوية المسكّنة للأوجاع وهي التي تخلط فيها المخدّرات للحسّ والمنوّمات لا ينبغي أن تتناول إلا في مواضع الأوجاع الشديدة الصعبة كالقولنج الصعب والحصى والسهر المقلّق يحلّ القوة أو لتسكين السعال الشديد الذي يعنف على صاحبه ويؤذيه بمنزلة ما يعرض لمن ينفث الدم أو لمن يصيبه نزلة تنحدر من رأسه صعبة شديدة. فأمّا ما يكون أقلّ غائلة من هذه التي ذكرناها فيكتفى فيها باستعمال أدوية غير مخدّرة. ثامنة الميامر.

٣٩. هذه الأدوية المؤلّفة لتسكين الأوجـاع التي تقع فيها المخدّرات ينبغي للرجل أن يقصد في تأليفه إلى ثلاثة خصال: أحدها أن يخدّر الحسّ والثانية أن لا يعقب استعمالها آفـة تبقى لابثة في العضو والثالثة أن يستنفع العضو العليـل بها منفعة عظيمة إمّا بتحليل الأخـلاط الفاعلة للعلّة أو تقطيعهـا وتلطيفها أو بتغيير طبيعة تلك الأخلاط وإصلاحها. وأحسـب أن يكون فيلون إنّما ألّف دواءه بعد أن نظر في هذه الثلاثة الخصال، وهو أقدم الأدوية وأشهرها. تاسعة الميامر.

٤٠. العرض متى كان معه أذى شـديد وأضرّ بالقوة اضطرّ الطبيب إلى ترك المرض والإقبال على العرض ليزيله أو يسكّن إضراره ولو بما يزيد في المرض ليسـتنقذ المريض من الهلاك. ثمّ يرجع يتلافى ما حصل من الأذية من أجل الاشتغال بطبّ الأعراض. وقد ترتفع تلك الأذية كلّها وقد تخلف ضعفا دائما في فعل من الأفعال أو بطلانه ويعيش المريض زمانا طويلا بزمانته تلك وهو الأولى. ثانية عشر الحيلة.

─────────────────────────

٣ فيهـا] بها ELOOxP ‖ ٤ الصعبـة] المبرحـة ELOOxP ‖ ٧ ذكرناها] ذكرنا add. ELOOxP ‖ ٩ والثانية] والثاني EL ‖ ١٢ أن يكون... ألّف] om. Ox ‖ فيلون] om. EGL ‖ في : om. EGL ‖ ألّف] om. EL ‖ أن نظر] النظر EL ‖ ١٦ الأذية] الأدوية G : إذاية L ‖ ١٧ الأذية] الأدوية G : إذاية L

41. Some symptoms are harmful to the strength and should be attended to [immediately] when they become urgent. In this case one discontinues the treatment of the disease itself and of its cause unless it happens that the remedy used to combat the symptom is also good for repelling the disease and its cause. These symptoms are sleeplessness, pain, and all the various kinds of evacuations. If one of these occurs to excess, it is taken over by syncope. *De methodo [medendi]* 12.[78]

42. When one draws blood or performs an evacuation or [tries to] to attract [the malignant humor] to the opposite side [of the body] but the pain persists, then the harmful substance has become fixed and settled in the organ and its treatment should consist of dissolving medications. In the same manner one should persistently treat those pains that arise from an inflating wind with refining foods and drinks, enemas, cataplasms, fomentations, and warm compresses. *De methodo [medendi]* 12.[79]

43. The method one should always apply is to seek the evacuation and dissolution of the unnatural [substance in the body]. If this is impossible because of the nature of the [affected] organ or because the illness is incurable, one should let the unnatural substance suppurate and putrefy. If this is unsuccessful, we excise and extirpate it either by operative treatment[80] or by caustic remedies. *De methodo [medendi]* 14.[81]

44. Weakness of the stomach, veins, arteries, and muscles and, in general, weakness of all the animal[82] and psychical systems[83] is caused by a bad temperament. *De [morborum] causis et symptomatibus* 1.[84]

45. A bad temperament occurring in any part of the body is an illness of that part.[85] It forms an obstruction and obstacle now for one and then another of that part's powers. Because of this, humors stream towards various parts at various times unequally and irregularly. *De [morborum] causis et symptomatibus* 3.[86]

46. Remedies with a strong heating effect weaken the strength of the body greatly and suddenly. As a result the body cannot tolerate treatment [anymore]. Therefore, the powers of the [various kinds] of food and drink that cut the thickness of the humors should be moderately hot. *De venae sectione.*[87]

٤١. الأعراض الضارّة بالقوّة التي ينبغي أن يقصد نحوها إذا حفزت جدّا ويترك الاشتغال بالمرض وبسببه ، إلا أن اتّفق أن يكون ما يقاوم به ذلك العرض ينفع أيضا في دفع المرض أو سببه ، هي السهر والوجع وأنواع الاستفراغ كلّها . إذا أفرط أحدها وأخذها الغشي .

٤٢. إذا فصدت أو استفرغت أو جذبت إلى خلاف الجهة وبقي الوجع لابثا فالشيء المـوذي قد لجّ ورسـخ في العضـو ، ومداواته تكون بأدوية محلّلة . وعلى هذا المثال تداوى الأوجاع الحادثة عن ريح نافخة بالمواظبة عليها بالأطعمة والأشـربة الملطّفة والحقن والأضمدة والنطولات والكمادات . ثانية عشر الحيلة .

٤٣. الطريـق الذي تسـلكه دائما هو أن تروم أن تسـتفرغ وتحلّل ما هو خـارج عن الطبع ، فإن لم يمكن بسبب طبيعة العضو أو بسبب أن العلّة علّة لا تبرأ فتقيح ذلك الشيء الخارج عن الطبيعة وتعفنه ، فإن لم ينجح قطعناه واستأصلناه إمّا بعلاج الحديد وإمّا بالأدوية التي تحرق وتكوي . أخيرة الحيلة .

٤٤. ضعـف المعدة والعروق والشـريانات والعضل وبالجملـة ضعف جميع الآلات الحيوانية والنفسانية يكون بسبب سوء المزاج . أولى العلل والأعراض .

٤٥. سوء المزاج الحادث في كلّ واحد من الأعضاء هو مرض من أمراض الأعضاء المتشابهة الأجزاء ويمنع وتعوق قوّة دون قوّة من قوى ذلك العضو فتنصبّ الرطوبات بسبب ذلك في أوقات مختلفة إلى أعضاء مختلفة على غير مساواة وعلى غير نظام . ثالثة العلل والأعراض .

٤٦. الأدوية التي تسـخن إسخانا شديدا ترخي القوّة إرخاء شديدا بغتة ، فيضعف البدن فلا يمكن فيه احتمال العلاج . ولذلك ينبغي أن تكون قوى الأطعمة والأشـربة التي تقطع غلظ الأخلاط معتدلة في حرارتها . في مقالته في الفصد .

٣ هـي] هـو EsG | أفرط] فـرط G ‖٥١،١٢–٥٤،٨ ضعـف المعـدة . . . أغلوق] أغلوق] om. P ‖ ١٥ وتعوق] G¹ ‖ ١٨ احتمال] G¹ : اختلاف G | ٥١،١٨–٥٧،٣ العلاج . . . ابيديميا] om. Ox | ولذلك] وكذلك G

47. Concerning the [various] steps of treatment, logical reasoning indicates and experience verifies that we should begin by cleansing the whole body from superfluities. Then we should be confident to treat the [ailing] part with a medication that has only a heating effect. If we do not evacuate the body first, [superfluous] matter is attracted to that part through the hot medication, analogous to the attraction of a cupping glass. *De methodo [medendi]* 4.[88]

48. When the illness is severe and difficult, one should hasten to evacuate [the body] through bleeding or relieving the bowels or emesis, even if overfilling is not indicated. The illness is severe and difficult when a major organ is endangered or when the illness itself is strong and severe, or bad and malignant, in quality, although not widespread [in the body].[89] *De methodo [medendi]* 4.[90]

49. He said: If you want to prevent the superfluity from increasing, you should attract it to the side opposite to where it tends [to stream]. And if you want to evacuate it, you should do so from the side where it is or from the side to which it is nearest. *In Hippocratis De natura hominis commentaria.*[91]

50. Those whose illness starts from many indigestions or from viscous thick foods and those who suffer from stretching or swelling in the hypochondria, or from an extremely severe heat [of the urine],[92] or from an inflamed tumor[93] in one of the viscera are not ready to be purged. *In Hippocratis Aphorismos commentarius* 1.[94]

51. Says Moses: When the indigestion has occurred a very long time ago and you have verified that its effects have worn off, and, similarly, when those humors have become fine and thin and you have ascertained that there was a complete coction, and you see that the patient needs evacuation, then you can evacuate him with peace of mind as long as he is free from tumors in the viscera and from afflictions in the hypochondria—but mind what I said here.

52. Take care not to apply a warm compress to the site of the illness before the evacuation, because then you attract more blood from the neighboring organs to it than the quantity that you dissolve. *In Hippocratis De acutorum morborum [victu et] Galeni commentarius* 2.[95]

٤٧ . الذي دلّ عليه القياس وصحّحته التجربة في مراتب العلاج أن نبتدئ أوّلا بتنقية جميع البدن من الفضول وبعد ذلك يوثق بمداواة العضو بدواء له حرارة وحده. وإن لم نتقدّم باستفراغ البدن جذبت إلى العضو مادّة بالدواء الحارّ كما تجذب المحجمة. رابعة الحيلة.

٤٨ . إذا كانت العلّة شـديدة صعبة فبادر واسـتفرغ بفصد أو بإسهال أو بقيء وإن لم تكن دلائل الامتلاء موجودة. والعلة تكون شـديدة صعبة إذا كانت في عضو شـريف ذي خطـر، أو تكون في نفسـها عظيمة كبيرة أو تكون رديئـة خبيثة الكيفية وإن كانت كمّيتها قليلة. رابعة الحيلة.

٤٩ . قـال إذا أردت أن تمنـع الفضل من التزيّد فينبغي أن تجذبـه إلى خلاف الجهة التـي مـال إليها. وإن أردت أن تسـتفرغه فمن الناحية التي هو فيها ومن التي هي إليه أقرب. في شرحه لطبيعة الإنسان.

٥٠ . الذيـن أوّل مرضهم من تخم كثيرة أو من أطعمة لزجة غليظة، والذين بهم فيما دون الشراسـيف تمدّد أو انتفاخ أو حرارة شـديدة مفرطة أو كان في بعض الأحشاء ورم فليس واحد من هؤلاء متهيّئ للإسهال. في شرحه للأولى من الفصول.

٥١ . قال موسـى: إذا بعد العهد بالتخمة جـدّا وتحقّقت بطلان أثارها وكذلك إذا رقّت تلك الأخلاط ولطفت وتبيّن لك النضج التامّ ورأيت أنّه يحتاج إلى استفراغ فاستفرغ بطمأنينة إذا سلم من أورام الأحشاء وأعراض ما دون الشراسيف فلا تغفل هذا.

٥٢ . احـذر أن تكمّد قبل الاسـتفراغ فإنّك تجذب إلى موضع العلّة من الأعضاء المجاورة له دما أكثر ممّا تحلّله. في شرحه لثانية الأمراض الحادّة.

---

١٣ للأولى] الأولى EsG || ١٥ تلك [G¹ || ١٧ أن] من أن EL

53. Sometimes a partial coction occurs that cannot be trusted, such as the coction of an abscess beneath the ears, for one assumes that the patient has recovered, yet he dies because the humors in the vessels were not cocted and they caused the illness. *In Hippocratis Epidemiarum* 1.2.[96]

54. [To apply] a cupping glass without scarification is very beneficial for the other pains that arise from a thick, inflating, cold wind that is retained in solid bodies and that cannot escape because of its own thickness and the solidity of those bodies. *In Hippocratis Epidemiarum* 2.6.[97]

55. When [superfluous] matter streams to the upper part of the mouth or the palate or the uvula, one should return it to the nostrils with sharp medications that are put in the nose. Similarly, the attraction of [superfluous] matter from the eyes to the mouth should take place through gargling with sharp medicines. *In Hippocratis De humoribus commentarius* 1.[98]

56. A loud voice widens the passages and eliminates the moisture in the stomach and the mouth and stimulates expectoration. It expels viscous bad phlegm and heats the body. For those who need their bodies to be warmed, the use of the voice is better than any medication or foodstuff, because it warms their bodies, stimulates their innate heat, and warms the cold parts of their bodies and dries the moist parts. But if someone has a dry and lean body, he should not use his voice [to expel superfluous moisture]. Similarly, if someone suffers from bad moistures in his stomach or suffers from indigestion, you should warn him about the use of a loud voice because it lets the malignant humor in the stomach pass into the whole body.[99] *De somno et vigilia.*[100]

57. If much blood streams to any part of the body, that part stretches and the vessels within it also stretch. This happens in the large vessels and in those small vessels which, initially hidden from the senses, become

٥٣ . قـد يحدث نضج جزئي لا يعتقد به مثل أن ينضج خراج تحت الأذن ، فيظنّ أنّ المريض قد برأ وهو يموت لأنّ الأخلاط التي داخل العروق لم تنضج وهي سـبب المرض . في الثانية من شرحه للأولى من ابيديميا .

٥٤ . المحجمة دون شـرط تنفع منفعة عظيمة في سـائر الأوجـاع الكائنة عن ريح غليظة نافخة باردة محتقنة في أجسام كثيفة فلا تجد مخلصا لغلظها وكثافة الأجسام . في سادسة شرحه لثانية ابيديميا .

٥٥ . إذا كانت المادّة تجري إلى أعلى الفم أو الحنك أو إلى اللهاة فتردّها إلى المنخرين بأدويــة حرّيفة تجعل في الأنف . وكذلك جذب المادّة عـن العينين ألى الفم يكون بالغرغرة بالأدوية الحرّيفة . في شرحه للأولى من الأخلاط .

٥٦ . الصوت الشـديد يوسـع المجاري ويفني الرطوبة الكائنة في المعدة والفم ويهيج النتخّـع ويخرج بلغما لزجا رديئا ويسـخن البدن . وأمّا الذين يحتـاجون إلى تسـخين أبدانهم فليس لهم دواء ولا غذاء أفضل من استعمال الصوت ، فإنّه يسخن أبدانهم ويهيج حرارتهم الغريزية ويسـخن أعضاءهم الباردة ويبّس أعضاءهم الرطبة . وأمّا من بدنه يابسـا نحيفا فـلا ينبغي أن يسـتعمل الصوت ، وكذلك من فـي معدته رطوبات رديئـة أو أهل التخم فحذّرهم من الصوت الشـديد فإنّه يسلك بالخلط الردئ الذي في المعدة في جميع البدن . في مقالته في النوم واليقظة .

٥٧ . إذا انحلـب إلـى عضو من الأعضاء دم كثير تمدّد ذلك العضو وتمدّد العروق التي فيه . ويعرض ذلك في العروق الكبار وفي العروق الصغار التي كانت أوّلا تخفى عن

___

٣ ابيديميا ] افيديميا EL ‖ ٤ عن ] من L ‖ ٦ ابيديميا ] افيديميا EL ‖ ٧ أو (1st) ] إلى add. EL ‖ ٧–٨ إلى المنخرين . . . العينين ] om. EL ‖ ١٤ الصوت الشديد ] add. ELO

visible structures because of their overfilling, just as we can see the vessels that often appear in the eyes because of the whiteness of their tunic. Perhaps there are other vessels smaller than those [of the eyes] that become visible when they stretch because of overfilling, but these are not seen due to their smallness. *De arte parva.*[101]

58. I know a man who relied upon bathing in waters mixed with salt or borax[102] or sulfur in order to evacuate his body [of yellow bile]. In the rest of his regimen he [equally] pursued the evacuation of the bile, but he did not know that every dominating unnatural [humoral] quality should be opposed by the opposite quality and that this is much better than evacuation. Nor did he listen to those who told him so. As a result the main organs [of his body] dried so much that he was afflicted by phthisis and marasmus and then died. *Ad Glauconem [de medendi methodo]* 1.[103]

59. When you treat tumors that are difficult to dissolve, you should mix some softening medications with the medications that have a strong dissolving effect in order to be sure that those tumors will not turn into the hard tumor called *skirros.*[104] *Ad Glauconem [de medendi methodo]* 2.[105]

60. When one is healthy, one should massage weak parts of the body more than the other parts, using dry massage especially. [When applied] during the times that the pains have eased, this kind of massage can prevent their occurrence in the weak parts, especially [when applied] two or three hours before the pains' actual attack. *De sanitate tuenda* 5.[106]

61. A change [of the temperament] to heat or cold can be treated most easily and cured most quickly. A change to moisture or dryness is harder to treat and to cure; to moisten what has become dry takes a long time. When the dryness becomes firmly settled, it is not susceptible to treatment, and when it becomes extremely well settled, it cannot be cured [anymore]. *De methodo [medendi]* 7.[107]

الحسّ ثمّ صارت آلات ظاهرة لامتلائها كما قد نرى تلك العروق تظهر في العين كثيرا لبياض غشائها . ولعلّ عروقا أخر أدقّ من تلك العروق التي تظهر بتمدّد بسبب امتلائها ولا تظهر لرقّتها . في الصناعة الصغيرة.

٥٨ . وإنّي لأعرف رجلا ركن إلى الاستحمام بهذه المياه التي يشوبها ملح أو بورق أو كبريت كي يستفرغ بدنه. وقد كان يجري في سائر تدبيره نحو استفراغ المرار، ولم يعلم أنّه ينبغي أن يدخل على كلّ كيفية تغلب وتخرج عن الأمر الطبيعي ضدّها ، وأنّ ذلك أصلح كثيرا من الاستفراغ. ولا قبل ممّن أمره بذلك فأورثه ذلك يبسا شديدا في أعضائه الأصلية حتّى أصابه السلّ والذبول ثمّ مات. أولى أغلوقن.

٥٩ . إذا عالجت الأورام العسرة التحلّل فينبغي أن تخلط في الأدوية التي تحلّل تحليلا قويا بعض الأدوية الملينة لتأمن انتقال تلك الأورام إلى الورم الصلب المسمّى سقيروس. ثانية أغلوقن.

٦٠ . الأعضاء الضعيفة في أوقات الصحّة ينبغي أن تدلك أكثر ممّا تدلك سائر الأعضاء ولا سيّما الدلك اليابس. ومن شأن هذا الدلك في أوقات الراحة أن يمنع حدوث الأوجاع في تلك الأعضاء الضعيفة وخاصّة قبل حدوث النوبة بساعتين أو ثلاث ساعات. فأمّا في أوقات التي تهيج العلل في تلك الأعضاء الضعيفة فينبغي أن يحذر استعمال دلكها . خامسة تدبير الصحّة.

٦١ . الاستحالة إلى الحرارة أو البرودة أسهل مداواة وأسرع بروء . والاستحالة إلى الرطوبة واليبوسة أعسر مداواة وأنكد بروء . ويحتاج ترطيب اليابس إلى زمان طويل . ومتى استحكم اليبس فهو غير قابلا للعلاج ممتنع البروء عند ما يستحكم في الغاية . سابعة الحيلة .

An incurable consolidation of dryness means that the very substance of the main parts[108] has dried up. The closer the degree of dryness is to this [degree of consolidation], the more difficult it is to heal and the more prolonged. Even the lowest degree of dryness [is difficult to cure]
5    because the moistening [process] is difficult and hard and requires a long time. *De methodo [medendi]* 7.[109]

62. There are four degrees of dryness: The first and the easiest to heal is when the dryness occurs in the small vessels that are specific to every part of the body and that provide nourishment to those parts
10   through their openings. The second degree is when the dryness reaches the point where it eliminates that moisture scattered through the parts of the body which is like drizzle.[110] This is the moisture whose property is to stream out of the openings of those thin vessels and adapt itself to a [particular] part to provide it with food.[111] The third degree is when
15   the dryness reaches the point where it eliminates the moisture in those parts of the body that are of a moist, nearly coagulated, and hardened substance—just like fat and flesh—that then liquefies and dissolves.[112] The fourth degree is when the main parts become dry, such as the substance of the heart and the liver and the like. *De methodo [medendi]* 7.[113]

20   63. When the temperament deviates from its balance towards cold, you should continue to heat it until it returns to its balance as long as you feel certain and confident about the result. But to cool a warm temperament is not the same matter—it should be done with caution and care and without taking any risk. If the area surrounding that part which one
25   wants to cool is not completely strong, one cannot be sure that it will not suffer great harm from the cooling substances. *De methodo [medendi]* 7.[114]

The stomach and liver need astringent substances [when superfluities stream into them] more than the other organs of the body, for these two organs are extremely eminent and important and each one of them
30   should—also in case of illness—carry out its specific function perfectly. *De methodo [medendi]* 11.[115]

64. Remedies that are applied to the liver should combine—according to what is needed—astringent ingredients with attenuating ones so that their astringency is like that of aromatic substances. The
35   best is when a remedy [for the liver] combines these two properties[116] so that it is both astringent and aromatic. *De arte parva.*[117]

استحكام اليبس الذي لا بروء له هو أن لا يكون نفس جوهر الأعضاء الأصلية قد
يبس، وكلّما كانت مرتبة اليبس أقرب من هذه كان بروءها أعسر وأطول، ولو أوّل مراتب
اليبس فإنّ ترطيبه عسر نكد مفتقر لطول الزمان. سابعة الحيلة.

٦٢. مراتب اليبس أربع: أوّلها وهو أسهلها بروء هو حدوث اليبس في العروق
الصغار الخاصّة بكل عضو وعضو الذي من فوهاتها تغتذي الأعضاء. والمرتبة الثانية هو
أن ينتهي اليبس الى فناء الرطوبة المبثوثة في أعضاء البدن بمنزلة الرذاذ. وهي التي من
شأنها أن تخرج من فواهات تلك العروق الدقيقة، وهي المشاكلة للعضو لغذائه. والمرتبة
الثالثة هي أن ينتهي اليبس إلى فناء رطوبة الأعضاء التي هي من جوهر رطب قريب
الانعقاد والجمود بمنزلة الشحم واللحم إذا ذابا وإنحلا. والمرتبة الرابعة هي أن تيبس وتجفّ
الأعضاء الأصلية بمنزلة جرم القلب والكبد وغيرهما. سابعة الحيلة.

٦٣. المزاج الذي قد خرج عن اعتداله إلى البرودة فأبت في إسخانه حتّى يرجع الى
الاعتدال على أمن عاقبة ووثاقة. وأمّا تبريد ما يسخن فليس الأمر فيه كذلك، بل افعل
ذلك بتوقّ وحذر ولا تجترئ. وإن لم يكن جميع ما حول العضو الذي تريد تبريده قويا لم
يؤمن عليه أن يناله من الأشياء الباردة مضرّة عظيمة. سابعة الحيلة.

المعدة والكبد أحوج من سائر الأعضاء إلى أشياء قابضة، فإنّ هذين العضوين في
غاية الشرف وجلالة الخطر. وينبغي أن يفعل كلّ واحد منهما فعله الخاصّ به على التمام
في حال المرض أيضا. حادية عشر الحيلة.

٦٤. الأدوية التي توضع على الكبد بحسب ما يحتاج ينبغي أن لا تخلو من قبض
يكون معه لطافة ليصل قبضه مثل الأشياء العطرة. والأجود أن يكون قد جمع هاتين القوتين
حتّى يكون قابضا عطرا. في الصناعة الصغيرة.

---

65. Quotidian fever hardly ever occurs without a stomach illness, just as quartan fever hardly ever occurs without an illness in the spleen. *Ad Glauconem [de medendi methodo]* 1.[118]

66. A compound remedy made up of many simple drugs is not more beneficial for every illness than one of the simple drugs it is compounded of; rather, the simple drug alone may be more beneficial for a particular illness. The intention of making a compound remedy is to have one single medication beneficial for many [individual] illnesses, each of which needs a simple remedy, although the benefits of such a compound drug are limited. *Mayāmir* 8.[119]

67. The application of a moist, hot compress is beneficial for tumors arising from bile, and the application of a dry, hot compress is beneficial for tumors arising from fine, watery blood. The application of a hot compress that holds the middle [between moisture and dryness], namely one that comes into contact with a moderately warm body, is beneficial for biting humors. The application of a biting, hot compress is good for thick, viscous humors in that it dilutes and cuts them. *In Hippocratis De acutorum morborum [victu et] Galeni commentarius* 2.[120]

68. It is only very rarely that one will see the illness of diabetes occur, for I have only seen it twice until now. *De locis affectis* 6.[121]

69. Says Moses: I too have not seen it in the Maghreb,[122] nor did any one of the elders under whom I studied inform me that he had seen it. However, here in Egypt I have seen more than twenty people affected by this disease in approximately ten years. This is to show you that this disease occurs mostly in hot countries. Perhaps the water of the Nile, because of its sweetness, plays a role in this.[123]

٦٥. إنّ الحمّى النائبة كلّ يوم فليس تكاد أن تحدث إلا مع علّة في المعدة، كما أنّ الربع ليس يكاد أن تحدث إلا مع علّة في الطحال. في الأولى من أغلوقن.

٦٦. الدواء المركّب من مفردات كثيرة ليست منفعته بليغة في كلّ علّة ينفع منها أحد تلك المفردات. بل ذلك المفرد وحده أنفع لتلك العلّة. وإنّما قصد بالتركيب في هذا الغرض ليكون دواء واحد ينفع من علل كثيرة يحتاج كلّ واحد منها لدواء مفرد وإن كانت منافعه مقصّرة. ثامنة الميامر.

٦٧. التكميد الرطب يستنفع به في الأورام الحادثة من المرار، والتكميد اليابس يستنفع به في الأورام الحادثة من الدم الرقيق المائي، والتكميد المعتدل وهو الكائن بملاقاة جسم حارّ باعتدال يستنفع به في الأخلاط اللذّاعة، والتكميد اللذّاع يستنفع به في الأخلاط الغليظة اللزجة إذ كان يلطّف ويقطع. في شرحه لثانية الأمراض الحادّة.

٦٨. علّة ديابيطس قلّ ما تراها تحدث إلا في الندرة. فإنّي أنا إلى هذا الوقت لم أرها إلا مرّتين فقط. في سادسة التعرّف.

٦٩. قال موسى: وكذلك لم أرها أنا في المغرب ولا حدّثني أحد من الشيوخ الذين قرأت عليهم أنّه راءها. لكنّي هنا بمصر رأيت من أصابتهم هذه العلّة في نحو العشر سنين أكثر من عشرين رجلا. فهذا يدلّك أنّ هذا المرض أكثر ما يتولّد في البلاد الحارّة. ولعلّ لماء النيل للذّته في ذلك أثر.

١ إنّ] ELP : om. O | النائبة] أمّا | في EEs²LOP add. ‖ ٢ في] (1st) ELOP om. ‖ ٤–٥ بالتركيب في هذا الغرض] في هذا التركيب L ‖ ٥ واحد] (2nd) علّة ELP ‖ ٦ ثامنة] ثانية EsG ‖ ٩–١٠ اللذّاعة . . . الأخلاط] om. L ‖ ١٢ فقط] om. EL ‖ ١٣ وكذلك لم أرها أنا] وكذلك أنا لم أرها ELOP ‖ ١٤ أنّه راءها] أنّهم راوها EsG | من] ممّن ELOP | هذه] تلك EL

70. The time of the morning can be compared to spring and the time that comes after it can be compared to summer. The time of the evening is similar to autumn and the nighttime resembles winter. Just as diseases are most severe and lethal in autumn, so their attacks are most severe in the evening. *In Hippocratis Epidemiarum* 2.1.[124]

71. The best wind is the one that blows from the high sea; the next best is the one that blows from the mountains; the worst is the one that blows from marshes or swamps or morasses. Intermediate between these is the wind that blows from other [directions]. *In Hippocratis De humoribus commentarius* 3.[125]

72. The eye and the cardia of the stomach: these two parts of the body cannot tolerate anything put on then and burdening them. The eye can tolerate this so much less than the stomach that we see it [already] irritated[126] by a medication put on it as a salve. *Ad Glauconem [de medendi methodo]* 2.[127]

73. Dissolution and dilution are in most cases a very successful treatment for any chronic disease. *Ad Glauconem [de medendi methodo]* 2.[128]

74. The first thing to take care of in the beginning of treatment is to expel that which dissolves and destroys the strength [of the body]. *De methodo [medendi]* 7.[129]

75. When the Greeks were in doubt about a disease, they left it to nature [to expel it].[130] They said: Nature knows the temperament of the organs, and sends to every organ the appropriate kind of food and looks after the health of living beings and treats them in the case of disease. *De clysteribus.*[131]

٧٠ . وقت الغداة يشــبـه للربيع والوقت الذي بعده يشبه للصيف ووقت العشاء شبيه
بالخريف ووقت الليل شـبـيـه بالشـتـاء ، فكما أحدّ ما تكون الأمراض وأقتلها في الخريف
كذلك أحدّ ما تكون نوائبها بالعشاء . في الأولى من شرحه لثانية ابيديميا .

٧١ . أفضــل الريـــاح ما يهبّ من لجج البحر ، وأقربـها إلى أفضلها مـا يهبّ من
الجبــال ، وأردأها ما يهبّ من غياض أو آجام أو وقائع، والمتوسّــطة منها ما يهبّ من غير
ذلك . في شرحه لثالثة الأخلاط .

٧٢ . العين وفم المعدة لا تحتمل هذان العضوان شيئًا يوضع عليهما ممّا يثقلهما . والعين أقلّ
احتمالا لذلك من المعدة حتّى أنّا رأيناها تستقل ما يطلى عليها من الأدوية . ثانية أغلوقن .

٧٣ . التحليــل والتقطيــع علاج منجح بالغ فـي كلّ علّة تطول علـى الأمر الأكثر .
ثانية أغلوقن .

٧٤ . أوّل شـــيء ينبغي أن يعنى به ويبتدأ بأمره في حال العلاج هو دفع الشيء الذي
يحلّ القوّة ويهدّها . سابعة الحيلة .

٧٥ . اليونانيون إذا أشــكل عليهم علاج المرض خلّوا بين الطبيعة وبينه وقالوا الطبيعة
تعلم مزاج الأعضاء وترسل إلى كلّ عضو ما يلائمه من الغذاء وهي القيّمة على الحيوان في
صحّته والمعالجة له في سقمه . في مقالته في الحقن .

---

١ للربيــع] الربيع ELOP | للصيـف] بالصيـف ELOP || ٢ الليــل] الليـل ¹G | فكما] أنّ
add. ELOP || ٣ ابيديميا] افيديميا ELP || ٦ لثالثة] الثالثة G || ٧ العضوان]
¹G || ٨ رأيناها] رأينـاه L || ١٣ اليونانيون] اليونانيـن EsG : اليونانين؟OOx | وقالوا]
¹G || ١٤ تعلم] تعني L | الحيوان] ¹G

76. Ibn Zuhr said: Every substance you want to use for cleansing the body, whether externally or internally, should be lukewarm. Every repelling or restraining substance should be cold, such as spring water. Every substance that opens should be hot and every substance that dissolves should be slightly warmer than [that used for] cleansing. When you want to alleviate internal or external pain, you should administer the remedy while it is lukewarm. But when you are afraid of syncope, you should give the medication with cold water.

77. Ibn Zuhr said: It has been proved by experiment that every astringent [substance] has some purgative effect, except for myrtle,[132] which has no purgative force at all. And every purgative has some sort of astringent quality.

*This is the end of the eighth treatise,*
*by the grace of God, praise be to Him.*

◆

٧٦ . قال بن زهر : كلّ ما تريد به الجلاء حملته على البدن أو ســقيته فليكن فاترا .
وكلّ دافع أو رادع فبارد مثل ماء الآبار . وكلّ مفتّح فسخن والمحلّل أسخن من الجلاء قليلا .
ومتى أردت تسكين وجع من داخل أو خارج فاستعمل الدواء فاترا . ومتى خشيت غشيا
فاسق أدويتك بماء بارد .

٥

٧٧ . قــال بن زهر : صحّ بالامتحان أنّ كلّ قابض فيه ما يسـهل إلا الآس فإنّه لا قوّة
مسهلة فيه أصلا . وكلّ مسهل ففيه ما يمسك قبضا .
تمّت المقالة الثامنة وللّه الحمد والمنّة .

---

١ رادع] ردّاع L ‖ ٣ أردت] رمـت ELOOxP ‖ ٤ فاسـق] فاسـقو G : فاسـقي
EsOOx?P ‖ ٥ بن] ابن G ‖ ٦ مسـهلة فيـه] inv. EsG ‖ ٧ تمّت . . . والمنّة] كملت
المقالــة الثامنة والحمد لله وعدد فصولها ثمانــون فصلا EL : كملت المقالة الثامنة الحمد لـ< . . . >
بالعقل وعدد فصولها ثمانون Ox : كملت المقالة الثامنة عدد فصولها ثمانين P

# The Ninth Treatise

5          *Containing aphorisms concerning specific diseases*

1. The humors that produce epilepsy are thick, cold, and viscous. Their improvement consists in the transformation of the [temperament of the young in] age from moisture into dryness, and in exercise, and a drying regimen together with evacuation by means of medications. *In*
10    *Hippocratis Aphorismos commentarius* 2.[1]

2. In the case of a nosebleed you should not wait for the strength [of the body] to collapse. Rather, if you see the blood streaming rapidly, you should bleed the vein at the inner side of the arm[2] on the same side as the hemorrhage, then you should tie the extremities with linen ban-
15    dages, and then you should apply a cupping glass to the hypochondria on the side opposite to[3] the nostril from which the blood flows. I have done all this and as a result the flowing of the blood stopped. As for the medications that are put into the nose or on the forehead as prescribed by the physicians,[4] we have tried them and found all of them to be weak.
20    *De venae sectione.*[5]

بسم الله الرحمن الرحيم ربّ يسّر

# المقالة التاسعة

تشتمل على فصول تتعلّق بأمراض مخصوصة

١ . الأخــلاط المولّــدة للصرع هــي غليظة بــاردة بلغمية وصلاحها يكـون بانتقال
السـن عن الرطوبة إلــى اليبس والرياضة والتدبير المجفّف مع الاسـتفراغ بالأدوية .
في شرحه لثانية الفصول .

٢ . لا تنتظر بالرعاف سقوط القوّة . بل إذا رأيت الدم يجري بحفز فافصد من مأبض
اليد من جهة السـيلان، ثمّ تشـدّ الأطراف بلفائف كتّان، ثمّ ضع المحجمة على ما دون
الشراسيف على محاذاة المنخر الذي يجري منه الدم . فجميع هذا عملناه فانقطع الدم الذي
كان يجري . فأمّا الأدوية التي توضع في الأنف أو تطلى على الجبهة ممّا رسمه الأطبّاء فقد
جرّبناها ووجدناها كلّها ضعيفة . في مقالته في الفصد .

---

١ بسم . . . يسّر] om. ELOP : بسم الله الرحمن الرحيم Ox ‖ ٩ محاذاة] محاداة
O ‖ ١٠ الأطبّاء] قدماء الأطبّاء ELOOxP

3. If someone's superfluities from the brain are usually evacuated through a discharge from the ear and if this suddenly stops and vertigo and dizziness occur to him, we observe that if we stimulate that evacuation and provoke it to the ears through opening medications, such a
5      patient immediately benefits therefrom. *In Hippocratis Epidemiarum* 6.2.[6]

4. People who suffer from severe pains caused by thick blood or internal cold, such as migraine and the like, clearly benefit from drinking pure wine either immediately after the meal or during the meal. Their pains are alleviated by the heating and diluting effect of the wine. Similarly,
10     one should soak bread or *sawīq*[7] in the pure wine because, by mixing the pure wine with food, one is protected from a hot vapor arising from it and harming the painful site. Rather, an even heat arises from it in all the parts of the painful organ. This heat then increases [in these parts] without vapor and dissolves the obstruction through the dilution of the
15     humors that got stuck. A long sleep follows and the parts that surround the painful organ become lighter; their pores widen, and that which causes the pain is dissolved. [For] it is in the nature of these things to occur as the result of an even heat. *In Hippocratis Epidemiarum* 6.6.[8]

5. If a nosebleed becomes excessive and does not stop with the appli-
20     cation of a cupping glass on the hypochondria, one should put a cupping glass on the nape of the neck and use something to cool the head. *In Hippocratis Epidemiarum* 6.7.[9]

6. If the mucous discharge from the nose is watery and uncocted, we stop it with things with which we foment the head in order to heat the
25     brain, and with those things that are inhaled through the nose, and with those things that are dripped into the ears. *In Hippocratis De humoribus commentarius* 1.[10]

7. All those suffering from defluxions are adversely affected in the beginning of their occurrence by sneezing because at that moment the
30     humors are raw and congested. Also, the heavy movement [of sneezing] increases the fullness of the head. Especially at that moment, the [various] parts of the head and chest need rest, tranquility, and moderate

٣ . من جرت عادته أن تستفرغ فضول دماغه بشيء يسيل من أذنه ، ثمّ انقطع ذلك دفعة وحدث به سدر ودوار فإنّا إذا هيّجنا ذلك الاستفراغ واستدعيناه إلى الأذنين بالأدوية المفتّحة رأينا صاحب تلك الحال ينتفع بذلك على المكان . في الثانية من شرحه لسادسة ابيديميا .

٤ . القوم الذين يجدون آلاما شديدة كالشقيقة ونحوها من غلظ دم أو عن برد في الباطن ينفعهم شرب الخمر الصرف بعقب الطعام أو مع الطعام منفعة بيّنة ، وتسكّن آلامهم بتسخين الخمر وتلطيفها . وكذلك انفع لهم خبزا أو سويقا في الخمر الصرف لأنّ باختلاط الخمر الصرف بالطعام تأمن أن يرتفع عنها بخار حارّ يضرّ الموضع الآلم ، وتحدث عنه سخونة مستوية في جميع أجزاء العضو الآلم . وتتزيّد تلك السخونة من غير بخار ويتحلّل السدد بتلطيف الأخلاط التي قد لحجت ويحدث النوم الطويل وتستخفّ الأعضاء المحيطة بالعضو الآلم وتتّسع مسامّها ويتحلّل منها ما يؤلّها لأنّ هذه الأشياء من شأنها أن تحدث عن الإسخان المستوي . في السادسة من شرحه لسادسة ابيديميا .

٥ . إذا أسرف الرعاف ولم ينقطع بتعليق المحجمة على ما دون الشراسيف فينبغي أن تعلق المحجمة على القفاء مع استعمال ما يبرد به الرأس . في السابعة من شرحه لسادسة ابيديميا .

٦ . متى كان المخاط مائيا غير نضيج فحسمنا له يكون بالأشياء التي تنطل على الرأس كيما تسخن الدماغ وبالأشياء التي تستنشق والتي تصبّ في الأذن . في الأولى من شرح الأخلاط .

٧ . جميع أصحاب النزلات يتأذّون في ابتداء حدوثها بالعطاس لأنّ الأخلاط حينئذ نيّة محتقنة ، وكذلك الحركة العنيفة يزداد بها امتلاء الرأس . وإنّما تحتاج أعضاء الرأس والصدر

---

٢ دفعة] واحدة ELOOxP add. ‖ ٤ ابيديميا] افيديميا ELOxP ‖ ٥ آلاما شديدة] ألما شديدا L ‖ ١٠ وتستخفّ] وتسكّن ELOOx : وتسخفّ P ‖ ١٢ ابيديميا] افيديميا ELOxP ‖ ١٤ ابيديميا] افيديميا ELP ‖ ٦٠،١٨ – ٦٤،١ محتقنة . . . ونحوهما] om. Ox

heat so that those raw humors are cocted. When a defluxion occurs [after such a period of rest], the humors are—because they have been cocted—dissolved and evacuated through sneezing. *In Hippocratis De humoribus commentarius* 1.[11]

5      8. The sparks that a person sees before his eyes result from humors whose consistency and color are contrary to the albuminoid humor that gathers between the crystalline humor and the hornlike [tunic]. *In Hippocratis De humoribus commentarius* 1.[12]

       9. Headaches are alleviated by bandaging[13] the head when the
10     humors that effect the headache need moderate heating. *In Hippocratis De humoribus commentarius* 1.[14]

       Sneezing is especially beneficial in the case of watery humors, but it is harmful in the case of bilious humors because it stimulates and increases them. *In Hippocratis De humoribus commentarius* 1.[15]

15     10. The treatment of sleeplessness [consists of] binding the hands and legs at the time when he [who suffers from it] usually goes to sleep, preventing him from sleeping, and making him open his eyes when he closes them[16] until he is languid and tired. Then the ligatures are loosened, the lamp is removed, and all sudden movements and speaking are
20     stopped, for then he will have a wholesome, deep sleep. *In Hippocratis De humoribus commentarius* 2.[17]

       11. If a person is overcome by a torpor, one should grasp the tip of the tongue and press it completely down. Then one should look for a receptacle with a narrow opening, and put some [moist] liquid food into
25     it, and put it into the mouth on the base [of the tongue], and pour the contents into the esophagus. *De motibus [manifestis et] obscuris.*[18]

حينئذٍ إلى الراحة والسكون والإسخان المعتدل لتنضج تلك الأخلاط النيّة . فإذا انحطّت النزلة
انحلّت بالعطاس لأنّ الأخلاط قد نضجت وتستفرغ بالعطاس . في شرحه لأولى الأخلاط .

٨ . اللمع الذي يراه الإنسان قدّام عينيه هو من أخلاط قوامها ولونها مخالف للرطوبة
البيضية تجتمع بين الجليدية والقرنية . في الأولى من الأخلاط .

٩ . أوجاع الرأس تنتفع بضغط الرأس متى كانت الأخلاط الفاعلة لوجع الرأس تحتاج
إلى إسخان معتدل . في الأولى من الأخلاط .

العطاس إنّما ينفع في الأخلاط المائية ويضرّ في الأخلاط المرارية ويهيّجها ويزيد
فيها . في الأولى من الأخلاط .

١٠ . علاج السهر شدّ اليدين والرجلين في الوقت الذي جرت العادة فيه أن ينام . ومنع
النوم وتغميض العين ويضطرّ العليل إلى فتحها حتّى إذا استرخى وتعب حلّت الرباطات
ورفعت السراج وقطعت الحركات والكلام بغتة ، فإنّه عند ذلك ينام نوما طيّبا مستغرقا .
في الثانية من شرح الأخلاط .

١١ . الناس إذا أصابهم السبات فإنّما تضبط طرف اللسان وتغمزه كلّه إلى الأسفل
وتعمد إلى إناء ضيق الفم فتجعل فيه بعض الأغذية الرطبة السيّالة . ثمّ توجره على أصل
فتصبّ ما في الإناء إلى المريء . في مقالته في الحركات المعتاصة .

---

١ تلك] بذلك ELOxP ‖ ٢ قد] om. G : Es² ‖ ٤ البيضية] البيضا L ‖ ١١ مستغرقا]
مستقرا G ‖ ١٣–١٥ الناس . . . المريء] فقد رأيت بعض البياطرة وهو يريد أن يصبّ في المريء
بعض ما توجره الدوابّ قد ضبط اللسان مع اللحي الأسفل ضبطا شديدا حتّى لا يتحرّك . فأذكرني ذلك
بما يوجره الناس إذا أصابهم السبات . وإنّا بحلق أيضا نعمد إلى إناء ضيّق فنجعل فيه بعض الأغذية الرطبة
السيّالة ثمّ نجوّزه أصل اللسان فنصبّ ما فيه إلى المريء Galen, Fī al-ḥarakāt ‖ ١٣–١٥ فإنّما
تضبط . . . وتغمزه . . . وتعمد . . . فتجعل . . . تؤخّره . . . فتصبّ] فإنّا نضبط . . .
ونغمزه . . . ونعمد . . . فنجعل . . . نوجره . . . فنصبّ ELO ‖ ١٤ الأغذية الرطبة السيّالة]
الأدوية الرطبة اليابسة Es G ‖ ١٥ إلى] في ELO : Es²

12. It sometimes happens to a person that he lies on his back[19] the entire night and that [when he arises in the morning] he is overtaken by a stroke, torpor,[20] or an epileptic fit, since the ventricles of his brain are filled with those superfluities. *De instrumentu odoratus.*[21]

13. For the treatment of a child suffering from epilepsy, after I cleansed his body, I often contented myself with a potion of vinegar and honey until I had completely healed him. There was no need for anything else but for this potion. *Puero epileptico [consilium].*[22]

14. If there is a nosebleed[23] from one of the nostrils and one puts cupping glasses [one at a time] on the liver or spleen on the same side as the bleeding nostril, the nosebleed stops. If the nosebleed is from both nostrils and is very severe, one should put cupping glasses on both spots at the same time. *Ad Glauconem [de medendi methodo]* 1.[24]

15. All the afflictions and diseases that occur to the leading activities[25] but do not include swellings [in the corresponding organs] originate from a bad temperament of the brain. [Such] a bad temperament sometimes occurs in the ventricles of the brain and sometimes in the pulsatile and nonpulsatile vessels that are scattered throughout them. Sometimes it occurs in the fluid that diffuses in the substance of the brain itself, or [sometimes] the temperament of the substance of the brain itself is corrupted. To find out which kind of bad temperament one is dealing with is not an easy job, but it is one for which a physician should love to exert himself. *De locis affectis* 3.[26]

16. Melancholic delusion occurs from the fact that all the blood in the vessels is melancholic, and the harm done to the brain is comparable to the general harm.[27] But the change in the blood can also be in the brain alone, either because a melancholic humor poured into it or because it developed in [the brain] as a result of the heat there, which roasts and burns the yellow bile or the thick blood. If the melancholic blood is common to the whole body, begin with phlebotomy, and if it is in the brain only, take care of the brain alone. *De locis affectis* 3.[28]

١٢ . ربّـما اتّفـق للإنسـان أن يكـون مسـتلقيا على قفـاه ليلته أجمـع ، فيسـبق حينئـذ إليه حدوث السكتة والإغمـاء والصرع عند امتـلاء بطون الدمـاغ من تلك الفضول . في مقالته في آلة الشمّ .

١٣ . وقد اكتفيت مرارا كثيرة بشراب الخلّ والعسل في علاج صبي كان يصرع حتّى أبرأته بروءا تامّا بعد أن أنقيت البدن من غير حاجة إلى شـيء آخر خلاء هذا الشراب . في مقالته في صبي يصرع .

١٤ . متى كان الاسـتفراغ من أحد المنخرين فوضعت المحاجم على الكبد والطحال بحسـب المنخر الذي يجري منه الدم انقطع الرعاف . ومتى كان من المنخرين غزيرا كثيرا فضع المحاجم على الموضعين جميعا . في الأولى من أغلوقن .

١٥ . جميـع مـا يحدث من الآفات والعلل في الأفعال السياسـية مـن غير ورم إنّما حدوثه من سـوء مزاج الدماغ . وسـوء المزاج مرّة يكون في بطون الدماغ ومرّة يكون في العروق الضـوارب وغير الضوارب المتفرّقة في جميعه . ومـرّة يكون في الرطوبة المبثوثة فـي نفـس جرمه أو يكون جرم الدماغ نفسـه يفسـد مزاجه . وأمّا الوقوف على ذلك السـوء مـزاج من أيّ نوع هو فليس ذلك بعمل صغير وهـو الذي ينبغي للطبيب أن يكون محبّا للتعب فيه . ثالثة التعرّف .

١٦ . الوسواس السوداوي قد يكون من قبل أنّ جميع ما في العروق من الدم سوداويا ويكـون ضـرر الدماغ من طريق الضرر العامّ . وقد يكون التغيّـر في الدم الذي في الدماغ وحده إمّا بأنّ خلطا سوداويا انصبّ إليه أو حدث فيه من أجل حرارة هناك تشيّط وتحرق المرّة الصفراء أو الدم الغليظ . فإن كان الدم السوداوي عامّا للبدن كلّه فابدأ بفصد العرق ، وإن كان ذلك خاصّا بالدماغ فتعنى بالدماغ وحده . ثالثة التعرّف .

---

٥ أنقيت] نقيت ELOP ‖ ١٢ المتفرّقة] المفرّقة L ‖ ١٧–١٨ ويكون . . . سـوداويا] المتفرّقة في (1st) Es ‖ ١٩ فابدأ] فابتدئ ELO ‖ من Es ‖ في (1st) | om. EL

17. The cold brain humor, namely lethargy, and the hot one, namely phrenitis, have in common that in the beginning both should be treated by phlebotomy and by the application of rose oil and vinegar in order to expel the harming humor—whatever humor it is—from the head. [This should be done] although one disease goes with sleeplessness and the other with torpor. Hereafter one should try to calm [the person suffering from] sleeplessness and to awaken and stimulate the person who suffers from torpor. *De methodo [medendi]* 13.[29]

18. When a brain tumor reaches its culmination, one should rub the head of the person whose illness is accompanied by sleeplessness and delirium with a salve prepared from poppy,[30] while the corner of the nostrils and face should be rubbed with substances that cool the brain. If someone's illness is accompanied by torpor, one should heat the thick humor. *De methodo [medendi]* 13.[31]

19. If either of these two diseases, namely lethargy or phrenitis, become chronic, we apply cupping glasses and castoreum for their treatment, because they coct both illnesses. When both are in a state of decline, their treatment should [also] be one and the same. *De methodo [medendi]* 13.[32]

20. When the lethargy stops getting worse,[33] smear strong and sharp medications on the palate and then apply those drugs that stimulate sneezing, and put similar drugs on the head, even mustard. *De methodo [medendi]* 13.[34]

21. When someone suffers from a headache caused by inebriety, he should try to sleep and rest for the entire day; in the evening he should enter the bathhouse and feed himself with foods that produce good blood and do not heat, such as barley groats. One should let him eat lettuce,[35] because it produces beneficial blood and has a cooling effect,[36] and cabbage,[37] because it eliminates and dries the vapors. From the pulses [he should eat] lentils,[38] and for a drink he should take water, and when his stomach becomes lax[39] because of the water he should suck

١٧ . يعـمّ ورم الدماغ البارد وهو لثيرغـس وورم الدماغ الحارّ وهو فرانيطس أنّ في أوّل الأمر تقصد و تستعمل دهن الورد والخلّ ليدفع عن الرأس الخلط المؤذّي أيّ خلط كان وعلى أنّ مع أحد المرضين السهر ومع الآخر السبات . ثمّ تروم تسكين السهر وهدوءه وتنبيه صاحب السبات وتحريكه . ثالثة عشر الحيلة .

١٨ . عند منتهى ورم الدماغ من كانت علّته مع سـهر واختـلاط تصبّ على رأسـه لطوخ الحشـحاش وتلطخ طرف منخريه ووجهه بما يبرّد الدماغ . من كانت علّته مع سبات فتسخن الخلط الغليظ . ثالثة عشر الحيلة .

١٩ . إذا طالت كلّ واحدة من هاتين العلّتين أعني ليثرغس وفرانيطس اسـتعملنا في علاجهما المحاجم والجندبادسـتر فإنّه ينضج هاتين العلّتـين . وإذا صارتا جميعا في حدّ الانحطاط صارت مداواتهما واحدة مشتركة . ثالثة عشر الحيلة .

٢٠ . ليثرغـس إذا تمّ تزيّـده لك أن تطلي الحنك بأدوية قوية حرّيفة واسـتعمل بعد ذلـك الأدويـة ألتي تهيج العطـاس وتضع على الرأس أدوية شـبيهة بهذه حتّـى إنّا نضع عليه الخردل . ثالثة عشر الحيلة .

٢١ . الصـداع العارض عن السـكر يلزم صاحبه بالنوم والهدوء فـي النهار أجمع ، ويدخل بالعشي إلى الحمّام ويغتذي بأغذية تولد دما جيّدا ولا تسخن مثل كشك الشعير . وتطعمـه الخسّ لأنّـه يولد دما محمودا ويطفئ ويطعم الكرنب أيضا لأنّه يفني البخارات ويجفّفها . ومن الحبوب العدس وشـرابه الماء فإن ارتخـت معدته من الماء فليمصّ الرمّان

pomegranate[40] and quince[41] and the like. The next day he should enter
the bathhouse and pour lots of hot water over his head in order to dissolve the vapors. [Just like] all the others suffering from a headache, he
should abstain from movement until the headache subsides, and then
5    he should move so that the rest [of the vapors] dissolve. *Mayāmir* 2.[42]

22. [For eye pain] one should apply to the eye a warm compress
with a sponge [dipped] in water in which melilot[43] and fenugreek[44] have
been cooked. When the pain is mild, apply the compress once or twice
a day, and when the pain is severe, apply it many times, especially dur-
10    ing the long [summer] days. *Mayāmir* 4.[45]

23. Epilepsy and torpor[46] only originate from the brain. A torpor
amongst the voluntary activities is comparable to a deep sleep amongst
the sensory activities, while an epileptic spasm amongst the voluntary
activities is like sleeplessness amongst the sensory activities. *De [morbo-
15    rum] causis et symptomatibus* 4.[47]

24. Says Moses: What he means is that both a torpor and a deep
sleep are a lack of activity, while an epileptic spasm and sleeplessness are
a disturbance.[48]

25. A severe headache occurs from heat or cold. The headache
20    caused by dryness is weak. Moisture does not cause any pain at all. A
surplus of humors in the head causes heaviness but not a headache,
except when an obstruction occurs from it. For then a headache occurs
that is proportional to the degree of obstruction. *Mayāmir* 2.[49]

26. Every substance used for treating the ears should be [moderately]
25    lukewarm; for this we use breast milk or egg white on its own. Amongst
the medications for alleviating ear pains caused by biting matters [are
such] as we apply for eye pain. *Mayāmir* 3.[50]

والسـفرجل ونحوهما . ويدخل من الغدّ الحمّام ويصبّ على رأسه ماء حارّا كثيرا لتتحلّل
الأخرة . وسـائر من يصيبه الصداع يمسـك عن الحركة حتّى يأخذ الصداع في الانحطاط
فإنّه يتحرّك حتّى يتحلّل ما بقي . ثانية الميامر .

٢٢ . ينبغي أن تكمّد العين بالأسـفنج بماء قد طبخ فيه إكليل الملك وحلبة . وإن كان
الوجع خفيفا فكمّدها مرّة أو مرّتين في اليوم . وإن كان الوجع شـديدا فتكمّدها مرارا كثيرة
وبخاصّة في الأيّام الطويلة . أربعة الميامر .

٢٣ . الصرع والسـبات إنّما يكونان من الدماغ . والسـبات منزلته من الأفعال الإرادية
بمنزلة النوم المسـتغرق من الأفعال الحسّية . ومنزلة تشنّج الصرع من الأفعال الإرادية بمنزلة
الأرق من الأفعال الحسّية . رابعة العلل والأعراض .

٢٤ . قـال موسـى يعنـي أنّ السـبات والنـوم المسـتغرق عـدم فعل وتشـنّج
الصرع والأرق جريان منكر .

٢٥ . الصداع الشـديد يعرض من الحـرارة والبرودة . أمّا الصداع العارض من قبل
اليبوسـة فهو ضعيـف . فأمّا الرطوبة فليس يعرض منها وجع البتّة ، وأمّا كثرة الأخلاط
فـي الـرأس فتحدث ثقـلا لا صداعـا إلا أن حدث عنها سـدد . فإنّ الصداع يكون
بحسب مقدار السدّة . ثانية الميامر .

٢٦ . ينبغي أن يكون كلّ شيء يعالج به الأذن مفتّرا تفتيرا معتدلا ونحن نستعمل ألبان
النساء وبياض البيض مفردة . ومع الأدوية في تسكين أوجاع الأذن الحادثة عن موّاد لذّاعة
كما نستعملها في وجع العين . ثالثة الميامر .

---

١ ونحوهمـا [ Es² : أو أحدهما [ EsG || ٤ فيه [ G¹ || ٥ فكمّدها [ فتكمّدها : EOOxP
فتكمّد L || ٧ الصرع [ الصداع E O || ١٤ حدث [ حدثت ELOOxP

27. I know from experience that the hole of the ear should not be touched at all with anything at the time of pain. Rather, one should trickle drops into it that are as warm as can be tolerated. One should suspend one's hand in the air until the medicine flows from the end of the probe to the inner hole of the ear. One should do this repeatedly and not stop until the hole of the ear is filled. Then one should wipe off that which streams out of it very gently without touching the ear itself or any of its parts. This is a very important matter one should be very careful about when one treats the ear in the case of pain. *Mayāmir* 3.[51]

28. The remedies with which the inside of the nose is treated are rapidly washed out because of the moisture streaming from the nose. Therefore, one should persist in its treatment with these remedies in the same way one persists in treating the eye. *Mayāmir* 3.[52]

29. Any warm compress applied to the teeth either outside or inside the mouth should be applied before having a meal, on an empty stomach, or after a long time following a meal. *Mayāmir* 5.[53]

30. Al-Tamīmī[54] said: Chinese snow,[55] which is a white, round, lustrous stone, Indian tutty,[56] cadmia,[57] glass slag,[58] glass of Pharaoh,[59] excrement of lizards, shells of turtledove eggs and musk—if one calculates the [proper] amounts of these remedies and then prepares an eye powder from them, the powder removes the white opacity of the eye[60] extremely well and cleanses it without irritation or harm.

31. Inhabitants of hot countries often suffer from ophthalmia but are rapidly cured. Inhabitants of cold countries rarely suffer from ophthalmia, but if they suffer from it, it is severe and hard whereby the eyes are ruptured. There is a similar analogy regarding ophthalmia occurring in the winter and that occurring in the summer. *In Hippocratis De aeris [aquis locis] commentarius* 1.[61]

٢٧ . قد علمت بالتجربة أنّه ليس ينبغي أن يمسّ ثقب الأذن في وقت الوجع بشيء بتّـة بل يقطّر فيه ما يقطّر وهو حارّ بقدر الاحتمال ويدك معلّقة والدواء يسـيل من طرف الميل حتّى يصل إلى الصماخ. تفعل ذلك مرارا لا تفتر حتّى يمتلئ ثقب الأذن وتمسح ما يفيض برفق عظيم من غير أن تمسّ الأذن ولا شـيء من أجزائها . فهذا باب عظيم يحترز
٥ منه عند علاج الأذن إذا كان فيها وجع . ثالثة الميامر .

٢٨ . الأدوية التي تعالج بها داخل الأنف تنغسل سريعا بسبب ما يجري من الأنف من الرطوبة ولهذا ينبغي لك أن تواظب عليها بالعلاج كما تواظب على العين بمداومة أدويتها . ثالثة الميامر .

٢٩ . كلّ تكميد تكمّد به الأسنان من خارج الفم أو من داخله ينبغي أن تستعمله قبل الطعام على الريق أو من بعد تناول الطعام بوقت طويل . خامسة الميامر .

١٠ ٣٠ . قال التميمي الثلج الصيني وهو حجر أبيض مدوّر بصّاص وتوتيا هندي وإقليميا ومسـحقونيا والزجاج الفرعوني وبعر الضبّ وقشر بيض اليمام ومسك، تدبّر مقادير هذه الأدوية وتّتخذ منها كحل فإنّه يقلع البياض قلعا قويا وتجلوه من غير لذع ولا أذى .

٣١ . أهل المدن الحارّة يرمدون منه كثيرا ويسـلمون منه سـريعا ، وأهل المدن الباردة قلّ ما يرمدون وإذا رمدوا كان رمدهم شديدا صعبا تتصدّع فيه العين وكذلك المقايسة بين
١٥ أرماد الشتاء والصيف . في شرحه للأولى من كتّاب الأهوية .

---

٣ الصماخ] السـماخ EsGOxP : السماع O ‖ ٤ تمسّ] تمسح EsG ‖ ٦–٧ الأدوية . . . الميامـر . ] G¹ ‖ ٩ الريـق] الرفق G ‖ ١٠ الثلج] البلـح L ‖ ١٣ أهل المدن الحارّة يرمدون] المـدن الحارّة يرمدون أهلها L : المدن الحارّة يرمدون E ‖ ١٣–١٥ أهل المدن . . . والصيف] قال جالينوس إنّ سـكان المدينة الأولى لمّا كانوا يرمدون ويسـلمون منه سـريعا فهؤلاء ضدّ أولئك لا يعرض لهم الرمد فمتى أصابهم تصدّعت أعينهم وإنّما قلّ الرمد فيهم لبرد بلادهم كما أنّه لا يعرض الرمد في الشتاء لكثير من الناس فإن عرض كان شديدا مؤلما . . . . 9–5v35 .C, fol

32. Angina is any illness of the throat whereby the patient has a feeling of narrowness during swallowing. The most deadly one of these is where the swelling or redness does not appear in the pharynx, but in the esophagus or larynx or in their muscles only. Sometimes angina originates from cold, viscous, raw humors. *In Hippocratis Epidemiarum* 2.2.[62]

33. When the swelling in the case of angina is severe, one should not be content with [applying] internal medications alone but should also [use] external ones. One should apply cataplasms, pour hot water over it and let the patient enter the bathhouse. However, this should only be done when the illness is abating. Angina patients should be fed with medicinal soups[63] so that, when the liquid passes the swollen places, it has the same effect as[64] a cataplasm. *In Hippocratis Epidemiarum* 2.6.[65]

34. Speech is a movement only occurring in the respiratory organs. Therefore, if someone is discharging blood from the larynx, the lungs, the chest, or the windpipe, he should not make a sound nor breathe heavily. To move his arms is not bad for him. Most appropriate for such a condition is a movement of the legs moderate enough that the pulse does not become frequent. *In Hippocratis De humoribus commentarius* 1.[66]

35. The plucking of hair attracts the humors from the depth of the body to its outside. Therefore, it is beneficial for someone who suffers from the disease of forgetfulness and torpor, or for someone in whose body a humor that is not sound streams from the outside of the body to one of his joints or ears. *In Hippocratis De humoribus commentarius* 1.[67]

36. Sometimes an irregular bad temperament occurs in the muscles of the chest followed by a mild cough, which is, as it were, a pain that provokes coughing, because the muscle trembles and shakes out of desire to expel the harmful substance. *De [morborum] causis et symptomatibus* 5.[68]

٣٢ . الذبحة كلّ علّة تحدث في الحلق فيحسّ صاحبها منها بضيق عند البلع ، وأقتلها
ما لا يظهر معه في الحلق ورم ولا حمرة بل يكون التورّم في المريء والحنجرة أو في عضلهما
فقط . وقد تكون الذبحة عن أخلاط باردة لزجة نيئة . في الثانية من شرحه لثانية ابيديميا .

٣٣ . إذا كان الـورم في الذبحة عظيما لا تقتصـر على الأدوية التي من داخل فقط
بل من خارج أيضا ، اضمدة وصبّ الماء المسخن والاستحمام ولا تستعمل ذلك إلا عند
انحطاط العلّة . وأغذية أصحاب الذبح أحساء دوائية حتّى إذا مرّت المواضع الوارمة تقوم
لها مقام الضماد . في سادسة شرحه لثانية ابيديميا .

٣٤ . الكلام حركة تخصّ آلات التنفّس ولذلك ليس ينبغي لمن ينبعث الدم من حنجرته
أو مـن رئته أو من صدره أو من قصبة رئته أن يكون منه صوت ولا تنفّس عظيم . وأمّا
تحريك اليدين فليس بردئ له ، وأحرى بذلك تحريك الرجلين حركة اعتدال حتّى لا يحدث
تواتر في النبض . في الأولى من شرح الأخلاط .

٣٥ . نتف الشـعر يجذب الأخلاط من عمق البدن إلى ظاهره فلذلك ينفع من به علّة
النسيان والسبات أو من ينصبّ من ظاهر بدنه إلى مفصل من المفاصل أو لأذنه خلط ليس
بمستحكم . في الأولى من الأخلاط .

٣٦ . قد يكون في عضل الصدر سـوء مزاج مختلف فيتبعه سعال يسير يكون كأنّه
مضض يدعو إلى السـعال لأنّ العضل يهتزّ ويرتعد تشـوّقا منه لدفع الشـيء الموذي له .
في خامسة العلل والأعراض .

٣ ابيديميا ] افيديميا ELP || ٤ لا ] لم LOx || ٥ المسخن ] السخن LOx || ٧ ابيديميا ]
افيديميا ELP || ٩ أو من صدره ] om. L || ٦٦,١٤ – ٦٨,١ الأولى من الأخلاط . . . من
om. Ox || ١٥ – ١٧ قد . . . والأعراض . ] G¹ . ] يكون ] حتّى G¹

37. Medications for the spitting of blood are composed of drugs that dry without biting, or drugs that are somewhat agglutinant, or astringent drugs. This is right for stopping the spitting of blood in general. But when the spitting of blood is from the lungs, chest, windpipe, or larynx, I mix these drugs with those that are hot and fine, even if they are maximally contrary to this illness. The objective of this is that they will lead those astringent drugs and bring them—while protecting them—[to the affected sites].[69] When the spitting of blood is from the region of the esophagus, stomach, abdomen, or intestines, there is no need to mix in these [hot and fine] drugs. *Mayāmir* 7.[70]

38. Sometimes the drugs for the spitting of blood should also be mixed with soporific ones in order to let those who suffer from it fall into a lethargic sleep.[71] This[72] is very beneficial for someone who is harmed and shaken by coughing. Moreover, because of their coldness, these drugs stop the blood and prevent it from streaming to the affected vessel. *Mayāmir* 7.[73]

39. The amelioration of bad humors in the case of those who say that their sputum tastes like seawater takes a long time. If someone is afflicted with an ulcer in the lungs because of these [bad humors], he cannot be healed at all. For in the long time that it takes for the humors to become better, the ulcer becomes so dried up and hard that it cannot be cured [anymore], or it becomes putrefied and then in turn causes putrefaction to the surrounding area until the entire lung has decayed. *De methodo medendi* 5.[74]

40. Sometimes hiccups occur from coldness of the air, for every coldness prevents dissolution [of humors], and for this reason an overfilling occurs in the nervous parts, which [then] causes hiccups. *In Hippocratis Aphorismos commentarius* 6.[75]

41. Especially in the case of stomach ailments, the amount [of food] that one takes should be extremely[76] moderate so that it does not become a burden to [the stomach]. The same holds true for liver [ailments]. *In Hippocratis Epidemiarum* 2.1.[77]

42. Distress originates from humors that are not as bad as those that produce syncope. Yawning comes from the relaxation of the muscles that move the jawbones so that the vapor can be dissolved. Wine mixed with an equal amount of water is beneficial for all these [cases]

٣٧. أدوية نفث الدم هي التي تؤلّف من أدوية تجفّف من غير لذع و أدوية فيه بعض إلزاق وأدوية قابضة. هذا هو القصد في قطع نفث الدم على العموم. أمّا إن كان نفث الدم من الرئة أو الصدر أو قصبة الرئة أو الحنجرة فأنا أخلط مع هذه الأدوية أدوية حارّة لطيفة وإن كانت في غاية المضادّة لهذه العلّة. القصد بذلك لتؤدّي تلك الأدوية القابضة وتوصلها وتبذرقها. فأمّا متى كان نفث الدم من ناحية المريء والمعدة والبطن والأمعاء فلا حاجة إلى خلط أمثال هذه الأدوية. سابعة الميامر.

٣٨. قد يخلط في أدوية نفث الدم أدوية مخدّرة أيضا لتنوّمهم نوما سباتيا لما في ذلك من عظم المنفعة لمن كان السعال يؤذيه ويقلقه ولتمنع ببرودتها مجيء الدم وتوقفه وتمنع جريته إلى العرق الذي به العلّة. سابعة الميامر.

٣٩. إصلاح الأخلاط الردئة وهم القوم الذين يقولون إنّ طعم ريقهم كطعم ماء البحر يحتاج إلى زمان طويل. ولذلك من أصابته من هؤلاء قرحة رئة فإنّه لا بروء له بتّة لأنّ بطول الزمان حتّى تصلح الأخلاط تجفّ القرحة وتصلب حتّى لا تقبل البروء أو تعفن وتعفن ما حولها حتّى تعفن الرئة بأسرها. في الخامسة من حيلة البرء.

٤٠. قد يعرض الفواق من برد الهواء إذ كلّ برودة تمنع التحلّل فيحدث بسبب ذلك امتلاء في الأجسام العصبية فيحدث الفواق. في شرحه لسادسة الفصول.

٤١. ينبغي في علل المعدة خاصّة أن يكون مقدار ما يتناول مقدارا معتدلا على استقصاء حتّى لا يثقل عليها وكذلك الكبد. في الأولى من شرحه لثالثة ابيديميا.

٤٢. الكرب يتولّد من أخلاط أقلّ رداءة من الأخلاط المولّدة للغشي. والتثاؤب يحدث من قبل استرخاء العضل الذي يحرّك اللحي لتحلّل البخار والخمر الممزوجة بمثلها ماء تنفع

---

٣ قصبة الرئة] القصبة L ‖ ٨ وتمنع] وتثغع EL ‖ ١٠ إصلاح] أصحاب L ‖ ١١ بتّة] البتّة EL ‖ ١٧ ابيديميا] افيديميا ELP ‖ ١٩ اللحي] اللحم G

because it balances the bad humors, heats the stomach, aids digestion, dissolves the cold vapor, and is good for shivering that originates from hot humors. But one should refrain from giving it as a drink in the case of shivering during which there is only a fever or an inflamed tumor. *In Hippocratis Epidemiarum* 2.6.[78]

43. I observed that people suffered from epileptic spasms that arose from the cardia of their stomachs when they suffered from severe indigestion, or when they drank wine that was too hot, or when they had too much sexual intercourse at the wrong time. I also saw patients with fever suffering from sudden spasms because of a bad humor that streamed to the cardia of the stomach and irritated it. When they vomited, they found immediate relief. Other persons, burdened by bad food they had eaten and then struck by torpor, only found relief when they had vomited all that which oppressed the cardia of their stomach. When the cardia of the stomach is affected, a sudden and rapid syncope may also arise from it. *De locis affectis* 5.[79]

44. A gassy[80] disease makes the patient suffering from it depressed, sad, hopeless, and despairing [of good]. In short, their condition is like that of those suffering from melancholic delusion because of the connection between the cardia of the stomach and the brain. Their afflictions become [even] more severe when they suffer from indigestion. Most of these patients suffer from an affection of the spleen, and this is one of the indications that serous moisture is streaming from the spleen to the cardia of the stomach. *De locis affectis* 5.[81]

45. If someone's food often putrefies in his stomach, he benefits from emesis before eating and from drinking sweet wine. He should eat those foods that are not quickly putrefied and should accustom himself to relieving the bowels from time to time with those substances that have a moderately relieving force, such as [hiera] picra.[82] But if one neglects the bad humor, healing is difficult. *De sanitate tuenda* 6.[83]

46. When a hot, bad temperament mixed with [either] a small amount of moisture [or with dryness][84] dominates the stomach but does not affect the substance [of the stomach], we treat it with cold water without fear or hesitation, for cold water is not harmful to the organs close to the stomach because they are in a state of balance. *De methodo medendi* 7.[85]

من جميع ذلك لأنّها تعدّل الأخلاط الرديئة وتسخّن المعدة وتعين على الهضم وتحلّل البخار البارد وتنفع من الاقشعرار الكائن من أخلاط حارّة . وإنّما يمتنع من إسقائه في الاقشعرار متى كانت حمّى أو ورم حارّ فقط . في سادسة شرحه لثانية ابيديميا .

٤٣ . رأيت قوما يتشنّجون تشنّج الصرع من قبل فم معدهم إذا هم تخموا تخمة شديدة أو شربوا شرابا له فضل سخونة أو أكثروا الجماع في غير وقته . ورأيت محمومين يتشنّجون بغتة من خلط رديئ انصبّ إلى فم معدهم للذعه ، فلمّا تقيّأوا نجوا من ساعتهم . وقوم ثقل عليهم طعام رديئ تناولوه فأصابهم سبات لم يقلع عنهم حتّى تقيّأوا جميع ما كان يضغط فم المعدة منهم . وإذا اعتلّ فم المعدة يعرض منه أيضا غشي حادّ مسرع . خامسة التعرّف .

٤٤ . العلّـة النافخـة تصيّر صاحبها كئيبا مغموما سـيّء الرجاء مأيّسا من الخير وبالجملة حاله كحال صاحب الوسـواس السوداوي لمشـاركة فم المعدة للدماغ . وتشتدّ أعراضهم أذا تخموا وجلّهـم مطحولون ، وهذا ممّا يدلّ أن رطوبـة صديدية تنصبّ من الطحال الى فم المعدة . خامسة التعرّف .

٤٥ . من كان الطعام يفسـد في معدته كثيرا فقد يسـتنفع بالقيء قبل الطعام ويشرب الخمر الحلو . ويجعل أغذيته ما لا يسـرع إليه الفسـاد ويتعاهد بين مدد من الزمان إسهال البطن بالأشـياء التي تحدره إحدارا معتدلا وتنقيه بمنزلة الفيقرا . وإن أنت أغفلت الخلط الرديئ عسر بروءه . سادسة تدبير الصحّة .

٤٦ . إن كان الغالب على المعدة سـوء مزاج حارّ أو تخالطه رطوبة يسـيرة من غير أن يكـون المزاج بمـادّة فإنّا نداويها بالماء البارد بلا تهيّب ولا توقّف ، فإنّ الأعضاء القريب موضعها من المعدة لا تضرّها الماء البارد لأنّها في حال اعتدال . سابعة الحيلة .

---

٣ ابيديميا] افيديميا ELP ‖ ٥ يتشنّجون] تشنّجوا ELOOxP ‖ ٦ للذعه] لذعه L ‖ ٧ سبات] سكاتا EL ‖ ٨ غشي] غثي G ‖ ١٠ فم المعدة للدماغ] فم الدماغ EsG : المعدة .Es² add ‖ ١١ أعراضهم] أمراضهم ELOOxP ‖ ١٢ الى فم] لفم ELOP

But if bad humors have entered into the substance of the coats of the stomach, the best kind of treatment is their evacuation with aloe[86] or hiera [picra] ingested with water. The composition of hiera [picra] is six *mithqāls*[87] each of Chinese cinnamon,[88] Indian nard,[89] saffron,[90] asarabacca,[91] mastic and balsam[92] wood, and one hundred *mithqāls* of aloe. The hiera should be prepared in two ways, with washed aloe and unwashed aloe. The washed type strengthens the stomach more, while the unwashed type is a stronger laxative. *De methodo medendi* 7.[93]

47. [In the case of] indigestion associated with diarrhea so severe that it harms one's strength, one should feed oneself with things that are astringent more and more. Often diarrhea goes with loss of appetite. In this case the patient should take a stomachic of quinces and the like. However, if indigestion is associated with constipation and either with a fever arising from the indigestion or without a fever, and if the spoiled food is in the upper parts of the abdomen, one should bring it down with the various kinds of pepper and the like. When the spoiled food has gone down, one should expel it either with a suppository or with an enema of honey, water, and olive oil. If the patient has a strong biting [sensation] there, administer to him an enema of olive oil in which duck fat has been melted. If duck fat is not available, use chicken fat instead. If this is not available, use goat's fat or olive oil and washed wax. If the patient suffers from flatulence, administer to him an enema of olive oil in which rue[94] was cooked or in which seeds that disperse the winds, such as cumin,[95] caraway,[96] celery seed,[97] and the like, were cooked. *De methodo medendi* 8.[98]

48. When the bowels of someone suffering from indigestion are relieved by means of a suppository or enema, feed him immediately thereafter with foods that are not at all astringent. Do the same on the second day and order the patient to go to the bathhouse when he is completely free of indigestion. When he sleeps well during the night following the bathhouse, he is completely healed. And if he suffers thereafter from a minor attack of fever, do not be worried or alarmed about it, but let him go to the bathhouse the next day and then let him eat. *De methodo medendi* 8.[99]

إذا كانت أخلاط رديئة مداخلة لجرم طبقات المعدة فأفضل أنواع علاجها استقراغها بصبر أو بإيارج يؤخذ سقّا بالماء . وصفة الإيارج : دار صيني وسنبل وزعفران وأسارون ومصطكى وعود بلسان من كلّ واحد ستّة مثاقيل ، صبر مائة مثقال . وينبغي أن تتخذ إيارج صنفان بصبر مغسول أو بغير مغسول ، إذ المغسول يقوّي المعدة أكثر والغير مغسول يسهل أكثر . سابعة الحيلة .

٤٧ . التخم الذي ينطلق معها الطبع حتّى يفرط ويجحف بالقوة يغذى فيه بالأشياء القابضة على التدريج وكثيرا ما تسقط مع الذرب شهوة الطعام فيتناول المريض جوارشن السفرجل ونحوه . أمّا التخم التي يمسك معها الطبع مع ذلك كان ذلك مع حمّى حادثة عن تلك التخمة أو بغير حمّى فإن كان الطعام الفاسد في أعالي البطن فاحدره بالفلافلي ونحوه ، وإن كان انحدر الطعام الفاسد إلى أسفل فاخرجه إمّا بشيافة أو بحقنة من عسل وماء وزيت . وإن كان هناك لذع قوي فتحقنه بزيت قد أذيب فيه شحم بطّ وإن عدم فشحم دجاج وإن لم يحضر فشحم ماعز أو زيت وشمع مغسول . فإن كانت هناك نفخة فتحقنه بزيت قد طبخ فيه سذاب أو البزور الطاردة للرياح كالكمّون والكرويا وبزر الكرفس ونحوها . ثامنة الحيلة .

٤٨ . إذا أطلقت طبيعة المتخوم بشيافة أو بحقنة فاغذوا العليل من ساعتك بما لا يقبض أصلا وافعل ذلك في اليوم الثاني وتقدّم للمريض في دخول الحمّام إن كان قد نقي من التخمة أصلا . فإن نام في ليلته بعد الحمّام نوما طيّبا فقد برأ بروءا تامّا . وإن وجد المريض مسّ شيء من الحمّى بعد ذلك فليس ينبغي لك أن تجزع من ذلك ولا تتخوّفه بل تدخله أيضا من غدّ النهار الحمّام وتغذوه . ثامنة الحيلة .

---

٧ المريض] G¹ ‖ ٩ أعالي] أعلى EL

49. If someone is struck by syncope caused by yellow bile that streamed to the cardia of his stomach, let him drink cold, fragrant, watery wine. When the syncope is caused by a surplus of crude humors, let him drink warm pale or yellowish wine,[100] if his head is strong. But let anyone struck by syncope drink fragrant wine.[101] *De methodo medendi* 12.[102]

50. Patients with illnesses occurring in the stomach and abdomen because of bad humors benefit from medications prepared with aloe. But astringent things, whether foods, beverages, or drugs, cause great harm. When the cardia of the stomach is steeped in [moist] humors that are not bad [in quality] but are simply harmful because of their quantity, then the use of astringent drugs, foods, and beverages is most beneficial. *Mayāmir* 8.[103]

51. Strong and difficult emesis occurs when there is druglike fluid[104] in the stomach that is incompatible with it and that inflicts serious harm upon it. When, in addition, the stomach is weak, the harm is twice as great. The aim of the treatment of someone with this condition is to eliminate that bad fluid and then to strengthen the stomach with fragrant spices and seeds with similar properties. Just as all malodorous [spices and seeds] upset the soul[105] and cause nausea, all fragrant ones strengthen the stomach, especially when they belong to the comestibles, for these are most suited to benefit a stomach upset because of that fluid. *Mayāmir* 8.[106]

52. If someone is attacked by hiccups because of overeating or an acrid humor, emesis will cure him. And when he is attacked by it because of cold, heating [will cure him]. A similar effect is achieved when one transforms the things that are acrid and eliminates and dissolves them through refining and drying remedies; this is most beneficial. *Mayāmir* 8.[107]

٤٩ . من أصابه غشـي بسـبب مرار أصفر ينصبّ إلى فم معدته فاسـقه شـرابا
باردا ريحانيا مائيا . وما كان من الغشـي عن كثرة الأخلاط الخام فاسـقه شـرابا حارّا
أشـقر أو أصفر إن كان رأسـه قويا . وينبغي أن يسـقى جميع من يصيبه الغشـي شـرابا
ريحانيا . ثانية عشر الحيلة .

٥٠ . العلـل الحادثة في المعدة والبطن من قبل أخـلاط رديئة ينتفع أصحابها بالأدوية
المتّخذة بالصبر . أمّا الأشـياء القابضة أطعمة كانت أو أشربة أو أدوية فإنّها تضرّهم مضرّة
عظيمة . ومتى استقع فم المعدة بأخلاط رطبة لا رداءة فيها وإنّما تضرّ بكمّيتها فإنّ استعمال
الأدوية القابضة والأطعمة والأشربة القابضة حينئذ من أنفع الأشياء . ثامنة الميامر .

٥١ . ما كان من القيء شديدا صعبا فإنّما يعرض عندما يكون في المعدة صديد منافرا
لها مجانسـا لطبائع الأدوية فتتأذّى به أذى شـديدا ، فإن كانت مع هذا ضعيفة تضاعف
عليها الشـرّ . والغرض في علاج من هذا حاله أن يفنى ذلك الصديد الردئ ويقوى المعدة
بعد ذلك بالأقاويه الطيّبة الروائح والبزور التي هي كذلك . وكما أنّ كلّ الأنواع المنتنة تقلب
النفس وتغثي كذلك كلّ الأنواع الطيّبة الروائح تقوي المعدة وبخاصّة إن كانت من الأشـياء
التي تؤكل ، فإنّها أحرى أن تنفع المعدة المنقلبة من قبل الصديد . ثامنة الميامر .

٥٢ . مـن يصيبـه فواق من كثرة طعام أو لذع خلط فالقيء يبرئه . وإن أصابه من برد
فالتسخين . وكذلك تغيير الأشياء التي تلذع وإزالتها أو تحليلها بالأدوية الملطفة المجفّفة من
أنفع الأشياء . ثامنة الميامر .

١ فاسـقه] فاسـقيه EsG || ٢ ومـا كان مـن] وإن كان L || ٣ جميـع] كلّ ELP : J
om.O || ٥ العلل] العلّة L || ٨ الأدوية القابضة] Es¹G || والأطعمة] الأطعمة EsG | حينئذ]
G¹ || ١٢ التي هـي كذلك] الكذلك G | أنّ] om.G || ١٦ وإزالتها] وإحالتها G

53. If someone is struck by bulimia, either suddenly or gradually, we restore his strength by making him smell vinegar, pennyroyal,[108] ashes, and peppermint[109] [steeped] in vinegar, or by letting him smell apples and similar fruits, or a piece of bread, which he should also be compelled to eat. We also give him roasted or cooked pork to smell. In general, [one should have him smell] every kind of foodstuff that has a fragrant smell. Similarly, all fragrant substances revive [bulimic] patients and restore their strength. One should tightly bandage their hands and feet, prick their chests,[110] and pull their hair. When they awaken from their syncope, one should feed them bread steeped in wine or something else that restores their strength. *Mayāmir* 8.[111]

54. A craving for bad and detestable beverages can also occur in the same way as it occurs for bad foods. This is the case when a bad humor, either salty or biliary, is congested in the coats of the stomach. This craving is excessive when this humor is boiling. The variation in the types of things one wants to drink is commensurate with the variation of the types of humors in quality and badness.[112] *De [morborum] causis et symptomatibus* 4.[113]

55. It is difficult to treat weakness of the cardia of the stomach and quick nausea associated with constipation because everything that relieves the bowels causes nausea and upsets the soul,[114] while that which strengthens the cardia of the stomach causes constipation. The most beneficial [therapy] I found [for such patients] is to eat vegetables spiced with olive oil and garum.[115] Then they should take a small amount of pear or quince or pomegranate, according to what they like most. *De sanitate tuenda* 6.[116]

56. If you want to strengthen the stomach of those suffering from indigestion and the like even if they have ephemeral fever, put strengthening substances upon the stomach—these should actually be extremely hot because anything lukewarm loosens and softens the cardia of the stomach. *De methodo medendi* 8.[117]

57. If someone suffers from indigestion and the like and from a burning in the stomach that is so severe that one imagines that there is an inflamed tumor there, he will benefit from a salve[118] prepared with quince oil.[119] It is my practice to heat the oils in a double vessel[120] because their strength is lost if they are heated in any other way.[121] *De methodo medendi* 8.[122]

٥٣ . من أصابه بوليموس بغتة أو على تدريج فإنّا نســترّد قوته بشــمّ الخلّ والفوذنّج البرّي ورماد ونعنع في خلّ أو بشمّ التّفاح وشبهه من الثمار أو بشمّ كسرة خبز ويضطرّ للأكل منها ، ونشــمّمهم لحم الخنازير مشويا ومطبوخا وبالجملة كلّ ما يغذوا ممّا له رائحة تعبق . وكذلك الروائح الطيّبة تنبّههم وترّد قوتهم . وتشدّ أيديهم وأرجلهم شدّا قويا وتنخس صدورهم وتجذب شعورهم . فإذا أفاقوا من غشيهم فنغذوهم بخبز منقوع في شراب أو بشيء آخر ممّا ينعش القوة . ثامنة الميامر .

٥٤ . قد تحدث أيضا شــهوة الأشربة الردئة الكرهة كما يحدث ذلك للأطعمة الردئة . وذلك عندما يكون في المعدة خلط ردئ محتقن في طبقاتها إمّا مالح وإمّا مراري . وتكون هذه الشهوة مفرطة عندما يغلي هذا الفضل . وبحســب اختلاف أنواع الخلط في كيفيته ورداته تختلف أنواع الأشياء التي تشتهى . رابعة العلل والأعراض .

٥٥ . يعسر علاج ضعف فم المعدة وسرعة الغثيان مع احتباس البطن لأنّ كلّ ما يطلق البطــن يغثي ويقلب النفس ، والذي يقوّي فم المعدة يمســك الطبع . وأجود ما وجدت أن يستوفوا طعامهم ببقول مطيّبة بزيت ومرّي . ويتناولون بعد ذلك قليل من كمّثرا أو سفرجل أو رمّان بحسب الألذّ عندهم . سادسة تدبير الصحّة .

٥٦ . إذا أردت تقويــة معدة المتخومــيم ونحوهم ولو كانت معهــم حمّى يوم فضع الأشــياء المقوّية على المعدة وهي فــي غاية الحــرارة بالفعل ، فإنّ كلّ شــيء فاتر يحلّ فم المعدة ويرخي . ثامنة الحيلة .

٥٧ . من كان من المتخومــيم ونحوهم يجد في معدته حرقة شــديدة حتّى يوهمك أنّ هناك ورم حارّ فالقيروطي المتّخذ بدهن السفرجل نافع . ومن عادتنا أن نسخن الأدهان في إناء مضاعف لأنّ قوتها تفسد إذا سخنت على غير هذا الوجه . ثامنة الحيلة .

---

٣ له] G¹ ‖ ٤ وتنخس] تلين Es² ‖ ٥ أفاقوا] فاقوا EsG ‖ ٧ الردئة (1st)] G¹ ‖ ١١ ضعف] om. EL

58. In those suffering from dropsy, water accumulates in those places that are between the intestines and the membrane covering them.[123] *In Hippocratis Epidemiarum* 1.2.[124]

59. [In the case of] dropsy of the flesh, one should apply that which expels the phlegm—first of all through relieving the bowels, then through emesis, and then through gargling, since gargling evacuates the phlegm from the head. When the phlegm is spread through the whole body, we set about to apply all [possible] methods in order to evacuate it. In this disease we also give [the patient] medications to drink with cutting and heating properties so that we stimulate diuresis and evacuate the body completely through the dissolution [of the phlegm]. *In Hippocratis De humoribus commentarius* 1.[125]

60. [ . . .] And we [should] cleanse the bodies of jaundice patients from the biles they contain in every possible manner so that we evacuate [the body] from above and below and through the urine and the palate and the nostrils. *In Hippocratis De humoribus commentarius* 1.[126]

61. Sometimes a jaundice patient benefits from [looking at] yellow colors because this dissolves the yellow bile. A patient with hemoptysis should be forbidden to look at colors that are primarily red, because this will make the blood stream forth. To evacuate any humor, it is proper to look at the colors of that humor; and to repel any humor into the depth of the body, it is proper to look at the colors opposite to the color of that humor. *In Hippocratis De humoribus commentarius* 2.[127]

62. I have often [successfully] treated a hard tumor in the liver at its inception. But when it existed for a longer time, I was unable to effect a cure, nor have I seen anyone else who achieved this. All those affected by this disease are also afflicted with dropsy and [most of them][128] die after a long time. But if one of them has diarrhea, he dies quickly. *Ad Glauconem [de medendi methodo]* 2.[129]

٥٨ . اجتماع الماء في المستسقيين يكون في المواضع التي بين الأمعاء وبين الغشاء الممدود عليها . في الثانية من شرحه للأولى من ابيديميا .

٥٩ . الاستسقاء اللحمي ينبغي أن يستعمل فيه ما يخرج البلغم أوّلا بالإسهال ، ثمّ بعد ذلك ما يخرجه بالقيء ، ثمّ بالغرغرة لأنّ الغرغرة تستفرغ البلغم من الرأس . ولمّا كان البلغم منبثًّا في البدن كلّه صرنا نستعمل فيه جميع أنحاء استفراغه . ونسقي أيضا في هذه العلّة أدوية شأنها التقطيع والإسخان لندرّ بها البول ونستفرغ البدن كلّه بالتحلّل . في شرحه للأولى من الأخلاط .

٦٠ . وننقي أبدان أصحاب اليرقان من المرار بكلّ وجه يمكننا ذلك حتّى نستفرغه من فوق ومن أسفل وبالبول وبالحنك وبالمنخرين . في شرحه للأولى من الأخلاط .

٦١ . قد ينتفع صاحب اليرقان بالألوان الصفر لأنّه يحلّل الصفراء . وينهى صاحب نفث الدم عن رؤية الألوان الأوّلي الحمر لأنّه ينبعث الدم . وكلّ خلط تريد استفراغه فيوافق ذلك رؤية ألوان ذلك الخلط ، وكلّ خلط تريد دفعه لعمق البدن فيوافق ذلك رؤية ألون المضادّ للون ذلك الخلط . في الثانية من شرحه للأخلاط .

٦٢ . الورم الصلب الذي يكون في الكبد قد عالجنا منه في أوائل حدوثه مرارا كثيرة . وأمّا ما قد تطاولت به الأيّام منه فلا أنا قدرت أتاتي لبرئه ولا رأيت غيري وصل إلى ذلك منه . وجميع من تصيبه هذه العلّة يلحقه الاستسقاء ويموت بعد مدّة طويلة . ومن أصابه منهم الاختلاف مات سريعا . ثانية أغلوقن .

٢ ابيديميا] افيديميا ELP || ٤ ثمّ] بعد ذلك add. L || ٦ والإسخان] والتسخين L || ٨ أبدان] G¹ || ١١ الأوّلي] om. ELOP | ينبعث] يبعث ELOP || ١٢ رؤية ألوان ذلك الخلط] om. G || ١١٤ أوائل] أوّل EL

63. The treatment of patients suffering from dropsy caused by a hard tumor in the viscera should be directed towards three goals: firstly, to succeed in healing the hard tumor in the viscera; secondly, to apply poultices that dissolve the moisture; and thirdly, to give [the patient] diuretic medications to drink. *Ad Glauconem [de medendi methodo]* 2.[130]

64. Transudation[131] of blood [occurs because of] the opening of small vessels or because of the evacuation of the watery part of the blood, as it occurs especially in the case of weakness of the liver or kidneys, for a patient suffering from this illness often urinates or defecates the watery part of the blood. *De [morborum] causis et symptomatibus* 6.[132]

65. In all [the various] types of dropsy, the liver itself fails to transform the food that reaches it into blood because of a cold bad temperament that dominates it. Sometimes this cold bad temperament dominates one of the digestive organs or one of the respiratory organs and passes from there on to the neighboring organs until it reaches the substance of the liver through the common vessels. As a result the illness settles in the substance of the liver and produces dropsy. Similarly, when an excessive loss of blood occurs in whatever way, the liver becomes cold and dropsy results. *De locis affectis* 5.[133]

66. Sometimes the liver is affected by such a dry bad temperament that it cannot transform the food into blood, and dropsy develops. Sometimes this happens because of a hard tumor in the spleen, because most illnesses of the spleen also affect the liver. *De locis affectis* 6.[134]

67. Obstructions of the liver should be treated with opening remedies, and congestion in the head, with walking before meals. Such patients should also walk slowly after meals. Everything that is good for opening obstructions is also appropriate for a slow digestion;[135] the best of these are oxymel and the various kinds of pepper. A thinning regimen is good for a slow digestion and relieves obstructions of the liver. *De sanitate tuenda* 6.[136]

٦٣. علاج أصحاب الاستسقاء الحادث عن ورم صلب في الأحشاء ينحا فيه نحو هذه الأغراض الثلاثة: أحدها أن تتأتّى لشفاء الورم الصلب الذي في الأحشاء والثاني أن تستعمل الأضمدة التي تحلّل الرطوبة والثالث أن تسقي أدوية تدرّ البول. ثانية أغلوقن.

٦٤. رشــح الدم انفتاح عروق صغار أو استفراغ مائية الدم كما يعرض ذلك خاصّة في ضعف الكبد والكلى. فإنّ صاحب هذه العلّة يعرض له مرارا كثيرة أن يبول أو يتبرّز مائية الدم. سادسة العلل والأعراض.

٦٥. في جميع أنواع الاستسقاء الكبد نفسها هي التي لا تغيّر ما يأتيها من الغذاء إلى الدم بسبب ســوء مزاج بارد يستولي عليها. وقد يكون ذلك الســوء مزاج البارد اســتولى علـى أحد آلات الغذاء أو أحد آلات التنفّس ويتعـدّى منه إلى ما قرب منه من الأعضاء حتّى يتّصل ذلك البرد بجرم الكبد بمشاركة العروق فتتمكّن العلّة في جرم الكبد فيحدث الاستســقاء. وكذلك إذا أفرط خروج الدم بأيّ وجه كان بردت الكبد فيحدث الاستسقاء. خامسة التعرّف.

٦٦. قد تنال الكبد مرارا كثيرة من سوء المزاج اليابس ما لا يمكها معه أن تغيّر الغذاء إلى الدم فيحدث الاستســقاء. وقد يحدث من أجل ورم صلب في الطحال لأنّ جلّ علل الطحال تعمّه مع الكبد. سادسة التعرّف.

٦٧. تعالج ســدد الكبد بالأشياء المفتّحة ويعالج الامتلاء العارض في الرأس بالمشي قبل الطعام ولا يمنع أيضا هؤلاء من المشـي برفق بعد الطعام. وكلّ ما يصلح لتفتيح السدد يوافق تخلّف الاســتمراء، وأجودها الســكبجين والفلافلي والتدبير الملطّف يستصلح به تخلّف الاستمراء وتشفى به سدد الكبد. سادسة تدبير الصحّة.

---

١ ينحا [Es²]: ينحو G Es ‖ ٥ كثيرة [om. EL ‖ ١٨–١٩ وأجودها . . . الاستمراء [om. EL

68. For [treating] tumors of the liver and stomach, I prefer absinthe.[137] When I think that the liver and stomach are in a bad condition, I immediately boil absinthe with olive oil and pour it over these parts of the body. If it is not at hand, [I use] quince oil or mastic oil. In case of a light fever, [I use] nard oil. *De methodo [medendi]* 11.[138]

69. When a tumor occurs in the liver, an extremely strict diet is required. No food is more beneficial to it than barley groats because they cleanse without biting, and there is no medication more beneficial for it than oxymel with cold water. But do not try to treat it[139] with pomegranate juice or apples or other astringent things that cause the openings of the vessels to contract and prevent the evacuation of bile. *De methodo [medendi]* 13.[140]

70. If there is a tumor on the convex side of the liver, it is time to purge it. One should do so by stimulating micturition. When it is on the concave side of the liver, one should purge it through relieving the bowels by mixing safflower,[141] Roman nettle seed,[142] and a moderate laxative into the food. When the tumor subsides, one should [continue to] do these things with confidence and trust. I have occasionally cooked common polypody[143] with barley groats and black hellebore.[144] One may also purge such patients with enemas initially prepared from water, honey, and borax or natron, and when the illness subsides, with something stronger such as mint,[145] pulp of the colocynth,[146] and small centaury.[147] *De methodo [medendi]* 13.[148]

[In the case of] a weak liver one should first of all take care to open its obstruction through cleansing and moderately dissolving remedies— such as resin from the turpentine tree[149]—so that the openings of the pulsatile and nonpulsatile vessels that the liver contains and that pass throughout it remain open without any obstruction, for an obstruction produces putrefaction. A medication prepared for the liver should not be strongly cooling but only moderately so. *Mayāmir* 8.[150]

71. Cultivated and wild chicory[151] have a temperament dominated by some cold and are also somewhat bitter, and together they have a moderately astringent effect. Because of the presence of these two qualities, they

٦٨. نختار لأورام الكبد والمعدة الأفسنتين، فأمّا متى توهّمنا أنّ الكبد والمعدة بحال رديئة طبخنا على المكان أفسنتين بزيت وصببناه على هذين العضوين. فإن لم يتهيّأ فدهن السفرجل ودهن المصطكى، وإن كانت الحمّى يسيرة فدهن الناردين. حادية عشر الحيلة.

٦٩. إذا حدث ورم في الكبد فهو يحتاج إلى تدبير مستقصى غاية الاستقصاء. ولا غذاء له أوفق من كشك الشعير لأنّه يجلو بلا لذع، ولا دواء له أوفق من السكنجبين بماء بارد. ولا تقربه لا بماء رمّان ولا تفّاح ولا غيرهما من القوابض لئلا تجمع فوهات العروق ويمنع المرار من الاستفراغ. ثالثة عشر الحيلة.

٧٠. متى كان الورم في محدّب الكبد فوقت أن ينبغي أن تستفرغه. تستفرغ بإدرار البول، وإذا كان في مقعّر الكبد فبإسهال البطن بأن تخلط في الطعام قرطما وبزر الأنجرة وما يطلق البطن باعتدال. وإذا انحطّ الورم فافعل هذه الأشياء بثقة واتكال. وأنا طبخت في بعض الأوقات بسبايج مع كشك الشعير وخربق أسود، واستفرغ هؤلاء أيضا بالحقن تكون أوّلا بماء وعسل وبورق أو نطرون. وأمّا عند انحطاط المرض فبما هو أقوى كالفوذنج وشحم الحنظل والقنطوريون الدقيق. ثالثة عشر الحيلة.

الكبد الضعيفة تعنى أبدا بتفتيح سددها بما يجلو ويحلّل تحليلا معتدلا كصمغ البطم لتبقى أفواه العروق الضوارب وغير الضوارب التي فيها النافذة من بعضها إلى بعض مفتّحة غير مسدودة، لأنّ السدد يحدث العفونة. وينبغي أن لا يكون الدواء المؤلّف للكبد قوي التبريد لكنّ يكون تبريده تبريدا معتدلا. ثامنة الميامر.

٧١. الهندباء البستاني والبرّي الغالب على مزاجهما برد يسير وفيهما مع هذا شيء من مرارة وهما جميعا يقبضان قبضا معتدلا. ولمكان هتين الكيفيتين صارا من جياد

---

١ فأمّا] فإنّه ELP : فإنّا O : مرخي O || فإن] متى E | add. E || ٧٤،٤–٧٦،١٠ غاية . . . الفصول إلا] om. Ox || ٥ من (1st)] ماء EOP add. || ٦ تقربه] تغذوه L || ٩ المرض] الورم EL || ١٥ مفتّحة] مفتوحة ELOP || ١٦ لا] G¹

are amongst the best remedies for the treatment of a hot, bad temperament of the liver. They are not as harmful for a cold, bad temperament
as are cold, moist remedies without astringency and without bitterness.
The reason for this is that they cool the liver moderately, and strengthen
5      it through their astringency, and cleanse it through their bitterness.
They are beneficial for the liver against a simple bad temperament and
against one combined with [serous] matter, for when they are mixed
with honey, they make those serous moistures and other moistures flow
and descend [from the body].[152] *Mayāmir* 8.[153]

10     72. Of the remedies for hardness of the liver, the softening ones
should be very weak, and those remedies that heat and refine should be
more predominant than in the case of the treatment of hardness of the
other organs. For the substance of the liver is indeed like congealed
moisture, and if those remedies soften it greatly, its powers dissolve.
15     *Mayāmir* 8.[154]

73. Among the remedies that are very effective for cleansing the
liver and for opening its narrow passages without visibly warming or
cooling it is fern,[155] which, because of its bitter taste,[156] strongly pre-
dominates. *Mayāmir* 8.[157]

20     74. The medications for a tumor in the stomach or liver should be
mixed with astringent fragrant substances;[158] one should not limit oneself to using only softening, slackening medications. If one does so, one
endangers the patient and puts him on the verge of death. *Mayāmir* 8.[159]

75. Astringent and biting substances are not as harmful for tumors
25     on the convex side of the liver as they are for tumors on the concave
side, because the powers of the substances that a person takes change
before they reach the convex side of the liver. Thus, an astringent substance is not as astringent as it was before, and a biting substance is not
as biting as it was before, and a viscous substance is less viscous. *De*
30     *methodo [medendi]* 13.[160]

76. When a tumor occurs in the spleen and the body contains superfluous melancholic humor, mixing astringent ingredients with the dissolving medications is unavoidable in order to preserve the [body's]
strength—the superfluities are thus attracted and the body can be
35     cleansed from them. When the body is clean, one should not mix anything at all astringent with [other] medications for its treatment, unless
the astringent [quality] is as weak as possible. *De methodo [medendi]* 11.[161]

الأدوية التي يعالج بها سوء مزاج الكبد الحارّ، ولا يضرّان بسوء المزاج البارد مضرّة شديدة كما تضرّ الأشياء الباردة الرطبة من غير قبض ولا مرارة، وذلك أنّهما يبرّدان تبريدا معتدلا ويقويان الكبد بقبضهما ويجلوان بمرارتهما. وهما ينفعان الكبد من سوء مزاج ساذج ومن سوء مزاج بمادّة، لأنّ إذا خلط بهما العسل يدرّان ويحدران تلك الرطوبات الصديدية وغيرها من الرطوبات. ثامنة الميامر.

٧٢. صلابة الكبد ينبغي أن تكون الأدوية المليّنة في أدويتها ضعيفة ضعفا كثيرا، وتغلب فيها الأشياء التي تسخن وتلطّف أكثر ممّا تغلب في علاج صلابة سائر الأعضاء، لأنّ جرم الكبد إنّما هو بمنزلة رطوبة جامدة فإن ليّنته تليينا قويا انحلّت قواه. ثامنة الميامر.

٧٣. ممّا يبلغ في تنقية الكبد وفتح الطرق الضيّقة التي فيها من غير أن يسخنها اسخانا ظاهرا أو يبرّدها السرخس لأنّ طعم المرارة غالب عليه غلبة قوية. ثامنة الميامر.

٧٤. الـورم الحادث في المعدة أو في الكبد يخلط في أدويتهما أدوية قابضة عطرية، ولا يقتصـر على الأدوية الملّينة المرخية وحدها. ومتى فعل ذلك كان صاحبها على خطر وشرف من التلف. ثامنة الميامر.

٧٥. أورام محدّب الكبد لا تضرّها الأشياء القابضة واللذّاعة كإضرارها بأورام مقعّر الكبد، لأنّ الأشياء التي يتناولها الإنسان تتغيّر قواها قبل وصولها لمحدب الكبد، والقابض لا يقبض مثل ما كان، واللاذع لا يلدغ كما كان واللزج تقلّ لزوجته. ثالثة عشر الحيلة.

٧٦. الطحال إذا ورم وكان في البدن فضل خلط ســوداوي فلا بدّ من أن نخلط مع الأدوية المحلّلة أدوية قابضة لتحفظ عليه قوته حتّى تجتذب الفضول وينقى منها البدن. أمّا إن كان البدن نقيا فلا تخلط شيئًا قابضا البتّة أو يكون القابض أقلّ ممّا يمكن.

---

١ الكبد] G¹ || ٧ علاج] om. G || ٨ ليّنته] ليّنتها EL || ٩ ممّا . . . ثامنة الميامر.] EL || ١٣ التلف] التلاف ELP || ١٤ بأورام] G¹ || ١٦ واللاذع] واللداغ EL || ١٧ البدن] بطن EL || ١٩ القابض] G¹ | ممّا ما] L

77. The best remedy for hardness of the spleen is a poultice prepared from roots of caper,[162] absinthe, vinegar, and honey. Be careful
not to apply a poultice with astringent remedies to the chest. *De methodo
[medendi]* 11.[163]

5          78. A constant use of vinegar together with dissolving remedies in
the case of illnesses of the spleen and of hard swelling in the fleshy part
of any muscle is a safe remedy. Simple gum ammoniac[164] with vinegar is
often sufficient for the treatment of tumors and hardness of the spleen.
*De methodo [medendi]* 14.[165]

10         79. Sometimes the distress of a melancholic delusion results from
an illness of the spleen and often arouses a very strong craving for food,
especially when a purely acid superfluity streams to the stomach. Often
an aversion and dislike of food occurs and the soul becomes upset[166]
when the craving is spoiled in another way.[167] *De locis affectis* 6.[168]

15         80. There is only one way to evacuate the superfluities that collect
in the spleen, namely [through] relieving [the bowels], because it is not in
[the spleen's] nature to expel its contents to the kidneys. Therefore, when
a tumor develops in the spleen, we stimulate it through laxatives, so that
it expels the superfluities that got stuck in it. *De methodo medendi* 13.[169]

20         81. Pleurisy should be treated through bleeding, the application of
a hot compress, and softening of the stool. Be careful not to administer
barley groats when the pleurisy reaches its climax so that a crisis is not
hindered.[170] *De acutorum morborum [victu et] Galeni commentarius* 1.[171]

82. If you want to apply a hot compress to [someone suffering from]
25    pleurisy, you should put soft wool or a folded garment or a small cushion
underneath the hot compress so that the contact of the hot compress
with the ribs is without pressure and without any harm whatsoever. *De
acutorum morborum [victu et] Galeni commentarius* 2.[172]

83. The [inhalation] of the vapor[173] of a hot compress is only benefi-
30    cial when the vapor is moist and when the pleurisy[174] is dry, without any
expectoration. *De acutorum morborum [victu et] Galeni commentarius* 2.[175]

٧٧ . أصلح ما يداوى به جساء الطحال بضماد يتّخذ بأصول الكبر والأفسنتين والخلّ والعسل وإيّاك أن تضمّد الصدر بأدوية قابضة . حادية عشر الحيلة .

٧٨ . مداومة استعمال الخلّ مع الأدوية المحلّلة في علل الطحال والجزء اللحمي من كلّ عضلة إذا حدث هناك ورم صلب مأمون العاقبة . والأشق مع الخلّ كثيرا ما يكتفى
٥ باستعماله وحده في مداواة أورام الطحال وصلابته . أخيرة الحيلة .

٧٩ . قد يحدث عن علل الطحال كأبة الوسواس السوداوي ويهيج مرارا كثيرة شهوات الأطعمة قوية جدًّا ، وخاصّة إذا صبّ إلى المعدة فضل خالص الحمضة . ومرارا كثيرة يحدث بغض الطعام وكراهته وتقلب النفس منه إذا كانت الشهوة فاسدة من وجه آخر . سادسة التعرّف .

٨٠ . ليس لاستفراغ ما يجتمع في الطحال من الفضول إلا طريقا واحدا وهو الإسهال ،
١٠ لأنّ ليس من شأنه أن يدفع ما فيه إلى الكليتين . ولذلك متى تورّم حرّكاه إلى أن تدفع الفضول المستكنة فيه بالإسهال . ثالثة عشر الحيلة .

٨١ . علاج ذات الجنب بالفصد والتكميد وتليين البطن واحذر أن تعطي كشك الشعير في وقت منتهى ذات الجنب لأن لا تعوق البحران . في شرحه لأولى الأمراض الحادّة .

٨٢ . إذا أردت أن تكمّد في ذات الجنب فينبغي أن تضع تحت ما تكمّد به صوفا
١٥ ليّنا أو ثيابا مطوية أو مخدّة صغيرة ليكون لقاء التكميد للأضلاع بلا ضغط ولا أذية بتّة . في شرحه لثانية الأمراض الحادّة .

٨٣ . إنّما ينتفع بخار الكماد متى كان رطبا وكانت الشوصة يابسة لا ينفث منها شيء . في شرحه لثانية الأمراض الحادّة .

---

١ يتّخذ [ G¹ ‖ ٥ أورام] أمراض EL ‖ ٦ عن] من ELO : ورم add. G ‖ علل] G¹ ‖ ٧ شهوات] شهوة L ‖ الأطعمة] للأطعمة ELOP ‖ ١٣ البطن] الطبع EL : الطبعية Ox

84. One should avoid phlebotomy when pleurisy is caused by a bilious, melancholic, or phlegmatic humor. It should also be avoided in pleurisy caused by a bloodlike humor when the time [of the year] is extremely hot, or when the humor that dominates the body of the patient consists of bile, or when the bloodlike humor has changed into bile—that is, when the patient spits up bile after spitting up blood. *In Hippocratis De humoribus commentarius* 3.[176]

85. Everything necessarily resulting from an inflammation of the nervous part of the diaphragm also results from severe inflammations of the membrane covering the ribs on the inside.[177] *De pulsu* 16.[178]

86. Drugs prepared with aromatic herbs are very beneficial for abscesses occurring deep inside the body and especially in the intestines, for these drugs dissolve and melt the humors accumulated in them. [There are many other similar remedies];[179] the best of these is the great theriac,[180] and less good are the drugs prepared with water mint.[181] *De methodo medendi* 14.[182]

87. An appropriate therapy in general for abscesses occurring deep inside the body is to treat them with refining and drying drugs. Also good for these patients is to drink a little bit of thin wine. *Mayāmir* 7.[183]

88. Says[184] Moses: Among the refining and drying remedies are vinegar, which is cold, and maidenhair,[185] a drug intermediate between hot and cold. The other well-known and often-applied remedies are all of them hot and dry. However, since most internal abscesses are followed by fever, it is necessary for a physician to remember those remedies that Galen has specified as attenuating and drying, next to their degrees of heat and dryness. Of the medications that dry and attenuate and are hot and dry in the first degree, there are four that are commonly used: agrimony,[186] lemon-grass,[187] tamarisk,[188] and pistachio.[189] Of the medications that are hot and dry in the second degree, there are eight: Roman nettle,[190] balsam,[191] birth-wort,[192] lily,[193] squirting cucumber,[194] rhubarb,[195] asphodel,[196] and gillyflower.[197] Of the medications that are hot and dry in the third degree, there are twenty: savin,[198] gentian,[199] wild carrot,[200] Chinese cinnamon,[201] hypericum,[202] sweet reed,[203] hyssop,[204] black poplar,[205]

٨٤. امتنـع من الفصد في ذات الجنب إذا كانت من خلط مراري أو سـوداوي أو بلغمي ، وكذلك تمتنع منه في ذات الجنب الدموية إذا كانت الوقت شـديد الحرارة أو كان الخلط الغالب على بدن المريض المرار أو كان الخلط الدموي قد اسـتحال مرارا وذلك بأن ينفث بعد النفث الدموي نفثا ماريا . في شرحه لثالثة الأخلاط.

٨٥. كلّ شـيء يلزم الورم الحادث في الجـزء العصباني من الحجاب فهو لازم للأورام العظام الحادثة في الغشاء المستبطن للأضلاع. سادسة عشر النبض . ٥

٨٦. الدبيلات التي تحدث في باطن البدن وبخاصّة في الأحشاء فإنّ الأدوية المتّخذة بالأقاويـه نافعة لهـا جـدّا لأنّها تحلّل وتذيب الرطوبات المجتمعـة فيها . وأحمد الأدوية لها الترياق الكبير ودونه الأدوية المتّخذة بالفوذنج النهري. أخيرة الحيلة.

٨٧. العلاج الموافق لجميع الدبيلات الحادثة في باطن البدن عامّة هو أن تعالج بأدوية ملطّفة تجفّف ويوافقهم أيضا شرب اليسير من الشراب اللطيف . سابعة الميامر . ١٠

٨٨. قال موسى : الأدوية الملطّفة التي تجفّف من جملتها الخلّ وهو بارد . وكزبرة بئر وهو دواء معتدل بين الحرارة والبرودة. وأمّا سائر الأدوية المشهورة الكثيرة الاستعمال فكلّها حارّة يابسـة. ولكون أكثر الدبيلات الباطنة تتبعها حمّـى ينبغي للطبيب أن يكون ذاكرا للأدوية التي نصّ جالينوس فيها بأنّها مجفّفة ملطّفة، ويذكر درجتها في الحرّ واليبس. من ١٥ ذلك الأدوية التي تجفّف وتلطّف وهي حارّة يابسة في الأولى من الكثيرة الاستعمال أربعة أدوية: غافت، إذخر، طرفاء، فستق. ومن الحارّة اليابسة في الثانية ثمانية أدوية: أنجرة، بلسـان، زراوند، سوسن، قثّاء حمار، راوند، خنثى، خيري. ومن الحارّة اليابسة في الثالثة عشرون دواء: أبهل، جنطيانا، دوقو، دار صاني، هيوفاريقون، وجّ، زوفا، جوز

---

١-٢ إذا . . . في ذات الجنب] om. ELOx ‖ ٧ وبخاصّة] وخاصّة ELOOxP ‖ ٨ الرطوبـات] الأخلاط ELOx ‖ الأدوية لها] أدويتها ELOP : أدويته Ox ‖ ١٠ هو] هي ELOOxP

amomum,[206] Cubeb pepper,[207] marjoram,[208] bishop's weed,[209] peppermint, thyme,[210] rue,[211] cinnamon,[212] sagapenum,[213] mint,[214] fennel,[215] and
nigella.[216] Of the remedies mentioned by later physicians that dry and
attenuate and that are hot and dry in the first degree, there are three
drugs that are commonly used: silk, rose chestnut tree,[217] and smaller
cardamom,[218] which is called *hāl*.[219] Altogether there are thirty-seven
drugs; of these, one should use whatever is available as a simple or compound remedy according to what one deems appropriate.

89. When internal ulcers do not come with an inflammation, they
can be healed quickly with astringent remedies. But those that come
with an inflammation and fever cannot be healed. Rather, their size
increases every day.[220] Watery vesicles occur more rapidly in the membrane surrounding the liver than in the other organs.[221] *In Hippocratis
Aphorismos commentarius* 7.

90. When in the case of malignant intestinal ulcers one of the
two membranes is so much eaten away[222] that it disappears completely,
the other membrane replaces the first and the person is saved. *De usu
partium* 5.[223]

91. The ancient physicians acted correctly in applying poultices and
hot compresses for a colic arising from a vitreous humor that settled
in the colon. If someone wants to use this [therapy], he should apply
warm packs and poultices continuously, for then he heals the disease
and relieves the patient from the bad symptoms [of the colic]. But if he
applies a warm pack only once or twice, he harms the patient severely
because the distension increases. *De clysteribus*.[224]

92. When intestinal pain occurs with fever, apply a hot compress
with common millet.[225] If the pain does not subside, take one of the
seeds that dissolve the flatulent winds and cook it in olive oil of a fine
consistency, strain it, and melt duck fat in it, and apply this as an enema.
If there is no duck fat available, [use] chicken fat that is unsalted and
not very old. If the pain [still] does not subside, melt some castoreum
into that oil and apply this as an enema. *De methodo [medendi]* 12.[226]

رومي ، حماما ، كبابة ، مرزنجوش ، نانخواه ، نعنع ، نمام ، سـذاب ، سـليخة ، سكبينج ،
فودنج ، رازيانج ، شونيز . وممّا ذكره المتأخّرون وهي أدوية تجفّف وتلطّف وهي حارّة يابسة
في الأولى كثيرة الاستعمال ثلاثة أدوية : حرير ، نارمشك ، قاقلّة صغيرة وهي الهال . الجملة
سبعة وثلاثون دواء ، تستعمل منها ما حضر مفردة ومركّبة بحسب ما تراه .

٨٩ . القروح الباطنة إن لم يكن معها ورم تبرأ سـريعا بالأشياء القابضة ، والتي تكون
معهـا ورم وحمّى ليس يمكـن أن تبرأ ، بل يزداد مقدارها كلّ يوم . ونفّاخات الماء يسـرع
حدوثها في الغشاء المحيط بالكبد أكثر من سائر الأعضاء . في شرحه لسابعة الفصول .

٩٠ . القـروح الردئة في الأمعاء إذا عقرت أحـد الصفاقين حتّى يذهب أصلا فيقوم
الصفاق الآخر مقامه ويسلم الإنسان . في خامسة المنافع .

٩١ . قد أصاب القدماء في اسـتعمالهم الضماد والتكميـد في القولنج الذي يكون
من خلط زجاجي يسـتكنّ في قولون . وينبغي لمن أراد اسـتعمال ذلك أن يديم التكميد
والضمـاد ، فإنّه إذا فعل ذلك أبرأ العلّة وأراح العليل من الأعراض الردئة . وإن كمّده مرّة أو
مرّتين أضرّ بالعليل إضرارا شديدا لأنّ الامتداد يتزيّد . في مقالته في الحقن .

٩٢ . إذا حدث وجع الأمعاء مع حمّى فاسـتعمل التكميد بالجاورس ، وإن لم يسكن
الوجع فاعمد إلى أحد البزور التي تحلّل الرياح فاطبخه بزيت لطيف الأجزاء وصفّه وأذب
فيه شـحم بطّ واحقن به . فإن لم يحضر شـحم بطّ فشـحم دجاج غير مملوح ولا عتيق
جدّا . وإن لم يسكن فأذب في ذلك الزيت يسير جندبادستر واحقن به . ثانية عشر الحيلة .

93. There are three kinds of abdominal worms: the kind similar to vinegar worms,[227] which originates in the region around the anus, the kind resembling gourd seeds,[228] [which form] in the large intestine, and the kind resembling snakes,[229] which form in the small intestine. They produce pain in the stomach when they ascend in its direction. Sometimes abdominal worms originate from a bad, biting humor. *In Hippocratis Epidemiarum* 2.1.[230]

94. Sometimes the humors dissolve in the [nonpulsatile] vessels[231] and a watery serum is formed in them. When the kidneys cleanse that serum from the [nonpulsatile] vessels and transport it to the urinary bladder, it is excreted with the urine. When the kidneys are too weak to attract this watery [serum], one of two things happens to it: the [nonpulsatile] vessels either expel it to the abdomen, or they disperse it and let it flow throughout the entire body, thereby causing dropsy. *De [morborum] causis et symptomatibus* 6.[232]

95. If an abscess[233] forms in a kidney and ripens and the patient micturates pus, he will find relief from his pain, but he should be wary of an ulcer in that kidney. Therefore, one should attempt its cicatrization[234] by all means. If it does not form a scar quickly, a cure will be very difficult. *De locis affectis* 6.[235]

96. Sometimes no urine at all comes to the bladder because the kidneys have stopped functioning; the urinary bladder is empty and nothing at all is retained in it. *De [morborum] causis et symptomatibus* 6.[236]

97. The diseases of the anus are difficult to heal because of four reasons: this part of the body is hypersensitive; it is the outlet for biting humors; drugs hardly stay there; and its temperament is warm and moist, so it needs remedies that are cool and dry. However, cooling and drying remedies are mostly astringent, and astringent [drugs] are biting, and the anus cannot tolerate biting. Therefore, the best medications consist of mineral substances that are not hot when they are washed.[237] *Mayāmir* 9.[238]

٩٣. أنـواع دود البطن ثلاثة: الشــبيهة بدود الخلّ تتولّد فيما يلي الدبر، والشــبيهة بحبّ القرع في المعاء الغلاظ، والشــبيهة بالحيات يكون في الأمعــاء الدقاق، فيحدث وجعــا في المعدة إذا ارتفع نحوها. وقـد يتولّد الدود في البطن من خلط ردئ لذّاع. في الأولى من شرحه لثانية ابيديميا.

٩٤. قـد تذوب الأخــلاط في العروق ويحدث فيها صديد مائ، وإن اســتنظفت الكليتان تلك المائية من العروق ويذهبان بذلك الصديد إلى المثانة خرج بالبول. وإن ضعفت الكليتان عن جذبه تلك المائية إلى أحد أمرين، إمّا أن تدفعها العروق إلى البطن وإمّا أن تبثّها وتصبّها إلى جميع البدن فيحدث من ذلك الاستسقاء. سادسة العلل والأعراض.

٩٥. إذا حصـل ورم في الكلية ونضج وبال العليل القيح فهو يجد راحة من الوجع، لكنّــه على وجل من قرحة الكلية فاحرص بــكلّ حيلة على إدمال تلك القرحة وختمها. فإنّه إن لم تندمل سريعا صارت عسرة البرء جدًّا. سادسة التعرّف.

٩٦. قد لا يجيء البول إلى المثانة أصلا لأنّ فعل الكلى يتعطّل، وتكون المثانة فارغة ليس فيها شيء محتقن البتّة. سادسة العلل والأعراض.

٩٧. علل المقعدة وهي السـفلى عسر ما تبرأ لأربعة أسباب وهي كثرة حسّ العضو وكونه مصبّ فضول تلذع وقلّة مكث الأدوية عليه وكون مزاجه حارًّا رطبا، فهو يحتاج ما يبرّد ويجفّف، والأدوية المبرّدة والمجفّفة في أكثر الأمر قابضة والقابض يلذع وهي لا تحمل اللذع، ولذلك أفضل أدويته المعدنية التي ليست بحارّة إذا صوّلت. تاسعة الميامر.

٧٩,١ - ٨١,١١ الشــبيهة بـدون ... من هذا [om. Ox ‖ ٢ المعاء الغــلاظ] الأمعاء الغليظة EL ‖ ٤ ابيديميا] افيديميا ELP ‖ ٧ البطن] الباطن EsG ‖ ٩-١٠ ونضج ... الكلية] om. OP ‖ ١٤ السفلى] السفل EL: السفلة OP ‖ ١٥ يحتاج] إلى add. EL: ل om. OP L

98. Among diseases of the skin due to black bile are mange and peeling of the skin. And when the illness occurs in the flesh or in the [nonpulsatile] vessels,[239] it is called cancer. Elephantiasis starts from melancholic humor. When much time passes, the black bile dominates the blood, and those suffering from this illness smell bad,[240] ulcers appear [on their bodies], and their complexion changes. *De tumoribus [praeter naturam].*[241]

99. The moisture in the joints is mucous. When it increases so much that it makes the flesh around the joints wet, it produces tumors similar to those in patients with dropsy. These tumors have misled[242] some physicians so that they have cut into them, believing that they would find pus in them. But they did not find pus; on the contrary, they found that all the flesh around the joint was full of mucous. *In Hippocratis Epidemiarum* 6.8.[243]

100. For marasmus occurring from a condition similar to old age, and for marasmus that is called parching,[244] and for marasmus that is accompanied by syncope[245]—for these three conditions—milk, barley gruel,[246] and groats of Roman wheat[247] cooked in vinegar are appropriate. But the groats should be cooked in the same way as the barley [gruel] so that it can be distributed throughout the organs. Hydromel is [only] beneficial in cold conditions. *De marcore.*[248]

101. Much flesh and fat is harmful and detrimental and gives the body an ugly appearance and hinders its activities and movements. Therefore, those suffering from it should travel a lot and do much walking in the sun. Travel over sea is especially good because the sea air dissolves the [superfluous] moistures. One should let them eat foods with little nourishment, such as vegetables, and that which contains heat, such as onions, garlic, and salted fish, and that which strengthens but does not moisten, such as lean roasted meat. One should not let them bathe in any hot water except that of thermal springs. One should keep them a little thirsty and make their bodies firm in any possible manner. *De extenuatione corporum pinguium.*[249]

٩٨ . من الأمراض السوداوية التي تحدث في الجلد الجرب وتقشّر الجلد . ومتى حدثت
في اللحم أو في العروق سُمّيت سـرطانا . والجذام ابتداء حدوثها عن خلط سوداوي .
فإذا امتدّ الزمان غلبت المرّة السوداء على الدم وحدث بأصحاب العلّة نتن وظهرت القروح
وتغيّر اللون . في مقالته في الأورام .

٩٩ . الرطوبــة التـي في المفاصل مخاطية ، وإذا كثرت حتّــى تبلّ اللحم التي حول
المفاصل أحدثت أوراما شبيهة بأورام أصحاب الاستسقاء . وقد عثّرت هذه الأورام قوما
من الأطبّاء حتّى بطّوها وظنّوا أنّ هناك مدّة . ولم يجدوها بل وجدوا اللحم كلّه الذي حول
المفصل مملوءا مخاطا . في الثامنة من شرحه لسادسة ابيديميا .

١٠٠ . الذبول الحاصل عن الحالة الشبيهة بالشيخوخة والذبول المسمّى المحترق
والذبول المسمّى ذا الغشي ، هذه الثلاثة حالات يلائمها اللبن وماء الشعير وطبيخ الخندروس
بالخلّ مثل ما يطبخ الشعير لينفـذ في الأعضاء . وأمّا ماء العسـل فإنّه نافع في الحالات
الباردة . في مقالته في الذبول .

١٠١ . كثرة اللحم والشحم مؤذية ضارّة يرى بها الجسم سمجا وتمنع الأفعال وتعوق
الحركات وينبغي لهم أن يسـتعملوا الأسفار وكثرة المشي في الشمس وخاصّة سفر البحر
لأنّ هـواء البحر يحلّل الرطوبات . وتغذوهم بأغذية قليلة الغذاء كالبقول وبما فيه حرارة
كالبصل والثوم والسمك المملوح . وبما يقوّي ولا يرطّب كالشـواء من لحوم غير سـمينة .
وتجنبهم الاستحمام بالماء الحارّ إلا ماء الحمّات وتعطشهم قليلا وتصلّب أبدانهم بكلّ وجه .
في مقالته في تهزيل الأجساد العبلة .

١ الجرب وتقشّـر الجلـد ] om. G || ٢ والجـذام ] أيضا add. ELOP || ٣ نـتن ] وهن
EsGOP || ٥ التـي ] الـذي ELOP || ٨ ابيديميا ] افيديميا ELP || ٩ والذبول المسمّى
المحترق ] om. L || ١٢ في مقالته في الذبول ] P¹ : في تلك المقالة ELP || ١٧ الاسـتحمام ]
الحميم EsGOP | الحمّات ] الحمّام O || ١٨ الأجساد ] الأجسام EL

102. Do not be frightened of the severity of illnesses when performing surgery; rather, consider whether these illnesses are dangerous and
serious or minor. For instance, you should not be frightened of a large
hernia and think that it is a serious illness. Rather, consider and know
that a hernia in which the membrane that covers the intestines and
stomach, namely the omentum, descends, is a serious and grave illness
although the size of the hernia may not be large. A hernia that encloses
water[250] is a minor illness, although it may reach a large size. And a hernia into which a portion of the intestines has descended is very grave and
serious. The same applies to the other illnesses. *De examinatione medici.*[251]

103. In order to stop the [superfluous] matters that stream to their
feet, patients suffering from podagra imbibe only the other medications
for their illness. But they do not cleanse the [superfluous] matters that
are [already] present in the painful limbs. And this is even worse for
them, for when the humors do not stream to that place, they circulate in
the body until they sometimes choke [that patient].[252] I have seen this
several times. Therefore, I advise anyone who suffers from this pain not
to drink those medications but rather to drink theriac. I have seen many
patients with this pain who constantly took this electuary and found
relief from their illness. *De theriaca ad Pisonem.*[253]

104. All dissolving medications have a hot temperament. One of
the effects of such a temperament is biting, and this occurs when the
medication is extremely hot. Therefore, be careful with using very hot
remedies amongst the remedies for dissolving [superfluous matter] in
the organ, especially when the affected organ is evidently cold.[254] For if
one uses such remedies to the extent that one adds biting to the illness of
the organ, not a small pain ensues from this, and every pain stimulates
and attracts [superfluous] matter. Therefore, [only] that remedy which is
moderately hot does not produce pain in such organs. When the organ
is markedly cold[255] or when it is deep inside the body and a strong dissolution is required, use an extremely hot remedy. *De arte parva.*[256]

١٠٢ . لا يهولك في أعمال اليد كبر الأمراض بل النظر في خطرها وقوتها وضعفها . من ذلك أنّه ليس ينبغي أن يهولك كبر القيلة وعظمها فتظنّها مرضا قويا بل تنظر وتعلم أنّ القيلة التي ينزل فيها الغشاء الذي على المعاء والمعدة وهو الثرب هو مرض قوي عظيم وإن كان حجمها ليس بعظيم . والقيلة التي هي ماء مرض يسير وإن كانت عظيمة الحجم . وأنّ القيلة التي نزل

٥ إليها شيء من الأمعاء أعظم وأقوى وكذلك في سائر الأمراض . في مقالته في محنة الطبيب .

١٠٣ . سائر الأدوية التي يستعملها أصحاب النقرس لمرضهم إنّما يشربوها لحسم الموادّ التي تنصبّ إلى أقدامهم . وليس ينقون بها ما يحصل من الموادّ في الأعضاء الآلة . وهذا عليهم أصعب لأنّ الأخلاط إذا لم تنصبّ إلى هناك تسري في البدن حتّى ربّما خنقت . وقد رأيت ذلك مرارا ولهذا أشير على من به هذا الوجع أن لا يشرب تلك الأدوية لكنّه

١٠ يشرب الترياق . وقد رأيت خلقا كثيرا ممّن به هذا الوجع شربوا هذا المعجون شربا دائما فاستراحوا من هذا السقم . في مقالته في الترياق إلى قيصر .

١٠٤ . الأدوية المحلّلة كلّها مزاجها حارّ ، ومن فعل هذا المزاج التلذيع إذا كان مفرط الحرارة . فقد ينبغي أن تحذر في الأدوية التي تحلّل بها في العضو استعمال الأدوية التي لها حرارة قوية ، لا سيّما إن كان العضو العليل باردا ظاهرا . فإنّك إن استعملت أشباه هذه الأدوية حتّى تجمع على العضو مع علّته التلذيع عرض فيه من الوجع أمر ليس باليسير . وكلّ

١٥ وجع يهيج ويجلب المادّة . فالدواء اذا الذي معه حرارة معتدلة هو الذي لا يحدث في مثل هذه الأعضاء وجعا وإن كان العضو البارز باردا أو كان في عمق البدن واحتجت إلى تحليل قوي ، فافعل بدواء شديد الحرارة . في الصناعة الصغيرة .

---

١ النظر] أنظر L || ٢ أنّ [(2nd)] بأنّ EL || ٣ وهو الثرب] والثرب EL | هو [(2nd)] هي EL || ٤ فيها] ed. Iskandar, p. 136, l.1 | ماء [om. ELO | سائر [om. G || ٥ محنة] امتحان EL | om. ELOOxP add. || ٦ سائر [om. L || ٧ وليس] ولا ELO || ١٦ وجع] فهو ELOOxP add.

105. The kind of shingles that is associated with corrosion[257] should be treated with remedies that are cooling but not moistening, just like the other kinds of shingles. But next to their cooling [properties] they should have drying [properties]. One should initially apply vine

5    tendrils[258] and offshoots of bramble[259] and plantain.[260] After this, one should mix these [same] ingredients with lentils and with some fine[261] honey and *sawīq* of barley.[262] *Ad Glauconem [de medendi methodo]* 2.[263]

106. The following noncorrosive remedies are applied for erysipelas and shingles: lettuce, knot-grass,[264] duckweed,[265] nenuphar,[266] seed of

10   fleawort,[267] purslane,[268] chicory, sempervivum,[269] and similarly, black nightshade.[270] *Ad Glauconem [de medendi methodo]* 2.[271]

107. Elephantiasis and a cancerous tumor can be healed at their onset by means of a constant evacuation of the melancholic humor and by prescribing the patient a regimen that produces good blood. The regi-

15   men plays a prominent role in this disease: for instance, we find that many people in Alexandria are stricken by elephantiasis because of their bad regimen and the heat of their place.[272] However, we do not find that this disease occurs in the land of Mysia save in an exceptional case. In the land of the Scyths, who feed themselves with milk, we have never seen

20   anyone afflicted by this disease. *Ad Glauconem [de medendi methodo]* 2.[273]

108. The nutrition of patients with elephantiasis or cancer should consist of barley gruel and whey, both of which should be consumed in abundance.[274] Of the vegetables they should eat marshmallow,[275] orache,[276] wild amaranth,[277] and gourd.[278] Among the fish they should

25   eat those that can be sighted amongst the rocks.[279] They may eat all [kinds of] birds, except water birds. The consumption of viper flesh is a wonderful remedy for patients suffering from elephantiasis, but it should be eaten once the head and tail have been severed, the abdomen cleansed, the skin stripped off, and the flesh boiled in a lot of water with some

30   olive oil, aneth,[280] and leek[281] until it is overdone. *Ad Glauconem [de medendi methodo]* 2.[282]

١٠٥ . مـا كان من النملـة معه تأكّل فتكون أدويته مبرّدة لا مرطّبة كسـائر أصناف النملـة ، بل يكون فيهـا مع تبريدهـا تجفيف . فتضـع عليها أوّلا أطـراف الكرم وأطراف العلّيق ولسـان الحمل ، ثمّ من بعد ذلك فاخلط بهذه العدس وشـيئا من العسـل في رقّته وسويق من الشعير . ثانية أغلوقن .

١٠٦ . الأدويـة التي توضع علـى الحمرة والنملة إلا أن تكون متأكّلة هي هذه : الخس وعصـا الراعي والطحلـب والنيلوفر وبزر قطونا والرجلة والهندبـاء وحيّ العالم وكذلك عنب الثعلب . ثانية أغلوقن .

١٠٧ . الجذام والورم السـرطاني في ابتدائهما يمكن بروئهما بمداومة استـقراغ الخلط السوداوي وتدبير صاحب العلّة تدبيرا يولد دما محمودا . فإنّ للتدبير في هذه العلّة أعظم حظّا . من ذلك أنّا نجد الجذام بإسـكندرية يصيب كثيرا من الناس لسوء تدبيرهم وحرارة بلدهـم ولا نجدها تحدث في بلاد موسـيا إلا في الفرط . وأمّا في بـلاد الصقالبة اللذين غذاءهم اللبن فلم نرى أحدا منهم أصابته هذه العلّة . ثانية أغلوقن .

١٠٨ . أغذية أصحاب الجذام والسـرطان أكثرها ماء كشك الشعير وماء الجبن ومن البقول الخبّاز والسرمق والبقلة اليمانية والقرع ومن السمك ما كان مراه في الصخور والطيور كلّهـا إلا طير الماء ، وأكل لحوم الأفاعى لأصحاب الجـذام دواء عجيب ينبغي أن يأكلوها بعد قطع رؤوسها وأذنابها وتنظيف بطونها وسلخها وطبخها بماء كثير وزيت يسير وشبثّ وكرّاث وتطبخ حتّى تتهرّأ . ثانية أغلوقن .

109. When someone is bitten by a scorpion and its sting gets fixed in[283] a nerve, or a pulsatile or nonpulsatile vessel, he is seized by very severe symptoms because the sting of the scorpion may penetrate deep into the body and pass through the entire skin. *De locis affectis* 3.[284]

5      110. I have often seen that the bodies of those who gave up sexual intercourse while they were used to it turned cold and that their movements became burdensome. Others were afflicted by sadness for no [evident] reason and evil thoughts.[285] The occurrence of this affliction is similar to what happens to those suffering from melancholic delusion.

10     All this occurs following the putrefaction of the retained sperm because it causes bad vapors to ascend. *De locis affectis* 6.[286]

111. When milk boiled in an iron vessel is mixed with heating substances such as tutty, it is beneficial for cancerous ulcers and alleviates their pain. *De [simplicium] medicamentorum [temperamentis ac facultatibus].*[287]

15     112. Amongst the most efficient oils for healing tautness of the skin is fresh aneth oil and oil of grape juice. They completely dissolve fatigue and relax [the skin] even if the fatigue is severe. Similarly, oil of pine seed is beneficial for severe fatigue. *De sanitate tuenda* 3.[288]

113. We have seen many perfectly healthy people—both young and

20     old—attacked by sudden heart palpitations. All of them benefited from venesection and a thinning diet. *De locis affectis* 5.[289]

114. I do not at all recommend treating organs from which blood is being emitted with cooling, astringent substances that are applied externally, because these substances push the blood inwards so that the

25     internal vessels are filled. I know people whose chests were cooled because of blood they spat up from the lungs; others, whose stomachs were cooled externally because of blood they vomited; and still others whose heads were cooled because of a nosebleed. [All] this clearly inflicted harm on them. One should only do this once the blood is tending to another

30     place or is attracted to the opposite side. *De methodo [medendi]* 5.[290]

١٠٩ . إذا لسعت إنسـانا عقرب ووقعت حمتها في عصبة أو في عرق ضارب أو غير ضارب عرضت لذلك الملسوع أعراض شديدة جدّا لأنّ حمة العقرب قد يمكن أن تبلغ إلى غور البدن وتنفذ الجلد كلّه . ثالثة التعرّف .

١١٠ . اللذيـن يتركون الجماع ممّن اعتـاده قد رأيتهم مرارا كثيرة تبرد أبدانهم وتعسر حركاتهم . ومنهم قوم حدثت لهم الكأبة بلا سـبب وسوء الفكر . وتوقّع البلاء مثل الذي يعرض لأصحاب الوسواس السوداوي . كلّ ذلك يتبع عفن ذلك المني المحتبس فإنّه قد يبخّر أبخرة رديئة . سادسة التعرّف .

١١١ . إذا خلط باللبن المطبوخ بالحديد بعض الأشياء المسخنة كالتوتيا نفع من القروح السرطانية وسكّن وجعها . عاشرة الأدوية .

١١٢ . من أبلغ الأدهان في شـفاء تكاثف الجلد دهن الشـبّث الطري ودهن عصير العنـب ، تحلّ الإعياء حلًّا تامّا وترخي ولو كان الإعياء قويا . وكذلك دهن حبّ الصنوبر يصلح للإعياء الشديد . ثالثة تدبير الصحّة .

١١٣ . اختلاج القلب رأيناه أصاب قوما بغتة أصحّاء لا يذمّ من صحّتهم شيئا شبابا وكهولا . وجميعهم انتفع بفصد العرق وتلطيف الغذاء . خامسة التعرّف .

١١٤ . لسـت أحمد حمدا مطلقا بتدبير الأعضاء التي ينبعث منها الدم بالأشياء المبـرّدة المقبّضة التي توضع من خارج لأنّها تدفع الدم للباطن فتملأ العروق الباطنة . وإنّي أعلـم قوما برّدوا صدورهم من أجل دم ينفثونه من الرئة ، وآخرين برّدوا معدهم من خارج من أجل دم يتقيّأونه ، وآخرين برّدوا روسهم من أجل الرعاف ، فأضرّ بهم ذلك ضررا بيّنا . وإنّما يعمل هذا بعد إمالة الدم إلى موضع آخر أو جذبه إلى خلاف الجهة . خامسة الحيلة .

115. When the affliction[291] of a nerve is accompanied by pain, one should treat it with a poultice prepared from bean[292] flour, vinegar, honey, and liquid pitch. This should be well cooked and applied while still hot. *De methodo [medendi]* 6.[293]

116. Those who are stricken by syncope because of the emaciation of their bodies and the severe weakening[294] of the pneuma should be nourished with foods that do not decay[295] rapidly, and bread and gruel from spelt, and astringent fruits that do not spoil easily, [given] sometimes alone and sometimes with bread. One should also feed them egg yolk and testicles of roosters. And finally one should thicken their humors and make their skin more dense. *De methodo [medendi]* 12.[296]

117. When an ulcer occurs on the side of a large vessel, whether it is pulsatile or not, the glands swell very rapidly,[297] and that vessel becomes completely visible in that part of the body; it is red and tense and painful upon touch. *De methodo [medendi]* 13.[298]

118. When glands begin to swell, begin from the first day to alleviate the pain and apply wool soaked in hot olive oil on them. When the body is full [of superfluities], heating substances attract them. If this is the case,[299] one should first of all use venesection or scarification on a part that is not affected and that is opposite to it.[300] When the illness is in the arm, the leg should be scarified; when it is in the leg, the arm should be scarified. But if one is slow[301] in purging the body, the glands will swell to the point of suppuration. *De methodo [medendi]* 13.[302]

١١٥ . إن كان مـع عـارض العصب وجـع فينبغي أن يـداوى بالضمـاد المتّخذ مـن دقيـق الباقلـى وخـلّ وعسـل وزفـت رطب ويطبـخ طبخـا جيّدا ويضمّد به وهو حارّ . سادسة الحيلة .

١١٦ . اللذين يعتريهم الغشي لسخافة أبدانهم وكثرة تحلّل الروح تغذوهم بأغذية لا تسرع التحلّل والخبز وحسو الخندروس ، والفاكهة القابضة التي يعسر فسادها مرّة وحدها ومـرّة بالخبـز . وتطعمه أيضا صفرة البيـض وخصى الديوك . وأتى أمـرك على أن تغلّظ الأخلاط وتكثّف الجلد . ثانية عشر الحيلة .

١١٧ . متـى حدثت قرحة إلى جانب عـرق عظيم ضاربـا كان أو غير ضارب فـإنّ اللحـم الرخو يرم في أسـرع الأوقات ويظهر ذلك العرق كلّه فـي العضو أحمر ممتدّا يوجع عند اللمس . ثالثة عشر الحيلة .

١١٨ . متـى ابتـدأ اللحم الرخو يرم فابتدئ من أوّل يوم بتسـكين الوجع وتضع عليه صوفا مبلولا بزيت حارّ . وإن كان البدن ممتلئا فالأشياء المسخنة تجذب له . ولذلك ينبغي أن يتقـدّم بفصد العرق أو بشرط عضو آخر ليس بعليل محاذيا له ، وإن كانت العلّة في اليد شرطت الساق أو في الساق شرطت اليد . ومتى فرّط في استفراغ البدن زاد ورم اللحم الرخو حتّى يؤول به الأمر إلى التقيّح . ثالثة عشر الحيلة .

---

١ مـع عـارض العصب] معرض العصب : OOxP عـرض فـي العصب L : يعـرض للعصب E ‖ ٤ تغذوهـم] فتغذوهـم ELOOxP ‖ ٥ والخبز] كالخبز ELOOxP ‖ ٦ وتطعمه] وتطعمهم ELO ‖ وأتى أمرك] وابني أمرك ELOxP : وأنا أمرك O ‖ ٨ عرق] Es² : عضو EsG ‖ ١١ من] في L ‖ يوم] om. G ‖ ١٤–١٥ في استفراغ . . . يؤول] G¹

119. The evacuation of a poison from someone bitten by an animal is effected by means of agents[303] that have a strong attractive force and that transform this poison.[304] Such a transformation is effected by medications that either change the quality of the poison or that dissolve its substance. Agents that have a strong attractive force without heating are cupping glasses and hollow horns.[305] Some people suck and attract the poison out of the bitten limb with their mouth. *De methodo [medendi]* 13.[306]

120. [For the treatment of] hard tumors, softening remedies should always be mixed with a discutient agent. Vinegar is good for that; it is the strongest remedy with which tendons and ligaments can be treated. But one should not use it continuously because an excessive use robs the humors from their thin and fine quality and makes that which remains as hard as stone. Moreover, when vinegar is used for a long time, it harms and damages the substance of the nerves. Therefore, it should not be used in the beginning of the disease nor for a prolonged time. *De methodo [medendi]* 14.[307]

When a cancer is in an initial stage, it can be cured especially by washed mineral remedies and by cleansing the body through purgation. But when the cancer[308] becomes large and this becomes evident, we try to prevent it from increasing [even further]. *De methodo [medendi]* 14.[309]

121. Gout and pains in the joints[310] should be treated first of all by the evacuation of the harmful chyme. Then one should first treat the hands and feet with detaining and restraining drugs.[311] But in the case of the hip joint, one should be careful not to use restraining and cooling remedies because it is situated at a deep spot and [this kind of treatment] would increase the overfilling.[312] Rather, following the evacuation, one should first of all alleviate the pain with agents that heat and do not cool, and the heat should not be [as] strong as [the heat of those agents that] one should apply in the end after excessive evacuation. *Mayāmir* 10.[313]

122. For ischias, emesis is more beneficial than purging [the bowels] because it attracts the matters that cause the disease. Do this first of all by means of food[314] and then give emetics—begin with the mildest and lightest. But if the humors get stuck there and are difficult to dissolve because of sharp medications that the physicians initially used and that hardened and roasted the [superfluous] matter, cupping glasses are very beneficial. The same holds good for purging [the bowels] by means of sharp purgative clysters that contain colocynth and the like. *Mayāmir* 10.[315]

١١٩. استفراغ ســمّ الحيوان من المنهوش بالأدوية التي تجذب جذبا شديدا وأحالته ونقله عمّا هو عليه إمّا بأدوية تغيّر كيفية السمّ أو بأدوية تحلّ جوهره. والذي يجذب جذبا قويا من غير إسخان المحاجم والقرون المجوّفة. ومن الناس من يمتصّ السمّ ويجذبه بفمه من العضو الملسوع. ثالثة عشر الحيلة.

١٢٠. الـورم الصلب يخلط مع أدويته الملّينة أبدا مـا يقطع. والخلّ جيّد لذلك وهو ٥ أقوى ما عولجت به الوترات والرباطات ولا تدمن استعماله فإنّ الخلّ إذا أفرط في استعماله ســلب من الأخلاط رقيقها ولطيفها ويحجّر البقية، مع أنّه إذا اسـتعمل زمانا طويلا أضرّ بجوهر العصب وأنكاه فلا تستعمله لا في ابتداء العلّة ولا زمانا طويلا. أخيرة الحيلة.

السـرطان في ابتداء كونه إنّما يبرأ بالأدوية المعدنية المغسـولة ونفض البدن بالإسهال.

وأمّا إذا عظم السرطان ويتبيّن أمره فقصدنا فيه أن نمنعه من التزيّد. أخيرة الحيلة. ١٠

١٢١. تبتدئ في علاج النقرس وأوجاع المفاصل باسـتفراغ الكيموس المؤذي وبعد ذلك تعالج اليدين والرجلين في أوّل الأمـر بالأدوية التي تمنع وتـردع. أمّا مفصل الورك فإيّـاك من ردعه وتبريده لأنّ موضعه غائـر ويزداد امتـلاء، بل تسـكّن الوجع أوّلا بعد الاسـتفراغ بما يسـخن ولا يبرّد ولا يسـخن إسـخانا قويا كما تفعل في آخر الأمر بعد المبالغة في الاستفراغ. عاشرة الميامر. ١٥

١٢٢. القيء أنفع في عرق النساء من الإسهال لجذبه المواد الفاعلة للعلّة. وتستعمله في أوّل الأمر بعد الطعام، ثمّ بعد ذلك بالأدوية التي تهيج القيء وتبتدئ بليّنها وأخفّها. وإن لجّت الأخلاط هناك وعسر انحلالها بسبب ما استعمله الأطبّاء في أوّل الأمر من الأدوية الحادّة التي حجّرت المادّة وشـوتها فالمجمجة تنفع حينئذ منفعة عظيمة جدّا، والإسـهال بالحقن المسهلة الحادّة التي يقع فيها شحم الحنظل ونحوه. عاشرة الميامر. ٢٠

---

٣ والقرون] والعروق G || ١٤ يسـخن] يسـكّن EsG || ٨٧,٧–٨٥,١٧ ثمّ . . . وللّه الحمد والمنّة [ELOOxP | بعد] من بعد P .om

123. In [his book entitled] *al-Murshid,* al-Tamīmī mentions the following way of treating a hernia before it becomes chronic. He said: Take two *mithqāls*[316] of savin fruit,[317] one *mithqāl* of its leaves, two *dirhams*[318] of fresh asphodel[319] flour, and one *mithqāl* of acacia. Knead these ingredients with dissolved fish glue and spread the [compound] while it is hot on a linen cloth. At the end of the bathhouse procedures, put it on the hernia on an empty stomach and lying down. On the cloth put padding, bandage it, and let the patient sleep on his back until the compress dries. Leave it bandaged for forty days. Every day let the patient drink [a potion prepared from] two parts of pulverized and strained savin fruit and one part of pulverized and strained savin leaves. From this [potion] he should drink two *dirham*s daily with one ounce[320] of myrtle[321] juice and sugar.

He further said: When one cooks extract of apricot leaves and uses this as a gargle, it is beneficial for a swelling of the uvula, throat, and tonsils. It dissolves and eliminates all the inflamed tumors occurring in the mouth, gums, and uvula.[322]

124. The therapy for a bone fracture should, after necessary surgery, consist of an extremely thinning diet. It is often first of all necessary to purge the bowels with a remedy. While the fracture heals, one should feed the patient with food that has good chymes and that is nutritious and viscous. The external remedies should be those that by their substance cause to adhere, cleave, and stick, and that heat slightly and dry moderately. *De methodo [medendi]* 6.[323]

125. If part of an inflamed tumor remains in an organ [after treatment], sharp remedies cause more irritation and swelling than dissolution. When the remaining part of an inflamed tumor has turned hard, use strong remedies with assurance and confidence. *De methodo [medendi]* 13.[324]

126. Sometimes, for tumors on hands and feet, it is sufficient to put a sponge on them with cold water and a little vinegar or astringent wine. As for tumors of the liver, do not put anything cold upon them; rather, cook quinces in wine and apply this lukewarm as a poultice in the beginning of the tumor. The same [benefit is derived] from a fomentation with quince oil or myrtle oil or mastic oil or nard oil or absinthe.

١٢٣ . ذكر التميمي في المرشد هذا النحو من علاج الفتق قبل أن يزمن . قال : يؤخذ جوز أبهل منقالان وورقه مثقال، إشراس حديث درهمين، أقاقيا مثقال . يعجن ذلك بغرى السمك محلولا ويبسط وهو حارّ على خرقة كتّان ويجعل على الفتق عند الخروج من الحمّام على الريق وهو مستلق . ويجعل على الخرقة رفادة ويقمط وينام على ظهره حتّى تجفّ اللزقة، ويبقى بقماطه أربعين يوم . ويشرب في كلّ يوم جوز أبهل جزء‌ان وورق أبهل جزء مسحوقين منخولين . يشرب منها وزن درهمين كلّ يوم بأوقية ماء آس وسكّر .

وقال إنّ عصير ورق المشمش إذا طبخ وتغرغر به نفع من ورم اللهاة والحلق واللوزتين ويحلّل جميع ما يعرض للفم واللثة واللهاة من الأورام الحارّة ويذهب بها .

١٢٤ . تدبير كسر العظام بعد ما تحتاج‌إليه من أعمال اليد أن تدبّر المريض بتدبير ملطّف في الغاية . وكثيرا ما تحتاج إلى إسهال البطن بدواء في الابتداء . فأمّا وقت تولّد الدشبد فتغذوه بغذاء جيّد الكيموس، كثير الغذاء لزج، والأدوية التي من خارج ما يتشبّث ويعلق ويشدّ بجوهره ويسخن قليلا ويجفّف باعتدال . سادسة الحيلة .

١٢٥ . متى بقي من الورم الحارّ في العضو بقيّة فإنّ الأدوية الحادّة تهيج وتنفر أكثر ممّا تحلّل . فإن كانت بقية الورم الحارّ قد صلبت فاستعمل الأدوية القوية بثقة واتكال . ثالثة عشر الحيلة .

١٢٦ . قد يكتفى في أورام اليدين والرجلين بأن يوضع عليها إسفنجة بماء بارد ويسير خلّ أو شراب قابض . أمّا أورام الكبد فلا يجعل عليها شيء بارد بل يطبخ سفرجل بشراب ويضمّد به وهو فاتر في ابتداء الورم . وكذلك نطول دهن السفرجل أو دهن آس أو دهن مصطكى

---

١٠ الدشبد] الجبر ELOOxP ‖ ١٢ من] في G ‖ ١٦ بماء بارد] Es² : باردة ESG

But none of these should be used cold, nor should any oily substance be used for tumors of the eyes or mouth. Sometimes rose oil and vinegar can be used as eardrops. *De methodo [medendi]* 13.[325]

127. Says Moses: In the ninth treatise of his *Book on Animals*, Aristotle has written a chapter that is very useful for medical practice. In my opinion Galen has not brought up the matter that I am going to mention now, nor has he drawn attention to it. It is the following statement of Aristotle. He said: Normally spasms mostly occur to babies, especially to those who are well nourished and who suck much milk that is very fat and whose wet-nurses are well-fleshed. In this case an excess of milk is harmful.[326]

*This is the end of the ninth treatise,*
*by the grace of God, praise be to Him.*

◆

أو دهن الناردين أو أفسنتين . ولا يستعمل شيء من ذلك باردا ولا يستعمل في مداواة أورام

العينين أو الفم شيء من الأدهان . وقد يقطّر في الأذنين دهن ورد وخلّ . ثالثة عشر الحيلة .

١٢٧ . قال موسى : قد ذكر أرسطوطاليس في آخر المقالة التاسعة من كتاب الحيوان

فصــلا نافعــا جدّا في أعمال الطبّ ولم أر جالينوس في ما أذكره الآن من كلامه ألمّ بذلك

المعنى ولا نبّه عليه . وهذا هو قول أرسطو قال : قد جرت العادة بأن يعرض لأكثر الصبيان

التشــنّج وخاصّة من كان منهم غذاءه غذاء جيّدا ويرضع لبنا كثيرا شديد السمن وكانت

مرضعاته خصبات الأبدان وكثرة اللبن تضرّ في ذلك . تمّت المقالة التاسعة ولله الحمد والمنّة .

---

٢ أو الفم] G¹ | دهن] G¹ | G¹ ‖ ٤ اذكره] ذكره O ‖ ٦ وكانت] وكانوا ELO ‖ ٧ تمّت . . .
والمنّة] om. O : كملت المقالة التاسعة والحمد لله كثيرا وعدد فصولها مائة واثنين وثلاثين فصلا EL

# Supplement

*Critical comparison of the Arabic text with the*
*Hebrew translations and the translation into English*

**6.4:** العطاس في الأمراض المزمنة عن أمراض الصدر والرئة علامة جيّدة ("Sneezing in the case of chronic diseases except for diseases of the chest and lungs is a good sign"). **N** translates this as: העטוש בחלאים הנושנים, לצד חליי החזה והריאה, הוא אות טוב. The translation of לצד for عن is explained by **m** in a note as meaning יוצא מן הכלל ("except for"). **R**, disregarding this note, interprets צד as: חולי הצד ("pleurisy") and translates: "Sneezing in chronic illnesses of the side ("pleuritis") and in illnesses of the chest and lungs is a favorable sign." **Z**, using בלתי for عن, translates the Arabic correctly as: העיטוש בחליים הארוכים בלתי חליי החזה והריאה הוא סימן טוב.

**6.11:** قد يتركّب الوسواس السوداوي والسرسام ("Sometimes melancholic delusion and phrenitis occur together"). **N**'s correct transcription for يتركّب, namely, יתרכב is read by **m** as: יתרבה ("to increase"). Following **m**, **R** translates: "Sometimes melancholic confusion of the mind is greatly increased and this is (called) phrenesia."

**6.17:** بالأغذية المغلّظة ("by means of fattening kinds of food"). **N** has: במזונות המעטים ("through a few foods") instead of the correct: במזונות המעבים. Thus **R** translates: "By eating little food." **Z** has a correct version: במזון אשר יעבה.

**6.21:** الحيات في البطن ("worms in the belly"). حيات can mean both "snakes" and "worms": **N**, translating it as: נחשים has obviously chosen the wrong meaning in our context. **Z** translates it correctly as: תולעים.

**6.26**: ينكر ("he will not believe it"). **N** transcribes the term as ינכר. **m** reads this incorrectly as יכבד. Consequently, **R** translates: "it is hard for him." **Z** translates it as: ירחיק.

**6.31**: الّذان لا يكون الغطيط إلا بهما ("which are the only ways through which snoring takes place"). Reading الغطيط إلا بهما as: لعادتهما **N** translates this sentence as: אשר לא תהיה על מנהגו. Consequently, **R** translates: "which is not usually one's habit." **Z** does not translate the terms misread by **N**.

**6.34**: ويدار بهم ("he is turned around"). **N**'s correct Hebrew translation: ויקף בהם is corrupted by **m** as: ויקיא בהם. This is translated by **R** as: "vomits."

**6.37**: فضل تهجّم وجرأة ("very aggressive and insolent behavior"). Reading لجاره instead of جرأة **N** translates the sentence as: יתרון גערה לשכניו. This is translated by **R** as: "search for conflict with neighbors." **Z** omits this section.

**Ibid.**: خشونة اللسان ("roughness of the tongue"). **N**'s correct translation: נחירות הלשון is corrupted by **m** as: לכידות הלשון. This is translated by **R** as: "licking of the tongue." **Z** translates: נסות הלשון.

**6.41**: حرّك الأعضاء ("it moves the organs"). **N**'s correct translation for حرّك, namely, מניע from a root נוע is read by **R** as: מונע from a root מנע. Hence his translation: "it prevents these organs."

**6.55**: معلّقا من الجانب الأيمن ("inherent to the right side"). **N** has a corrupt version תחלה for معلّقا that has been corrected in the margin as: תתלה. **m** adopting the corrupt version reads: תחלה מן הצד הימני. This is translated by **R** as: "first . . . on the right side." **Z** has the correct version: תלוי.

**Ibid.**: في خلقتها ("in its natural structure"). **N** translates this as: ביציאתו and **R** as: "its exits." **Z** has the correct version: בטבעו.

**6.78**: وإن كان الدم صديدا ("if the blood is serous"). **N** reading the Arabic صديدي as صدئ ("rusty") translates: וכשיהיה הדם חלודי. Accordingly, **R** translates: "If the blood is rust-colored." **Z** translates the term correctly as: מוגליי ("cf. Supplement, *Medical Aphorisms* 5.11").

**6.79**: Idem.

**6.83:** وهذان علامتان لا يكونان في شيء من قروح الأمعاء ("These two prognostic signs do not occur in any intestinal ulcer"). **N** translates: ואלו הם שני אותות שאינן כלום מנגעי המעים. It is clear that he has not translated the particle في. Therefore, **R** misunderstands the sentence as: "These two diagnostic signs indicate there is no affliction in the intestines."

**6.94:** وبذلت أخسّ الأفعال ("and gives up the activity that is least important"). Reading وبذلت as بدلت and أخسّ as الحقّ **N** translates: ויחליף משפט הפעולות. This is translated by **R** as: "which then reverses these (adverse) effects." **Z** reads وبذلت, just like **N** as بدلت and أخسّ as أخصّ, and accordingly translates: והחליף המיוחד שבפעולות.

**7.7:** يجلبها للعضو دما وروحا معا ("by attracting blood and air together to the [affected] organ"). Not reading يجلبها but يغلبها **N** translates: בהתגבר על האבר דם ורוח יחד. This is translated by **R** as: "in that blood and pneuma overpower the affected organ." **Z** gives a similar version as **N**—namely, בגבור.

**7.8:** وأعجب من هذا ("And [even] more amazing than this"). Not reading أعجب as a comparative but as an Imperfect 1 comm. sing. **N** translates: ואני מופלא מזה and **R**: "I am greatly astonished." **Z** translates the term correctly as: ויותר זר מזה.

**7.15:** ويزيل الكدر عن روحه ("and to remove the turbidity from its air"). Translating الكدر faultily as הסתימה **N** reads: ומסיר הסתימה מכלי הרוח. This is translated by **R** as: "and clear the obstruction from the respiratory passages." **Z** has a correct translation: ויסיר העכירות מרוחו.

**7.29:** كما أنّ خلط البلغم الغليظ قد يحدث عنه الصرع كذلك الخلط السوداوي قد يحدث عنه الصرع ("Just as a thick phlegmatic humor can produce epilepsy, so a melancholic humor can produce epilepsy"). Reading الصداع ("headache") instead of الصرع ("epilepsy"), **N** translates it as כאב הראש ("headache") and **R** has: "Thick, viscous humor causes headache. And all thick black humors cause headaches." **Z** has the correct version חולי האלצרע בלעז וויציאו ("the disease of epilepsy called **vicio** in Romance").

**7.35:** كان اتّباع الأخلاط له أسرع ("it is followed by delirium more quickly"). Reading الأخلاط as الأخلاط ("humors") **N** translates: ליחות. Consequently, **R** translates: "humors are attracted to it . . . more rapidly"). **Z** translates the term correctly as: בלבול.

**7.36:** فيحدث التّمانع ("and because he cannot . . ."). N's faulty translation: ויתחדש התנועה is probably a copyist's mistake for: ויתחדש המניעה. R translates it as: "and this movement." Z has the correct version: ויתחדש המניעה.

**7.37:** عسى أن يكون منشأ كلّ واحد من الأعصاب يبّل بتلك الرطوبة الغليظة اللزجة ("possibly occurring when the origin of each nerve is moistened by that thick and viscous moisture"). Taking a secondary meaning of يبّل, "to be healed," N translates it as מתרפא and R translates: "It is as if the sprouting of every nerve is healed by those viscous humors." Galen's text actually intends to convey the opposite message, that spasms are caused by moisture affecting the origin of the nerves. Z translates يبّل as יתבטל ("to be abolished"), thus deriving it from بطل.

**7.47:** وإمّا ضيق وضغط في طريق الهواء ومخّرقه ("narrowness and pressure in the respiratory passages"). N, reading ومخّرقه as ومختّنقه ("and its choking"), translates: בדרך האויר ומחנקו as في طريق الهواء ومخّرقه, and R translates, following N: "and compression of the respiratory passages causing choking." Z, regarding طريق and مخّرق as synonymous, translates correctly: בדרך האויר ("in the respiratory passage").

**7.69:** وإن غلظت نقصت خلوص البصر ("When this humor becomes thick, the clarity of vision is diminished"). N, reading خروج instead of خلوص, translates this sentence as וכשתתעבה יחסר יציאות הראות, and R translates this as "If it becomes thick, outgoing vision is diminished." Z's translation החסר הראות ("vision is impaired"), although more accurate than that of N, does not account for خلوص.

**Ibid.:** عاقت البصر ("it makes vision impossible"). N corrupts this as: שיצר הראות. This is translated by R as: "which gives rise to vision." Z translates correctly: ימנע הראות.

**8.7:** المرض الذي يعسر نضجه ليس يظهر لما يعالجه به منفعة بتّة إلا بعد زمان طويل ("When a disease is hard to cook, the benefit of the therapy becomes apparent only after a long time"). N translates the first part as החולי אשר יקשה לבטלו ("A disease that is hard to eliminate"). N's reading לבטלו ("to annul it") for نضجه is probably a corruption of לבשלו ("to cook it"). Following N, R translates: "Concerning a protracted illness [a note here reads, 'Literally: which is difficult to eliminate'] one does not observe any immediate benefit from the therapy employed but only after a prolonged period." **Z** translates this part correctly as החולי אשר יקשה להתבשל ("A disease that is hard to cook").

**8.9**: وإن جهلت ذلك فليس تخلو من أن تضرّ المريض مضرّة عظيمة ("For if one does not know this, one is not free from inflicting great harm upon the patient"). **N** reads تضرّ as تُضادّ ("to oppose") or تُضادّ, and مضرّة as مضادّة, and translates the second part of the sentence as לא תמנע מלנגד לחולה התנגדות גדולה ("one will unavoidably greatly oppose the patient"). Although **m** gives a correct interpretation of this sentence, "you cannot prevent causing great pain to the patient," **R** corrupts it as: "If one pays heed thereto, one will not at any given time withhold a powerful antidote from the patient," interpreting התנגדות as "antidote." **Z** translates this part correctly as לא תמלט מהיותך מזיק לחולה הזק גדול ("You will unavoidably cause great harm to the patient").

**9.4**: السدد ("the obstruction"). **N**, reading السدر ("vertigo") instead of السدد ("the obstruction"), translates: ערבוב הראש, and **R** translates this as: "mental perturbation." **Z** translates السدد correctly as הסיתומים.

**9.23**: الصرع والسبات إنّما تكون من الدماغ ("Epilepsy and torpor only originate from the brain"). **N** does not read الصرع but الصداع ("headache"), and thus translates: כאב הראש והתרדמה הם ההווים מן המוח, and **R**, following **N**, translates the text wrongly as "Headache and stupor originate in the brain." **Z** translates الصرع correctly as הוויציאו (see 7.29).

**9.24**: وتشنّج الصرع والأرق جريان منكر ("while an epileptic spasm and sleeplessness are a disturbance"). **N** reads جريان as جيران and accordingly translates: שכנים ("neighbors"), while **Z**, reading it as غريبان, translates: זרים ורחוקים ("strange and distant"). Following **N**, **R** translates: "and epileptic seizures and insomnia are neighbors."

**9.30**: الثلج الصيني ("saltpeter"). **N** faultily transcribes the Arabic term as אלבלח אל צ'יני which is interpreted by **m** as referring to the element called "beryllium" (p. 129, n. 98); **R** transcribes the Hebrew as "elbalach elsini." **Z** corrupts the Arabic term as הבלוח הצ'יני.

**Ibid.**: الزجاج الفرعوني ("glass of Pharaoh"). **N** corrupts this as (= פרעוני) זהנ פרפוני and **m** (p. 130, n. 102) interprets this as "zibaq" ("mercury"), "zāj" ("vitriol"), or "zāj qubruṣi" ("Cyper vitriol"). **R** translates this as "types of vitriol of cyper." **Z** correctly translates the first part of the term as זכוכית and transcribes the second term as פרעוני.

**9.31:** وأهل المدن الباردة قلّ ما يرمدون وإذا رمدوا كان رمدهم شديدا صعبا تتصدّع فيه العين ("Inhab-itants of cold countries rarely suffer from ophthalmia, but if they suffer from it, it is severe and hard whereby the eyes are ruptured"). **N**, reading تتصدّع as تتصعّب, translates the last part as וחזק ממנה העין ("the eye is strengthened by this"); **m** (p. 130, n. 110) interprets this as: יתחדשו כיבים ("ulcers will arise"). **R**, following **m**, translates: "People in cold lands seldom suffer from ophthalmia but, when it does occur, it is strong and hard and produces ulcers in the eye."

**9.39:** إصلاح الأخلاط الردئة وهم القوم الذين يقولون إنّ طعم ريقهم كطعم ماء البحر يحتاج إلى زمان طويل . ولذلك من أصابته من هؤلاء قرحة رئة فإنّه لا بروء له بتّة لأنّ بطول الزمان حتّى تصلح الأخلاط تجفّ القرحة وتصلب حتّى لا تقبل البروء: ("The amelioration of bad humors in the case of those who say that their sputum tastes like sea water takes a long time. Therefore, if someone is because of these [bad humors] afflicted with an ulcer in the lungs he cannot be healed at all. For in the long time that it takes for the humors to become better, the ulcer becomes so dried up and hardened that it cannot be cured [any more]"). **N** does not read لأنّ بطول الزمان ("because...") but إلا بطول الزمان, and accordingly translates it as: אלא באורך הזמן ("except after a long time"), thereby upsetting the central meaning of the sentence. The same holds true for **R**'s translation, dependent on **N**: "The amelioration of bad humors at the time when people claim that the taste of their sputum is like the taste of sea water requires a prolonged period. There-fore, one who is afflicted with sores of the lung cannot be healed except after a long time, until the liquids become localized and the ulcers and boils become dried up and hard." **Z** translates the crucial Arabic لأنّ بطول الزمان correctly as כי באורך הזמן ("because in the lengthy period").

**9.53:** وتنخس صدورهم ("and prick their chests"). **N**'s reading: ותנשב חזיהם is probably a corruption by a copyist of ותנשך חזיהם. It is translated by **R** as: "apply pressure on their chests" ("note 132: 'artificial respiration'"). **Z** translates correctly: ותנשוך חזיהם.

**9.114:** لست أحمد حمدا مطلقا بتدبير الأعضاء التي ينبعث منها الدم بالأشياء المبرّدة المقبّضة ("I do not at all commend to treat the organs from which blood is being

emitted with cooling, astringent substances that are applied externally"). **N**'s version אני משבח ("I do commend") instead of איני משבח
("I do not approve of") disregards the central لست. It is the basis for
**R**'s faulty translation: "I completely agree to cool the limbs from which
blood was removed with the external application of cooling substances
that are also astringent." The next part of the text clearly shows why
Galen condemns such a treatment, because in some cases it can be
very harmful: "I know people whose chests were cooled because of
blood they spitted up from the lungs; others whose stomachs were
cooled because of blood they vomited; still others whose heads were
cooled because of a nosebleed. [All] this clearly inflicted harm on
them." The translation "from which blood was removed," which is
explained by **R** as occurring by "hemorrhage and venesection" (n. 316),
and which is based on **m**'s note 424 (p. 148), is incorrect. The loss of
blood is the result of an internal affliction, as the text clearly shows.
**Z** translates لست أحمد حمدا مطلقا correctly as איני משבח שבח מוחלט.[1]

**9.115**: إن كان مع رض العصب وجع ("When an affliction of a nerve is accompanied by pain"). **N** does not read رض but عرض ("width") and thus translates: רוחב (העצב) ("the width of the nerve"); **m** interprets this as
"neuritis or pain in the length of the nerve" (p. 149, n. 431). Following **N** and **m**'s interpretation, **R** translates: "If the length of a nerve
is painful." **Z**'s translation of the Arabic אם יהיה עם ריצוץ העצבים כאב
("When a contusion of the nerves is accompanied by pain"), shows
that he consulted an Arabic manuscript that preserved the correct
version رض.

**9.118**: ومتى فرط في استفراغ البدن زاد ورم اللحم الرخو ("But if one is slow in purging
the body, the glands will swell"). The Arabic term *farraṭa* can mean
both to "be slow" and to "be excessive" in something. Since in our text
it stands for the Greek βραδύνω, it cannot mean anything else but "to
be slow." However, both Nathan and Zeraḥyah understand this term
as "to be excessive" by translating: וכשתפליג and וכשיתרבה respectively.
Following **N**, **R** translates: "If one excessively purges the body, soft
tissue abscess formation becomes worse."

---

1. A marginal gloss reads נמוד for מוחלט.

# Notes to the English Text

## Translator's Introduction

1. See Maimonides, *Aphorisms: Treatises 1–5*, ed. Bos, xx.
2. See Langermann, "Fūṣūl Mūsā."
3. Davidson, *Moses Maimonides*, 443–52.
4. I thank Dr. Binyamin Richler for this information.
5. See Maimonides, *Shemirat ha-beriʾut leha-Rambam*, ed. Amar.
6. For Maimonides' biographical and bibliographical data, see the introductions to Maimonides, *On Asthma*, ed. Bos, and Maimonides, *Aphorisms: Treatises 1–5*, ed. Bos.
7. For another aphorism based on this text, see aphorism 7.71 in this volume; see as well the introduction to Maimonides, *Aphorisms: Treatises 1–5*, ed. Bos.
8. Cf. Larrain, "Galen, *De motibus dubiis*."
9. See Muntner's edition of the Hebrew translation by Nathan ha-Meʾati: Maimonides, *Pirḳe Mosheh*, aphorism 1.
10. Cf. Maimonides, *Aphorisms*, trans. Rosner, aphorism 1.
11. Galen, "Die ps.-galenische," ed. Nabielek, 29.
12. See comparative table in Nabielek, "Über Schlaf und Wachsein," 33–34.
13. Cf. Galen, *De libris propriis* (ed. Kühn, 19:8–48); Ibn Isḥāq, *Galen-Übersetzungen;* idem, *Galen-Bibliographie;* Steinschneider, "Griechischen Ärzte"; Meyerhof, "Schriften Galens"; Strohmaier, "Syrische und arabische Galen."
14. Galen, *De victu attenuante*, ed. Kalbfleisch.
15. For other quotations from this treatise, see aphorisms 6.24, 70, 71 in this volume.
16. Cf. note 6.
17. See Bos, "Recovered Fragment."
18. Deichgräber, *Hippokrates' De humoribus*, 43.
19. Deichgräber, *Hippokrates' De humoribus*, 45.
20. Cf. aphorism 8.55, this volume; Deichgräber, *Hippokrates' De humoribus*, 51.
21. See "Die Exzerpte des Moses Maimonides aus den Epidemienkommentaren des Galen," in addenda to the various volumes of Galen, *In Hippocratis Epidemiarum*, ed. Wenkebach.

22. See aphorism 7.59 in this volume.

23. I.e., a bain-marie.

24. Cf. Goitein, *Community,* 2:253.

25. See the introduction to Maimonides, *On Asthma,* ed. Bos. For the meaning of the term *Maghreb* in Maimonides' works, see aphorism 8.69 in this volume.

26. Maimonides, *On Asthma,* ed. Bos, 13.33.

27. See Maimonides, *On Asthma,* ed. Bos, 12.9, 12.10.

28. Galen, *De methodo medendi* (ed. Kühn, 10:844).

29. Galen, *De methodo medendi* (ed. Kühn, 10:850).

30. See Pertsch, *Orientalischen Handschriften,* 3:477–78; Kahle, "Aphoris-morum Praefatio et Excerpta," 89–90.

31. Other sections missing are 20.30–33 and 25.56–58.

32. See the remark by the scribe at the end of **G**, treatise 24 (fol. 239a): "Something like the following was written at the end of this treatise: This is what I found in the copy written by Abū [ . . . ]: I did not make a fair copy of this treatise until after his death, may God have mercy on him, and [A]bū al-Zakāt the physician wrote: Praise be to God, who is exalted."

33. See Pertsch, *Orientalischen Handschriften,* 3:477–78; Kahle, "Aphorismo-rum praefatio et excerpta," 90; Kaufmann, "Neveu de Maïmonide," 152–53; Sirat, "Liste de manuscrits," 112; Meyerhof, "Medical Work," 276; Kraemer, "Maimonides Letters," 2:79–80 n. 93; Maimonides, *"Treatise to a Prince,"* ed. Stern, 18.

34. Cf. Schacht and Meyerhof, "Maimonides against Galen," 59; Mai-monides, *Aphorisms,* trans. Rosner, xiv.

35. See Voorhoeve, comp., *Handlist,* 85.

36. See Dozy, *Supplément aux dictionnaires arabes,* 1:836; Kahle, "Praefatio et Excerpta," 90–91.

37. Zotenberg, ed., *Catalogues des Manuscrits,* 223; Vajda, *Index general,* 345.

38. See Derenbourg and Renaud, *Medécine et histoire,* vol. 2, fasc. 2, pp. 74–75; Cano Ledesma, *Manuscritos árabes,* p. 65, no. 33; Koningsveld, "Andalusian-Arabic Manuscripts," 102 n. 87.

39. See Derenbourg and Renaud, *Medécine et histoire,* vol. 2, fasc. 2, p. 76; Cano Ledesma, *Manuscritos árabes,* p. 65, no. 33.

40. See Neubauer, *Hebrew Manuscripts,* no. 2113 (p. 721); see also Beit-Arié and May, *Supplement,* col. 392.

41. Beit-Arié and May, *Supplement,* col. 392, states that Steinschneider refers to "a physician by the name of Makhluf of Marsala, Syracuse (Sicily)."

42. Galen, *De usu partium* 12.3 (ed. Helmreich, 2:188 line 4).

43. See Neubauer, *Hebrew Manuscripts,* no. 2114 (p. 721); Beit-Arié and May, *Supplement,* col. 392.

44. See Neubauer, *Hebrew Manuscripts,* no. 2115 (p. 722); Beit-Arié and May, *Supplement,* col. 392.

45. See Langermann, *Synochous Fever,* 185 n. 24.

46. See Kahle, *Aphorismorum praefatio et excerpta,* 89.

47. See Ullmann, *Medizin im Islam,* 167 n. 4. I was unable to obtain photo-copies of this manuscript.

48. Maimonides, *Treatise to a Prince*, ed. Stern, 18; cf. comments by Joshua Blau, ibid., n. 6.

49. See Hopkins, *Languages of Maimonides*, 90.

50. Meyerhof, "Medical Works," 272.

51. Blau, *Judaeo-Arabic*, 41; cf. Baron, *High Middle Ages*, 403 n. 42.

52. Langermann, "Arabic Writings," 139.

53. Ibn Sahl, *Dispensatorium parvum*, ed. Kahl, 35–38.

54. Maimonides, *Pirke Mosheh*, ed. Muntner.

55. Nathan ha-Meʾati (from Cento) prepared this translation in Rome between 1279 and 1283. For his data see Vogelstein and Rieger, *Juden in Rom*, 1:398–400; Steinschneider, *Hebräischen Übersetzungen*, 766.

56. Maimonides, *Aphorisms*, trans. Rosner.

57. See Zotenberg, *Catalogues*, 215.

58. For Zeraḥyah's versions I consulted manuscripts Berlin, Or. Qu 512, and Munich 111. On Zeraḥyah, who was active as a translator in Rome and who prepared the translation of the *Medical Aphorisms* in 1279, see Vogelstein and Rieger, *Juden in Rom*, 1:271–75, 409–18; Ravitzky, "Mishnato shel R. Zeraḥyah," 69–75; Aristotle, *De Anima*, ed. Bos, ch. 7: "Zeraḥyah's Technique of Translation."

## The Sixth Treatise

1. "fastest [killing]": "severest," in **O**.

2. "difficulty": lit., "aversion, coercion." Cf. Galen, *In Hippocratis Aphorismos commentarius* 2.42 (ed. Kühn, 17B:541), which reads μετὰ βίας (with violence); and see Endress and Gutas, *GALex*, 2:188–89, par. 8: "ᶜasirun muʾdin."

3. Galen, *In Hippocratis Aphorismos commentarius* 2.42 (ed. Kühn, 17B:541).

4. Cf. Galen, *In Hippocratis Aphorismos commentarius* 4.34 (ed. Kühn, 17B:703), which reads ἢ διὰ ψύξιν ἰσχυρὰν τῆς ζωτικῆς ἀρχῆς.

5. Galen, *In Hippocratis Aphorismos commentarius* 4.34 (ed. Kühn, 17B:703).

6. Greek παραφρόσυνη. Galen, *In Hippocratis Aphorismos commentarius* 6.53 (ed. Kühn, 18A:91).

7. "by worry and fear": μετὰ σπουδῆς, in Galen, *In Hippocratis Aphorismos commentarius* 6.53 (ed. Kühn, 18A:91). See also Hippocrates, *Aphorisms* 6.53 (trans. Jones): "seriousness."

8. Galen, *In Hippocratis Aphorismos commentarius* 6.53 (ed. Kühn, 18A:91).

9. Galen, *In Hippocratis Prognostica commentarius* 2.39 (ed. Kühn, 18B:181–82).

10. Galen, *De curandi ratione per venae sectionem* 7 (ed. Kühn, 11:268). Cf. Steinschneider, "Griechischen Ärzte," 289 (341), no. 45; *Ḥunayn ibn Isḥāq*, ed. and trans. Bergsträsser, no. 71. For this text compare the translation by Brain, *Galen on Bloodletting*, 75: "The quantity of any plethos is estimated from the magnitude of its characteristic signs. To whatever extent the patient has a sensation of heaviness, it is clear that dynamic plethos has increased to that degree; similarly, to whatever extent the sensation of tension has increased, to that extent also the other kind of plethos has increased, which, as I said, is called by some plethos by filling." See as well Brain's explanation (n. 24): "The

essence of dynamic plethos is that the faculties are weak so that the peccant humor oppresses them; hence the sensation of weight. The other variety, plethos by filling, physically distends the vessels, so that the patient feels swollen." Cf. *Medical Aphorisms* 25.52.

11. Galen, *De plenitudine* 10 (ed. Kühn, 7:565).

12. "a sensation of ulceration": cf. Galen, *De plenitudine* 8 (ed. Kühn, 7:552), which reads ἑλκώδη δὲ αἴσθησιν. Galen gives a different order of the effects of increased pungency of the chymes: (1) itch; (2) sensation of ulceration; (3) shivering; (4) rigor.

13. Galen, *De plenitudine* 8 (ed. Kühn, 7:552).

14. Galen, *De tremore, palpitatione, rigore et convulsione*. Instead of Maimonides' *riʿda* for "tremor" we find *riʿsha* in the bibliographical literature (cf. *Ḥunayn ibn Isḥāq*, ed. and trans. Bergsträsser, no. 60; Sezgin, *Medizin-Pharmazie*, 3:135, no. 139).

15. Cf. Galen, *De tremore, palpitatione, rigore et convulsione* 6 (ed. Kühn, 7:612; trans. Sider and McVaugh, 197).

16. Galen, *De plenitudine* 10 (ed. Kühn, 7:576).

17. Galen, *In Hippocratis Epidemiarum* 3.1 (ed. Wenkebach [CMG 5.10.2.1], 39 lines 21–30; Deller translation, 529, no. 44); cf. Anastassiou and Irmer, eds., *Testimonien*, 90; and Hippocrates (ed. Littré, 4.482.17).

18. "melancholic delusion" (*al-waswās al-sawdāwī*): see Dols, Majnūn, 50.

19. "phrenitis" *(sirsām):* see Richter-Bernburg, trans., *"De Theriaca ad Pisonem,"* 155; Dols, Majnūn, 57.

20. Galen, *In Hippocratis Epidemiarum* 3.3 (ed. Wenkebach [CMG 5.10.2.1], 184 line 23–185 line 2; 186 line 5; Deller translation, 531, no. 53).

21. "the feces are retained": lit., "when the belly is retained."

22. Galen, *In Hippocratis Epidemiarum* 6.1 (ed. Wenkebach and Pfaff [CMG 5.10.2.2], 32 lines 24–29; Deller translation, 533, no. 63).

23. Galen, *In Hippocratis Epidemiarum* 6.1 (ed. Wenkebach and Pfaff [CMG 5.10.2.2], 42 lines 1–8; Deller translation, 533, no. 65).

24. Cf. Galen, *In Hippocratis Epidemiarum* 6.2 (ed. Wenkebach and Pfaff [CMG 5.10.2.2], 102 line 1), which reads ἐπὶ τοῖς μεγάλοις κακοῖς (in severe ailments [harmful states]).

25. "whether symptoms or diseases": cf. Galen, *In Hippocratis Epidemiarum* 6.1–8 (ed. Wenkebach and Pfaff [CMG 5.10.2.2], 102 lines 1–2), which has εἴτ᾽ οὖν πάθεσιν ἢ συμπτώμασιν. Also compare Deller translation, 534, no. 71: "seien sie nun symptomatischer oder kausaler Art (arab. hat wörtlich: akzidentiell oder krankhaft)."

26. Cf. Galen, *In Hippocratis Epidemiarum* 6.1–8 (ed. Wenkebach and Pfaff [CMG 5.10.2.2], 102 line 3): ἐπὶ δὲ τοῖς μικροῖς (in minor [illnesses]).

27. Galen, *In Hippocratis Epidemiarum* 6.1–8 (ed. Wenkebach and Pfaff [CMG 5.10.2.2], 102 lines 1–5; Deller translation, 534–35, no. 71).

28. Galen, *In Hippocratis Epidemiarum* 6.1–8 (ed. Wenkebach and Pfaff [CMG 5.10.2.2], 139 lines 5–10; Deller translation, 535, no. 75).

29. This definition of the term *melancholy* does not feature in the abovementioned treatise by Galen.

30. "starch" (amylum): *nashāstaj*, from Persian *nashāstah;* cf. Schmucker, *Materia medica*, no. 769.

31. "Roman wheat" *(Triticum dicoccum):* cf. Dietrich, ed. and trans., *Dioscurides triumphans*, 2:80, from Greek χόνδρος.

32. "young": lit., moist. Cf. Galen, *In Hippocratis Epidemiarum* 6.1–8 (ed. Wenkebach and Pfaff [CMG 5.10.2.2], 160 line 21): νέον.

33. Galen, *In Hippocratis Epidemiarum* 6.3 (ed. Wenkebach and Pfaff [CMG 5.10.2.2], 160 line 17–161 line 1; Deller translation, 536, no. 76).

34. "opens them and looks at them": lit., "looks at them and opens them."

35. Cf. Galen, *In Hippocratis Epidemiarum* 6.1–8 (ed. Wenkebach and Pfaff [CMG 5.10.2.2], 246 lines 20–22): ὅπως ἄν τις ἀπὸ τῶν ὀφθαλμῶν διαγινώσκοι περὶ τῆς ἐν ὅλῳ τῷ σώματι διαθέσεως, ἐπειδὴ μάλισθ' οὗτοι τὴν βεβαιοτάτην ἐνδείκνυνται διάγνωσιν (. . .that from the eyes one can form a diagnosis of the condition of the whole body, since especially the eyes provide a most firm diagnosis). The Deller translation, 537, no. 85, renders this "Wenn sie schauen und sich öffnen, [weisen sie] auf den Zustand der Gesundheit."

36. Galen, *In Hippocratis Epidemiarum* 6.4 (ed. Wenkebach and Pfaff [CMG 5.10.2.2], 246 lines 20–22; Deller translation, 537, no. 85).

37. Galen, *In Hippocratis Epidemiarum* 6.5 (ed. Wenkebach and Pfaff [CMG 5.10.2.2], 284 line 11ff.; Deller translation, 538, no. 88).

38. Galen, *In Hippocratis Epidemiarum* 6.5 (ed. Wenkebach and Pfaff [CMG 5.10.2.2], 285 lines 17–20; Deller translation, 538, no. 89).

39. "animal faculty"; i.e., vital faculty. The Greek term ζωτικός, esp. in combination with πνεῦμα, has become in Arabic, as a result of a wrong translation, *ḥayawānī* (animal); see Ullmann, *Islamic Medicine*, 63.

40. "which are partly putrefied": lit., mixed with putrefaction.

41. See aphorism 9.93 in this volume.

42. Galen, *In Hippocratis Epidemiarum* 6.7 (ed. Wenkebach and Pfaff [CMG 5.10.2.2], 408 lines 13–16; 410 lines 25–26; Deller translation, 542, no. 107).

43. Galen, *In Hippocratis De humoribus* 1.1 (ed. Kühn, 16:10). This commentary published by Kühn is, according to Deichgräber, *Hippokrates' De humoribus*, 42–55, a forgery dating from the Renaissance, probably from the hand of Rasarius. Deichgräber pointed out that Maimonides' quotations—in the form of the old Latin translation—were used by Rasarius for reconstructing part of the text. By comparing these quotations with parallels from Oribasius, Deichgräber also showed how problematic it is to distinguish between the Maimonidean and the genuine Galenic elements. Maimonides held Galen's commentary to this book in low esteem. Thus, he remarks in his introduction to his *Commentary on Hippocrates' Aphorisms* that Galen offers explanations that have no relation to the text.

44. "a very deadly [sign]": cf. Galen, *In Hippocratis De humoribus commentarius* 2.1 (ed. Kühn, 16:218): πάνυ θανάσιμον σημεῖον.

45. Galen, *In Hippocratis De humoribus commentarius* 2.1 (ed. Kühn, 16:218).

46. *Ricinus communis.*

47. *Vicia ervilia.*

48. See the translator's introduction to this volume.

49. Galen, *De atra bile* (ed. Kühn, 5:112; ed. de Boer, 75); cf. Maimonides, *Aphorisms: Treatises 22–25*, ed. Bos, 25.39.

50. Galen, *De atra bile* (ed. Kühn, 5:113; ed. de Boer, p. 75); cf. Maimonides, *Aphorisms: Treatises 22–25*, ed. Bos, 25.39.

51. Galen, *De morborum temporibus* (ed. Kühn, 7:406–39). The quotation is not found in this treatise.

52. "tumors" *(khurājāt)*: Galen, *De crisibus* 1.7 (ed. Kühn, 9:577; ed. Alexanderson, 86 line 12), has παρωτίδες; cf. Durling, *Medical Terms*, s.v. παρωτίς "tumor of the parotid gland."

53. Galen, *De crisibus* 1.7 (ed. Kühn, 9:577; ed. Alexanderson, 86 lines 11–14).

54. Galen, *De crisibus* 1.7 (ed. Kühn, 9:579; ed. Alexanderson, 87 line 20–88 line 3).

55. Galen, *De crisibus* 1.7 (ed. Kühn, 9:577; ed. Alexanderson, 86 lines 7–10).

56. "relaxation" *(istirkhāʾ)*: cf. Galen, *De motu musculorum* 2.4 (ed. Kühn, 4:437): ῥᾳθυμία.

57. Galen, *De motu musculorum* 2.4 (ed. Kühn, 4:437).

58. Galen, *In Hippocratis Aphorismos commentarius* 6.56 (ed. Kühn, 18A:95).

59. "delusion and delirium": cf. Galen, *De locis affectis* 3.9 (ed. Kühn, 8:178), which has παραφροσύνας. For "delusion" *(waswās)*, see aphorism 6.; for "delirium" *(ikhtilāṭ)*, cf. Dols, Majnūn, 57: "mental confusion."

60. "with fever": lit., heat. Cf. Galen, *De locis affectis* 3.9 (ed. Kühn, 8:178): "without or with fever."

61. Galen, *De locis affectis* 3.9 (ed. Kühn, 8:178).

62. "on minor occasions": lit., his dizziness is caused by small things. Cf. Galen, *De locis affectis* 3.12 (ed. Kühn, 8:202): ἐπὶ σμικραῖς προφάσεσιν.

63. "when he is turned around": cf. Galen, *De locis affectis* 3.12 (ed. Kühn, 8:202), which reads ὅταν αὐτοί ποτε ἐν κύκλῳ περιστραφῶσιν.

64. "palpitation of the heart": cf. Galen, *De locis affectis* 3.12 (ed. Kühn, 8:204), which has καρδιώγμους (heartburns).

65. Galen, *De locis affectis* 3.12 (ed. Kühn, 8:202–4).

66. Galen, *De locis affectis* 3.13 (ed. Kühn, 8:206); cf. Maimonides, *Aphorisms: Treatises 22–25*, ed. Bos, 25.52.

67. "is in danger of suffering a stroke" *(sakta)*: cf. Galen, *De locis affectis* 4.3 (ed. Kühn, 8:230), which reads τοὺς ἀποπληκτικοὺς ἐπιφέρει κινδύνους.

68. "paralysis" *(istirkhāʾ)*: cf. Kamal, *Islamic Medicine*, 843, no. 62: "Slackening, loosening of ligaments, paralysis, prostration." Also cf. Richter-Bernburg, *De Theriaca ad Pisonem*, 204–5; and Galen, *De locis affectis* 4.3 (ed. Kühn, 8:230), which has παραπληγίαν.

69. Galen, *De locis affectis* 4.3 (ed. Kühn, 8:229–30; trans. Siegel, 109).

70. "short-term memory loss": cf. Galen, *De locis affectis* 5.4 (ed. Kühn, 8:330; trans. Siegel, 148–49): "Sometimes we observe an irrational forgetfulness, when, for instance, the patients ask for the urinal but do not pass their water, or forget to surrender the urinal after having voided"; cf. the introduction.

71. "very aggressive and insolent behavior": cf. Galen, *De locis affectis* 5.4 (ed. Kühn, 8:330), which has θορυβωδέστερον ἤ ὅλως θράσύτερον ἀποκρίνασθαι

(very noisy and insolent answers). Also cf. Arabic trans. Ḥunayn (MS Wellcome Or. 14a, fol. 129b): ‎ويكون جوابه لمن كلمه جوابا مضطربا مشوشا وبالجملة جواب له فضل جراّة وتهجّم‎.

72. Cf. Galen, *De locis affectis* 5.4 (ed. Kühn, 8:330): καὶ μέγα καὶ ἀραιὸν ἀναπνέουσι. Trans. Siegel, 149, renders this "have a deep and fast respiration."

73. "picking flocks from garments or straw from walls": cf. Galen, *De locis affectis* 5.4 (ed. Kühn, 8:330): κροκυδίζουσι τε καὶ καρφολογοῦσι. Trans. Siegel, 149, has "they pick at little pieces of wool or straw."

74. "a dry discharge from the eyes": cf. Galen, *De locis affectis* 5.4 (ed. Kühn, 8:330), which reads αὐχμηροὺς ἱκανῶς ἴσχουσι τοὺς ὀφθαλμούς. See also the Arabic translation by Ḥunayn (MS Wellcome Or. 14a, fol. 129b): ‎ويكون أعينهم يابسة كثيرا... ثمّ يصير في العينين رمص‎.

75. "acoustic hallucinations": lit., false hearing. Cf. Galen, *De locis affectis* 5.4 (ed. Kühn, 8:331): παρακούειν.

76. "loss of the sensation of touch throughout the body even [when one is touched] with force": cf. Galen, *De locis affectis* 5.4 (ed. Kühn, 8:331), which has ἢ μέρους τινὸς ὀδυνηρὰν ἔχοντος διάθεσιν οὐδ' ὅλως αἰσθάνεσθαι, κἂν σφοδρότερον τις αὐτοῦ θίγῃ. Trans. Siegel has: "or they have a painful condition in parts of the body or no feeling at all even if somebody touches them with great force." Also cf. the Arabic translation by Ḥunayn: ‎وفي وقت آخر يكون في واحد من أعضايه علّة ولا تحسّ وجعا ولو أنّ إنسانا غمز على ذلك العضو الذي به الوجع غمزا شديدا‎.

77. Galen, *De locis affectis* 5.4 (ed. Kühn, 8:329–31; trans. Siegel, 148–49).

78. Galen, *De crisibus* 3.11 (ed. Kühn, 9:766; ed. Alexanderson, 210 lines 17–18).

79. *In Hippocratis Epidemiarum* 1.3 (ed. Wenkebach and Pfaff [CMG 5.10.1], 165 line 18ff.; 166 lines 27–30; Deller translation, 523 no. 14).

80. "stream": cf. Galen, *In Hippocratis Epidemiarum* 3.3 (ed. Wenkebach [CMG 5.10.2.1] 5 line 6): ῥυέντων. Deller translation, 529, no. 43: "lösen sich . . . auf" follows Maimonides, MS **L**: ‎يتحلّل‎.

81. Galen, *In Hippocratis Epidemiarum* 3.3 (ed. Wenkebach [CMG 5.10.2.1], 5 lines 4–8). Cf. the translator's introduction to this volume.

82. "abscess" *(khurāj):* Galen, *In Hippocratis Epidemiarum* 6.2 (ed. Wenkebach and Pfaff [CMG 5.10.2.2], 89 lines 20–21), reads ἀποστήμα (cf. aphorism 6.28 above).

83. "a bad temperament": i.e., dyscrasy.

84. "at long intervals": cf. Galen, *In Hippocratis Epidemiarum* 6.2 (ed. Wenkebach and Pfaff [CMG 5.10.2.2], 89 line 4), which reads ἐκ διαλειμμάτων τε μακροτέρων. The translation by Deller, 534, no. 67, "lange Zeit (anhaltend)," is incorrect.

85. Galen, *In Hippocratis Epidemiarum* 6.2 (ed. Wenkebach and Pfaff [CMG 5.10.2.2], 89 lines 18–23; Deller translation, 534, no. 67).

86. "of the power [that moves the muscles of the chest]": cf. Galen, *De locis affectis* 4.7 (ed. Kühn, 8:251), which has τῆς κινούσης δυνάμεως τοὺς μῦς τοῦ θώρακος.

87. "leaves": cf. Galen, *De locis affectis* 4.7 (ed. Kühn, 8:253), which reads πτερυγία (wings).

88. Galen, *De locis affectis* 4.7 (ed. Kühn, 8:251–53).
89. "usual or unusual": cf. Galen, *De locis affectis* 4.11 (ed. Kühn, 8:286), which has ἀνώμαλον ἢ ὁμαλήν.
90. "the lungs": cf. Galen, *De locis affectis* 4.11 (ed. Kühn, 8:287), which reads τὸ σπλάγχνον (the viscera).
91. Galen, *De locis affectis* 4.11 (ed. Kühn, 8:286–87).
92. "culmination" *(muntahā):* cf. Galen, *In Hippocratis De acutorum morborum victu et Galeni commentarius* 1.32 (ed. Helmreich [CMG 5.9.1], 150 line 18): ἀκμάζειν.
93. Galen, *In Hippocratis De acutorum morborum victu et Galeni commentarius* 1.32 (ed. Helmreich [CMG 5.9.1], 150 lines 19–23).
94. Galen, *In Hippocratis Epidemiarum* 6.7 (ed. Wenkebach and Pfaff [CMG 5.10.2.2], 426 line 44–427 line 7); this text does not appear in Deller's translation.
95. "troubled" *(qaliq):* cf. Galen, *In Hippocratis Epidemiarum librum* 3.3 (ed. Wenkebach [CMG 5.10.2.1], 186 line 20), which reads ταραχώδης.
96. Galen, *In Hippocratis Epidemiarum* 3.3 (ed. Wenkebach [CMG 5.10.2.1], 186 lines 19–21; Deller translation, 531, no. 54).
97. Cf. Galen, *In Hippocratis De humoribus commentarius* 3.25 (ed. Kühn, 16:450–51).
98. **S** and **B** add "are bad."
99. "tremors" *(kuzāz):* cf. Lane, *Arabic-English Lexicon* 7:2008: "A contraction and tremor arising from cold"; Ullmann, *WKAS* 1:166 "bad cold, shivers, ague"; Dozy, *Dictionnaires arabes,* 2:462: "spasme, tétanos"; Richter-Bernburg, *De Theriaca ad Pisonem,* 75: "Starrkrampf"; see as well the note at ibid., 148–49.
100. See aphorism 6.24, above.
101. "palpitation": Galen, *De praesagitione ex pulsu* 3.4 (ed. Kühn, 9:352), reads παλμός.
102. Galen's *De pulsu* [*magna*] (*Megapulsus*) encompasses four books consisting of sixteen treatises: *De differentia pulsuum* (four treatises), *De dignoscendis pulsibus* (four treatises), *De causis pulsuum* (four treatises), and *De praesagitione ex pulsu* (four treatises). Maimonides' quote appears in *De praesagitione ex pulsu* 3.4 (ed. Kühn, 9:352) which is the fifteenth treatise of the *De pulsu* [*magna*]. (See Ullmann, *Medizin im Islam,* 43; Steinschneider, *"Die griechischen Ärzte in arabischen Übersetzungen",* 282 [334]).
103. "Marasmus" *(dhubūl):* cf. Galen, *De febrium differentiis* 1.12 (ed. Kühn, 7:326), which has μαρασμός (withering, wasting).
104. "[inflamed] tumors": cf. Galen, *De febrium differentiis* 1.12 (ed. Kühn, 7:326), which reads φλεγμοναί.
105. Galen, *De febrium differentiis* 1.12 (ed. Kühn, 7:326). The Arabic *Fī l-ḥummayāt* or *Kitāb al-ḥummayāt* appears next to *K. aṣnāf al-ḥummayāt* for Galen's *De febrium differentiis.*
106. Cf. Galen, *De locis affectis* 1.5 (ed. Kühn, 8:47; trans. Siegel, 34): "The nails become bent in wasting diseases. A chill of no [evident] reason and followed by fever is a sign that an inflammation changes into an abscess."
107. Galen, *De locis affectis* 1.5 (ed. Kühn, 8:47).

108. "hypochondriac melancholia" *(murāqqīya):* cf. Dols, *Majnūn,* 50, which says "The third type of melancholic delusion, originating in the epigastrium, was known in Arabic as *murāqan* or *murāqīya,* 'ascending,' or hypochondriac melancholia."

109. Lit., moist. Cf. Galen, *De locis affectis* 3.10 (ed. Kühn, 8:186): ὑγραί.

110. "a gurgling sound" *(qarqara):* cf. Galen, *De locis affectis* 3.10 (ed. Kühn, 8:186), which reads ἐγκλύδαξις.

111. "Despondency" *(khabath al-nafs):* cf. Galen, *De locis affectis* 3.10 (ed. Kühn, 8:188), which has δυστυμίη.

112. Galen, *De locis affectis* 3.10 (ed. Kühn, 8:186–92).

113. "Contraction": lit., pulling up *(injidhāb ilā fawqu).* Cf. Galen, *De locis affectis* 5.4 (ed. Kühn, 8:332): ἀνασπᾶσθαι.

114. "an inflammation of the diaphragm" *(waram al-ḥijāb):* Galen, *De locis affectis* 5.4 (ed. Kühn, 8:332), reads: αὐτῶν τῶν φρενῶν πασχουσῶν. Trans. Siegel, 149, renders this: "when the patients suffer from a disease involving the diaphragm." Cf. Arabic translation by Ḥunayn (MS Wellcome Or. 14a, fol. 130a): علة الحجاب.

115. "when phrenitis has been established": cf. Galen, *De locis affectis* 5.4 (ed. Kühn, 8:332), which has ἐπ' ἐγκεφάλου δὲ ἕν τι τῶν ὕστερον ἐπιγενομένων ἤδη κατασκευαζομένου τοῦ πάθους καὶ οὐκ ἀρχομένου. Trans. Siegel, 149, has: "or when the disease spreads later to the brain, since the illness has then already been established and is not in its early stage." Cf. Arabic translation by Ḥunayn (MS Wellcome Or. 14a, fol. 130b): فإذا كانت العلة في الدماغ فهو من العلامات التي تظهر في آخر الأمر إذا استحكم العلة لا إذا كانت في ابتدائها (when the disease is in the brain, it is a symptom that appears at its end, once the disease has been established, and is not in its beginning).

116. "shallow": lit., small.

117. "deep and similar to groaning": cf. Galen, *De locis affectis* 5.4 (ed. Kühn, 8:331), which reads μέγα καὶ στεναγματῶδης.

118. Galen, *De locis affectis* 5.4 (ed. Kühn, 8:331–32).

119. Galen, *De locis affectis* 5.3 (ed. Kühn, 8:326).

120. "an inflammation in the liver" *(waram [ḥārr]):* Galen, *De locis affectis* 5.7 (ed. Kühn, 8:348), speaks of an illness of the liver (πεπονθέναι τὸ ἧπαρ) and of an inflamed tumor (φλεγμοναί). Cf. Arabic translation by Ḥunayn (MS Wellcome Or. 14a, fol. 136a): ورما حارّا أعني الورم المسمّى فلغموني.

121. "sensation of heaviness inherent to the right side": Galen, *De locis affectis* 5.7 (ed. Kühn, 8:348), speaks of a "heaviness in the right hypochondria."

122. "he often complains of [pain in] the ribs of the back if the liver is in its natural structure attached to those ribs": cf. Galen, *De locis affectis* 5.7 (ed. Kühn, 8:349), which reads αἱ νόθαι δὲ πλευραὶ συναλγοῦσι ἀμφοτέροις ἐνίοτε, καὶ τοῦτ' αὐτοῖς κοινὸν εἰκότως ἐστί, συμβαῖνον οὐ πᾶσι, ὅτι μὴ συνῆπται πᾶσι δι' ὑμένων τὸ ἧπαρ ταῖς πλευραῖς. Trans. Siegel, 156, reads this: "Sometimes the false ribs are painful on both sides. In these patients this symptom is naturally common but does not occur in each case, since the liver is not always attached to the ribs by ligaments."

123. "the patient suffers from constipation": lit., the nature of the patient is withheld. Cf. Galen, *De locis affectis* 5.7 (ed. Kühn, 8:348): ἐπίσχεται δ' αὐτοῖς καὶ ἡ γαστήρ. The translation by Ḥunayn is more correct than that by Siegel, 156: "The abdominal [wall] in these cases is retracted."

124. Galen, *De locis affectis* 5.7 (ed. Kühn, 8:348–49).

125. Galen, *De locis affectis* 5.5 (ed. Kühn, 8:337).

126. "inflammation" *(waram [ḥārr]):* cf. Galen, *De locis affectis* 5.7 (ed. Kühn, 8:349), which reads φλεγμοναί.

127. Galen, *De locis affectis* 5.7 (ed. Kühn, 8:349).

128. Galen, *De locis affectis* 5.8 (ed. Kühn, 8:360).

129. "the pulsatile vessels": lit., the species *(jins)* of pulsatile vessels.

130. Galen, *De compositione medicamentorum secundum locos* 2.1 (ed. Kühn, 12:500). For the Arabic *mayāmir* coined after the Syriac *mēmra*, see Ullmann, *Medizin im Islam*, 48, no. 50.

131. "stabbing pain": cf. Galen, *De locis affectis* 2.8 (ed. Kühn, 8:94), which has ὁ δὲ διαΐσσων πόνος. Trans. Siegel, 53, has "shooting pain."

132. "one-sided headache": i.e., migraine.

133. "inveterate headache": cf. Galen, *De locis affectis* 2.8 (ed. Kühn, 8:94), which has κεφαλαία.

134. "the membrane that lies under the skin": i.e., subcutaneous membrane. Cf. Galen, *De locis affectis* 2.8 (ed. Kühn, 8:103): ὁ μὲν οὖν ὑπὸ τῷ δέρματι τεταμένος ὑμήν.

135. "tensive numb pain": cf. Galen, *De locis affectis* 2.8 (ed. Kühn, 8:103), which reads τονώδεις τε καὶ ναρκώδεις.

136. Galen, *De locis affectis* 2.8 (ed. Kühn, 8:94, 99, 103).

137. "bone-piercing" *(muthaqqiba al-ʿiẓām):* cf. Galen, *De locis affectis* 2.8 (ed. Kühn, 8:104), which has ὀστοκόπους.

138. Galen, *De locis affectis* 2.8 (ed. Kühn, 8:104)

139. Galen, *De locis affectis* 2.8 (ed. Kühn, 8:104).

140. Galen, *De locis affectis* 2.8 (ed. Kühn, 8:91).

141. Galen, *In Hippocratis Aphorismos commentarius* 4.37 (ed. Kühn, 17B:715–17). Cf. Anastassiou and Irmer, eds., *Testimonien* 66 (ed. Littré, 4.466.8, 15).

142. Galen, *In Hippocratis Aphorismos commentarius* 4.46 (ed. Kühn, 17B:724–25).

143. Galen, *In Hippocratis Epidemiarum* 1.3 (ed. Wenkebach and Pfaff [CMG 5.10.1], 193 lines 1–6; Deller translation, 524, no. 18).

144. Galen, *In Hippocratis Epidemiarum* 1.3 (ed. Wenkebach and Pfaff [CMG 5.10.1], 398 lines 11–19; Deller translation, 528, no. 18).

145. "loss": lit., death: cf. Galen, *In Hippocratis Epidemiarum* 3.1 (ed. Wenkebach [CMG 5.10.2.1], 43 line 8), which has νέκρωσις.

146. Galen, *In Hippocratis Epidemiarum* 3.1 (ed. Wenkebach [CMG 5.10.2.1] 43 lines 5–8, 46 lines 15–16; Deller translation, 529, no. 45).

147. "tumors" *(awrām):* cf. Galen, *In Hippocratis Epidemiarum* 6.1 (ed. Wenkebach and Pfaff [CMG 5.10.2.2], 35 line 3), which reads φύματα.

148. "which have a pointed head": cf. Galen, *In Hippocratis Epidemiarum* 6.1 (ed. Wenkebach and Pfaff [CMG 5.10.2.2], 35 line 19), which has ἐ··Აᴱᴦα.

149. "the ones with a [less pointed] head": cf. Galen, *In Hippocratis Epidemiarum* 6.1 (ed. Wenkebach and Pfaff [CMG 5.10.2.2], 35 line 19), which reads κορυφώδη.

150. "tumors that tend downwards": cf. Galen, *In Hippocratis Epidemiarum* 6.1 (ed. Wenkebach and Pfaff [CMG 5.10.2.2], 36 line 9), which reads τὰ κατάρροπα φύματα.

151. "that do not have two heads": cf. Galen, *In Hippocratis Epidemiarum* 6.1 (ed. Wenkebach and Pfaff [CMG 5.10.2.2], 36 line 15), which has τὰ μὴ δίκραια (those which are not split).

152. "those which suppurate evenly": cf. Galen, *In Hippocratis Epidemiarum* 6.1 (ed. Wenkebach and Pfaff [CMG 5.10.2.2], 36 line 1), which reads τὰ ὁμαλῶς ἐκπυϊσκόμενα.

153. "and are not very hard": lit., and do not have hardness around them *(wa-lā jakūnu ḥawlahu ṣalāba)*. The Arabic is a literal translation of the Greek term περίσκληρος; Galen, *In Hippocratis Epidemiarum* 6.1 (ed. Wenkebach and Pfaff [CMG 5.10.2.2], 36 line 6).

154. Galen, *In Hippocratis Epidemiarum* 6.1 (ed. Wenkebach and Pfaff [CMG 5.10.2.2], 35 line 3–36 line 15; Deller translation, 533 n. 64).

155. Cf. Galen, *In Hippocratis Prognostica commentarius* 2.60 (ed. Kühn, 18B:204): "In all chronic diseases the fingers turn cold. But in hectic fevers they stay warm, since these fevers mostly occupy the solid parts of the body. That the fingers appear warmer until their very ends does not come from the external parts but from the internal fleshy parts."

156. The text quoted by Maimonides does not feature in book 3 but in book 2.

157. Cf. aphorism 6.24, above.

158. Cf. aphorism 6.24, above.

159. Galen, *De atra bile* (ed. Kühn, 5:122; ed. de Boer, 80 lines 15–17).

160. "cohesive": cf. Galen, *De crisibus* 1.11 (ed. Kühn, 9:587; ed. Alexanderson, 93 line 1), which has συνεστηκός.

161. Galen, *De crisibus* 1.11 (ed. Kühn, 9:587–88; ed. Alexanderson, 93).

162. "softer": cf. Galen, *De crisibus* 1.11 (ed. Kühn, 9:588; ed. Alexanderson, 93 lines 18), has ὑγρότερον (more moist).

163. "biting": cf. Galen, *De crisibus* 1.11 (ed. Kühn, 9:590; ed. Alexanderson, 94 line 19): δῆξις.

164. Galen, *De crisibus* 1.11 (ed. Kühn, 9:588–90; ed. Alexanderson, 93–95).

165. Galen, *De crisibus* 1.11 (ed. Kühn, 9:590–91; ed. Alexanderson, 94–95).

166. Cf. Galen, *De crisibus* 1.11 (ed Kühn, 9:592; ed. Alexanderson, 96 lines 1–3): τὸ δὲ ἄπεπτον διαχώρημα τὸ λεπτὸν καὶ τραχὺ καὶ ἀχύμωτόν ἐστι, καὶ τὴν τῶν ἐδεδεσμένων διαφυλάττον ποιότητα.

167. Galen, *De crisibus* 1.12 (ed. Kühn, 9:604; Alexanderson, 103 lines 16–19).

168. See Maimonides, *Aphorisms: Treatises 1–5*, ed. Bos, 2.2.

169. "serous" *(ṣadīd):* cf. Galen, *De locis affectis* 5.8 (ed. Kühn, 8:359), which reads ἰχωροειδές.

170. Galen, *De locis affectis* 5.8 (ed. Kühn, 8:359).

171. "thick": the Arabic text reads "pure" or "fresh." The correction is based on an emendation of عبط as غلظ; cf. Galen, *De locis affectis* 5.8 (ed. Kühn, 8:359), which reads παχύ; Nathan ha-Meʾati, *Sefer ha-Perakim* (MS Paris, Bibliothèque Nationale, héb. 1173), which has סג; and Zeraḥyah (untitled Hebrew translation, MS Berlin, Staatsbibliothek Preussisc her Kulturbesitz, Or. Qu. 512), which reads עב.

172. Galen, *De locis affectis* 5.8 (ed. Kühn, 8:359).

173. Galen, *De locis affectis* 5.8 (ed. Kühn, 8:371).

174. Galen, *De locis affectis* 5.8 (ed. Kühn, 8:370).

175. "Bloody diarrhea": cf. Galen, *De locis affectis* 6.2 (ed. Kühn, 8:381), which reads δυσεντερία (dysentery).

176. "shreds" *(khurāṭa):* cf. Galen, *De locis affectis* 6.2 (ed. Kühn, 8:382), which has ξύσματα.

177. Galen, *De locis affectis* 6.2 (ed. Kühn, 8:382).

178. Galen, *De locis affectis* 6.2 (ed. Kühn, 8:383).

179. "deep" *(mushabbaʿ):* lit., satiated; cf. Galen, *De crisibus* 1.11 (ed. Kühn, 9:592; ed. Alexanderson, 96 line 6): πυρρός.

180. Galen, *De crisibus* 1.11 (ed. Kühn, 9:592–93; ed. Alexanderson, 96).

181. I.e., the different qualities of the stool.

182. Galen, *De crisibus* 1.11 (ed. Kühn, 9:593; ed. Alexanderson, 96).

183. "boiled": lit., melted.

184. "from an anomalous disturbance": cf. Galen, *De crisibus* 1.11 (ed. Kühn, 9:594; ed. Alexanderson, 97 line 6), which reads ἀνωμάλου ταραχῆς.

185. "from the struggle between thick flatulence and moisture": cf. Galen, *De crisibus* 1.11 (ed. Kühn, 9:594; ed. Alexanderson, 97 lines 4–5), which has φυσώδους πνεύματος ὑγρῷ μαχομένου γίγνεται.

186. Galen, *De crisibus* 1.11 (ed. Kühn, 9:594; ed. Alexanderson, 97).

187. Galen, *De crisibus* 1.11 (ed. Kühn, 9:594; ed. Alexanderson, 97).

188. "the diseases and symptoms" *(aʿrāḍ):* cf. Galen, *De symptomatum causis* 3.2 (ed. Kühn, 7:216), which reads τά τε νοσήματα καὶ τὰ συμπτώματα.

189. "wrong": Galen, *De symptomatum causis* 3.2 (ed. Kühn, 7:216), reads πλημμελεῖς.

190. Galen, *De symptomatum causis* 3.2 (ed. Kühn, 7:216). *De morborum causis et symptomatibus* consists of the following treatises: (1) *De morborum differentiis,* (2) *De causis morborum,* (3) *De symptomatum differentiis,* (4–6) *De symptomatum causis* 1–3 (see Ullmann, *Medizin im Islam,* 42).

191. Galen, *In Hippocratis Aphorismos commentarius* 4.21 (ed. Kühn, 17B:683). See also Anastassiou and Irmer, eds. *Testimonien,* 112 (ed. Littré, 4.510.3–4) and 205 (ed. Littré, 5.76.4). **S, B, P, L** add "A black stool that is discharged in the beginning of the disease indicates terrible harm that occurred to the liver, but when it is discharged after the culmination of the disease, it is often a good sign, since its discharge means that nature is expelling those sickening superfluities."

192. "bloody diarrhea": cf. Galen, *In Hippocratis Aphorismos commentarius* 6.3 (ed. Kühn, 18A:11), which has δυσεντερία; see as well aphorism 6.82 above.

193. Galen, *In Hippocratis Aphorismos commentarius* 6.3 (ed. Kühn, 18A:11).

194. "pallor": lit., a yellow complexion. Cf. Galen, *De locis affectis* 6.4 (ed. Kühn, 8:409): ὠχριᾶν.

195. "becomes hot" *(yaskhun):* Galen, *De locis affectis* 6.4 (ed. Kühn, 8:409), reads ἀλύειν (to be restless). S and L read "becomes calm" *(yaskun).*

196. "most dear to nature": cf. Galen, *De locis affectis* 6.4 (ed. Kühn, 8:409), which has τὸ πάντων οἰκειότατον ἡμῖν. Trans. Siegel, 180, renders this "best adapted to the organism." Also cf. Arabic translation by Ḥunayn (MS Wellcome Or. 14a, fol. 160a): أقرب الأشياء كلها مشاكلة وموافقة للبدن.

197. Galen, *De locis affectis* 6.4 (ed. Kühn, 8:408–9).

198. Galen, *De locis affectis* 1.5 (ed. Kühn, 8:47).

199. "conjecture": cf. Galen, *De compositione medicamentorum secundum locos* 2.1 (ed. Kühn, 12:546), which has στοχαστικὸς.

200. "certain knowledge": cf. Galen, *De compositione medicamentorum secundum locos* 2.1 (ed. Kühn, 12:546), which reads ἐπιστημονικῶς.

201. Galen, *De compositione medicamentorum secundum locos* 2.1 (ed. Kühn, 12:546). For the Arabic *mayāmir* coined after the Syriac *mēmra*, see Ullmann, *Medizin im Islam*, 48, no. 50.

202. "distinction" *(tamyīz):* this faculty probably stands as a *pars pro toto* for the human mind in general *(dhihn)*, which encompasses all the faculties and dispositions, even imagination; cf. Munk, ed., *Guide des égarés*, 1:175–76 n. 5; Scheyer, *Psychologische system*, 60ff.

203. "homonym": cf. Maimonides, *Dalālat al-ḥāʾirin*, ed. Munk, introduction to chapter 1.

204. Cf. translator's introduction; for the concept of nature in ancient medicine, cf. Deichgräber, *Medicus gratiosus*, 51; Temkin, *Galenism*, 25; Brock, *Greek Medicine*, 25–29; Savage-Smith, trans., *Galen on Nerves*, 44ff; see as well Maimonides, *On the Regimen of Health*, ed. and trans. Bos, 2.2.

205. "If it finds it difficult to do so" *(idhā ghulibat ʿan dhālika):* cf. Dozy, *Dictionnaires arabes*, 2:220, s.v. *ghuliba min:* "s'embarrasser de, éprouver de la peine de."

206. Cf. Maimonides, *Aphorisms: Treatises 1–5*, ed. Bos, 2.42.

207. "mental activity": The text reads "amentia"; cf. Nathan ha-Meʾati, *Pirke Moshe*: טוב השכל (proper mental activity), Latin translation (starting with: Incipiunt Aphorismi excellentissimi Raby Moyses secundam doctrinam Galieni medicorum principis), ed. Bologna 1489: "mens." The Latin translation is discussed in J. O. Leibowitz, "The Latin translations of Maimonides' Aphorisms," *Korot* 6, fasc. 5–6 (1973): 273–281, in Hebrew, with an abridged version in English, ibid., xciii–xcix.

208. "suffering from madness": cf. Dols, Majnūn, 3.

209. "it indicates that the general strength is weak": lit., it comes from the weakness of the general strength.

210. "symptoms": "Erscheinungen," in Galen, *Platonis Timaeum*, trans. Schröder, 8).

211. "there is reason for suspicion": lit., there is place for suspicion.

212. Galen, *Platonis Timaeum*, trans. Schröder 8–9; cf. Larrain, *Galens Kommentar*, 211.

## The Seventh Treatise

1. "Anger": cf. Galen, *De praesagitione ex pulsibus* 1 (ed. Kühn, 9:268): θυμός.

2. Galen, *De praesagitione ex pulsibus* 1 (ed. Kühn, 9:267–68).

3. Galen, *De praesagitione ex pulsibus* 1 (ed. Kühn, 9:268).

4. "affected by anxiety, joy, or anger": Galen, *Ad Glauconem de methodo medendi* 1.15 (ed. Kühn, 11:49): θυμωθέντες.

5. Galen, *Ad Glauconem de methodo medendi* 1.15 (ed. Kühn, 11:49).

6. This passage from the lost commentary on humors does not feature in the pseudo-Galenic text published by Kühn (see aphorism 6.22 above), nor is it discussed by Deichgräber in his *Hippokrates' De humoribus*.

7. Galen, *In Hippocratis Epidemiarum* 1.3 (ed. Wenkebach and Pfaff [CMG 5.10.1], 385 line 37–386 line 3; Deller translation, 527, no. 32.)

8. "a dissolution of continuity": cf. Galen, *De methodo medendi* 12.6 (ed. Kühn, 10:852): συνεχείας λυσίς; also cf. Maimonides, *Aphorisms: Treatises 22–25*, ed. Bos, 25.21.

9. "that occurs to the organ through coercion and harshness": cf. Galen, *De methodo medendi* 12.6 (ed. Kühn, 10:853): βιαίαν γίνεσθαι τὴν μεταβολὴν.

10. Galen, *De methodo medendi* 12.7 (ed. Kühn, 10:851–53).

11. "activated": lit., moved.

12. Galen, *De methodo medendi* 13.3 (ed. Kühn, 10:879).

13. "describe": lit., encompass.

14. Cf. Galen, *De methodo medendi* 12.5 (ed. Kühn, 10:844).

15. Galen, *De methodo medendi* 12.7 (ed. Kühn, 10:850).

16. "serious": lit., oppressive.

17. Abū Marwān b. Zuhr (d. 1162), known in the West as Avenzoar, was one of the foremost physicians of the Western Caliphate. He was born in Seville, where he spent most of his life, and he is frequently quoted by Maimonides, who regarded him highly. In Maimonides, *On the Elucidation of Some Symptoms* (ed. and trans. Bos, forthcoming) he praises him as "unique in his generation and one of the greatest observers," and in *On Poisons* (MS Paris 1211, fol. 147b; ed. and trans. Bos, forthcoming) he remarks: "All this is mentioned and verified by Abū Marwān ibn Zuhr with his vast experience. For he was the greatest amongst men in testing drugs and was one who occupied himself with this more than any other. He was able to do so more than any other because of his great wealth and his skill in the medical art."

18. "is undoubtedly responsible for the death of the patient": lit., causes the patient to die. See also the introduction to this volume.

19. Cf. Maimonides, *Aphorisms: Treatises 1–5*, introduction, 2 line 27–3 line 4: "Rather, most of the aphorisms that I have selected are in the very words of Galen, or in his words and the words of Hippocrates, because the words of both are mixed in Galen's commentaries to Hippocrates' books; [in the case of] others, the idea [expressed] in the aphorism is partly in Galen's words and partly in my own; [in the case of] yet other aphorisms, my own words express the idea that Galen mentioned."

20. See the introduction to this volume.

21. "a quick collapse" *(suqūṭ ... bi-ḥadda wa-surᶜa):* cf. Galen, *De methodo medendi* 12.5 (ed. Kühn, 10:837), which has κατάπτωσίς ἐστιν ὀξεῖα. The Arabic *bi-ḥadda* is a literal translation of the Greek ὀξεῖα, which has the basic meaning of "sharp" but can also mean "quick."

22. Maimonides' discussion is basically a summary of Galen's lengthy exposition in *De methodo medendi* 12.5 (ed. Kühn, 10:837–45).

23. See the introduction to this volume.

24. "because of wasting fevers": cf. Galen, *De methodo medendi* 12.5 (ed. Kühn, 10:840): ἐν τοῖς συντηκτικοῖς πυρετοῖς.

25. "movements of the soul": i.e., emotions; cf. Maimonides, *On Asthma*, ed. Bos, 8.2.

26. "intense joy, which is called 'exultation'": cf. Galen, *De methodo medendi* 12.5 (ed. Kühn, 10:841), which reads ἡδοναὶ μέγισται, καλοῦσι δὲ καὶ ταύτας περιχαρείας.

27. Galen, *De methodo medendi* 12.5 (ed. Kühn, 10:841).

28. Galen, *De methodo medendi* 12.5 (ed. Kühn, 10:841).

29. "fainting" *(khumūlan):* cf. Galen, *De methodo medendi* 12.5 (ed. Kühn, 10:845), which reads τὰς καλουμένας λειποψυχίας. The standard Arabic dictionaries do not give this specific meaning of this term.

30. "interaction": lit., participation, collaboration.

31. Or from its pneuma, i.e., the animal (= vital) pneuma prepared in the heart from the fine, pure vapor of the blood and the inhaled air.

32. See Moshe Narboni (ca. 1300–1362), *Sefer Oraḥ Ḥayyim* (MS Munich 276, fol. 30b). For this medical compendium, see Bos, *R. Moshe Narboni: Philosopher and Physician.*

33. Cf. Galen, *De methodo medendi* 12.3 (ed. Kühn, 10:826); Galen, *In Hippocratis De aeris [aquis locis] commentarius* 2.2.1; forthcoming ed. Strohmaier: "For he (i.e., Hippocrates) would not have a grain of common sense if he did not know that putrid foods and beverages produce corruption similar to that produced by fatal poisons"; see as well Maimonides, *Aphorisms: Treatises* 16–21, ed. Bos (forthcoming), 20.10; Maimonides, *On Hemorrhoids,* ed. Bos (forthcoming), 1.3.

34. *Cucumis melo.*

35. *Cucumis sativus and var.*

36. *Cucurbita maxima* Duch.

37. I.e., to leave the body, to be excreted.

38. See Moshe Narboni, *Sefer Oraḥ Ḥayyim* (MS Munich 276, fol. 30b.)

39. Cf. **C**: "and when the body is nourished, the spleen attracts most of the food to it and does not let the body be nourished. As a necessary consequence, the body becomes emaciated. Therefore he says that the flesh is dissolved in the spleen and that the spleen is the cause of the emaciation of the body. But this is not the only way that the spleen emaciates the entire body. Because of its nearness to the liver, it corrupts and weakens the digestive faculty in it, and when the liver does not adequately digest the food, the body becomes emaciated and it dissolves." See also the Hebrew translation by Solomon ha-Meᵓati, *Airs, Waters, Places,* ed. Wasserstein, 44–45 ([228–29]). I thank

Professor Strohmaier for providing me with the text of the Arabic translation of Galen's *De aeris aquis locis*.

40. Galen, *In Hippocratis Epidemiarum* 6.4 (ed. Wenkebach and Pfaff [CMG 5.10.2.2], 137 lines 2–4; Deller translation, 535, no. 74).

41. Galen, *In Hippocratis Epidemiarum* 6.4 (ed. Wenkebach and Pfaff [CMG 5.10.2.2], 168 lines 16–19; cf. Deller translation, 536, no. 78).

42. "biting and corrosion": Pseudo-Galen, *In Hippocratis De humoribus commentarius* 1 (ed. Kühn, 16:54), reads δακνότης.

43. Pseudo-Galen, *In Hippocratis De humoribus commentarius* 1 (ed. Kühn, 16:54).

44. I could not locate this quotation in the mentioned book. The discussion bears some resemblance to Galen, *De plenitudine* 8 (ed. Kühn, 7:551); see next aphorism.

45. I.e., itching of the skin.

46. "movement . . . which occurs when moving the fingers in the region of the armpit": i.e., the body movements resulting from tickling the armpit. This quotation does not appear in the text edited by Kühn (ed. Kühn, 15:251–373), which is a Renaissance forgery.

47. Galen, *De plenitudine* 8 (ed. Kühn, 7:552).

48. Cf. aphorism 6.7 above.

49. Mentha *(fūdhanj):* cf. Galen, *De tremore, palpitatione, rigore et convulsione* 7.7 (ed. Kühn, 7:636), which has καλαμίνθη.

50. Galen, *De tremore, palpitatione, rigore et convulsione* 7.7 (ed. Kühn, 7:634–36; trans. Sider and McVaugh, 207–8); cf. aphorism 6.8 above.

51. Galen, *Ad Glauconem de methodo medendi* 2.12 (ed. Kühn, 11:140–41).

52. "caries" *(nakhz):* cf. Galen, *De causis morborum* 7 (ed. Kühn, 7:34), which reads τερηδών.

53. Galen, *De causis morborum* 7 (ed. Kühn, 7:33–34).

54. "dementia": cf. Galen, *De symptomatum causis* 2.7 (ed. Kühn, 7:201), which has μώρωσις.

55. Galen, *De symptomatum causis* 2.7 (ed. Kühn, 7:201–2).

56. Galen remarks that only under certain conditions is pain in membranes dissimilar. Galen, *De locis affectis* 2.8 (ed. Kühn, 8:101). Cf. translation by Ḥunayn (MS Wellcome Or. 14a, fol. 40b): متى امتدّت وأقبلت الأجزاء التي حول الجزء الذي به الآفة منها إليه وجب ضرورة أن يكون وجعا غير مَساوٍ لأنّ الموضع الذي يكون فيه الجزء المَتمدّد أكثرَ حسّا يكون الوجع فيه أشدّ والموضع الذي هو أقل حسّا يكون الوجع فيه أقل (When the parts that surround the painful spot are pulled and drawn near to it, the pain must necessarily become dissimilar, because when the spot of the part that is pulled is more sensitive, the pain is more severe, and when that spot is less sensitive, the pain is less severe).

57. Galen, *De locis affectis* 2.8 (ed. Kühn, 8:101).

58. Galen, *De locis affectis* 2.4 (ed. Kühn, 8:76–77).

59. "when it increases and becomes dominant": lit., when it becomes dominant and increases.

60. Galen, *De locis affectis* 3.9 (ed. Kühn, 8:174, 177–78).

61. "a [pulsatile] vessel": cf. Galen, *De praesagitione ex pulsu* 1.4 (ed. Kühn, 9:247), which reads ἀρτηρία.

62. Galen, *De praesagitione ex pulsu* 1.4 (ed. Kühn, 9:247–48).

63. "Tapeworms": cf. Galen, *De Theriaca ad Pisonem* (ed. Kühn, 14:15, p. 272), which has πλατεῖα ἕλμις; see also the Arabic translation, "Eine arabische Version," ed. Richter-Bernburg, 124a3.

64. Galen, *De Theriaca ad Pisonem* (ed. Kühn, 14:15, p. 272); Arabic translation, "Eine arabische Version," ed. Richter-Bernburg 124a3–4; "ad Pisonem": the Arabic title *ilā Qaysar* is a corruption of *ilā Fīṣun;* cf. Steinschneider, *"Die griechischen Ärzte in arabischen Übersetzungen,"* 292 (344), no. 55; Ullmann, *Die Medizin im Islam,* 49 no. 51.

65. Galen, *De symptomatum causis* 2.6 (ed. Kühn, 7:199).

66. Galen, *De compositione medicamentorum secundum locos* 5.4 (ed. Kühn, 12:850).

67. "livid": cf. Galen, *De compositione medicamentorum secundum locos* 5.4 (ed. Kühn, 12:850), which has πελιδνουμένους.

68. Galen, *De compositione medicamentorum secundum locos* 5.4 (ed. Kühn, 12:849–50).

69. "delirium": cf. Galen, *De locis affectis* 3.9 (ed. Kühn, 8:179), which reads παραφροσύναι.

70. "with a vaporous or smoky gas": cf. Galen, *De locis affectis* 3.9 (ed. Kühn, 8:179), which has πνεύματος ἀτμώδους ἢ καπνώδους.

71. Galen, *De locis affectis* 3.9 (ed. Kühn, 8:179).

72. Galen, *De tremore, palpitatione, rigore et convulsione* 3.3 (ed. Kühn, 7:586–87; trans. Sider and McVaugh, 186–87).

73. "thick and viscous moisture": The moisture which Galen has in mind is that which obstructs the outlets of the pneuma in the cerebral cavities (*De locis affectis* 3.9 [ed. Kühn, 8:173]).

74. Galen, *De locis affectis* 3.8, 9, 12 (ed. Kühn, 8:172–73, 199).

75. Galen, *De symptomatum causis* 2.2 (ed. Kühn, 7:152–53).

76. Galen, *De tremore, palpitatione, rigore et convulsione* 3.8 (ed. Kühn, 7:639–41; trans. Sider and McVaugh, 209).

77. "a thick wind": cf. Galen, *De tremore, palpitatione, rigore et convulsione* 3.5 (ed. Kühn, 7:599), which reads ἀτμῶδες πνεῦμα.

78. "it causes the mentioned palpitation": lit., it moves that which [thus] has that movement.

79. Castoreum, i.e., a desiccated excretion of the glands of the castor fiber.

80. Galen, *De tremore, palpitatione, rigore et convulsione* 3.5 (ed. Kühn, 7:596, 599–601; trans. Sider and McVaugh, 192–93).

81. Galen, *In Hippocratis Epidemiarum* 6.3 (ed. Wenkebach and Pfaff [CMG 5.10.2.2], 164 lines 7–9; Deller translation, 536, no. 77).

82. "animal faculty": i.e., vital faculty; cf. aphorism 6.21 above.

83. Galen, *De tremore, palpitatione, rigore et convulsione* 3.5 (ed. Kühn, 7:601), speaks about the dissolution of the vital force, as in stomachic and cardiac weaknesses; see aphorism 6.21 above.

84. Galen, *De tremore, palpitatione, rigore et convulsione* 3.5 (ed. Kühn, 7:601–2; trans. Sider and McVaugh, 192–93).

85. Galen, *De tremore, palpitatione, rigore et convulsione* 3.6 (ed. Kühn, 7:620–24, 629; trans. Sider and McVaugh, 201–3, 205).

86. Galen, *De tremore, palpitatione, rigore et convulsione* 3.6 (ed. Kühn, 7:606–9; trans. Sider and McVaugh, 195–96).

87. Galen, *De tremore, palpitatione, rigore et convulsione* 3.6 (ed. Kühn, 7:612; trans. Sider and McVaugh, 197).

88. Galen, *De febribus* 2.7 (ed. Kühn, 7:357–58).

89. Galen, *De tremore, palpitatione, rigore et convulsione* 3.7 (ed. Kühn, 7:633–36; trans. Sider and McVaugh, 207–8).

90. Galen, *De symptomatum causis* 2.5 (ed. Kühn, 7:194–95).

91. "narrowness and pressure": cf. Galen, *De locis affectis* 4.7 (ed. Kühn, 8:251), which reads στενοχωρία.

92. Lit., air passages.

93. Galen, *De locis affectis* 4.7 (ed. Kühn, 8:251).

94. "at intervals": cf. Galen, *In Hippocratis Epidemiarum* 1.3 (ed. Wenkebach and Pfaff [CMG 5.10.1], 130, line 9) which reads ἀραιός (thin).

95. "[and] in great gasps" (ʿazīman): Galen, *In Hippocratis Epidemiarum* 1.3 (ed. Wenkebach and Pfaff [CMG 5.10.1], 130, line 9): καὶ μέγα.

96. Galen, *In Hippocratis Epidemiarum* 1.3 (ed. Wenkebach and Pfaff [CMG 5.10.1], 130 lines 9–12; Deller translation, 522, no. 11).

97. Galen, *In Hippocratis Epidemiarum* 1.3 (ed. Wenkebach and Pfaff [CMG 5.10.1], 172 line 34–173 line 5; Deller translation, 523, no. 15). This text does not appear in the Hebrew translation by Nathan ha-Meʾati, which is the basis for the text numbering that Muntner and subsequently Rosner used and that I have adopted for this edition as well.

98. Galen, *In Hippocratis Epidemiarum* 1.3 (ed. Wenkebach and Pfaff [CMG 5.10.1], 352 lines 27–32; Deller translation, 526, no. 28).

99. Galen, *De locis affectis* 4.11 (ed. Kühn, 8:285).

100. This treatise only survives in an Arabic translation that has been edited and translated by Nabielek ("Schlaf und Wachsein"). Cf. Strohmaier, "Syrische und arabische Galen," 2015, no. 13. Maimonides' quotation does not appear in the Arabic translation; accordingly, Nabielek (p. 29) concludes that the original text of this treatise must have been more extensive. At the same time he concludes that, because of the similarity between Maimonides' text and the relevant passage from Oribasius's *Collectiones medicae* (see Nabielek's comparative table, 33–34), the latter must have been the source Maimonides copied from. See the introduction to this volume.

101. "by foods": cf. Galen, *De locis affectis* 5.6 (ed. Kühn, 8:344), which specifies "by the irregular [consumption] of foods or their excessive quantity or [bad] quality."

102. Galen, *De locis affectis* 5.6 (ed. Kühn, 8:344).

103. Or flatulent.

104. "leads to": lit., adheres to.

105. Galen, *De locis affectis* 3.10 (ed. Kühn, 8:187, 189).

106. Galen, *De locis affectis* 2.8 (ed. Kühn, 8:101–2).

107. "intestinal rumblings" (qarqara): cf. Galen, *De symptomatum differentiis* 4 (ed. Kühn, 7:69), which has κλύδων.

108. "discomfort" (karb): cf. Galen, *De symptomatum differentiis* 4 (ed. Kühn, 7:69), which reads ἀπορία.

109. "in a trembling way": cf. Galen, *De symptomatum differentiis* 4 (ed. Kühn, 7:69), which reads τρομωδῶς.

110. Galen, *De symptomatum differentiis* 4 (ed. Kühn, 7:69).

111. Galen, *In Hippocratis Epidemiarum* 1.3 (ed. Wenkebach and Pfaff [CMG 5.10.1], 191 lines 12–18; Deller translation, 524, no. 17).

112. "diabetes" *(istitlāq al-bawl):* Galen, *De locis affectis* 6.3 (ed. Kühn, 8:401), has διαβήτης. Cf. Maimonides, *Aphorisms: Treatises 1–5,* ed. Bos, 5.13.

113. Galen, *De locis affectis* 6.3; (ed. Kühn, 8:401).

114. I.e., sleep.

115. I.e., sleep.

116. Galen, *In Hippocratis Epidemiarum* 6.4 (ed. Wenkebach and Pfaff [CMG 5.10.2.2], 224 line 22–225 line 4; Deller translation, 536–37, no. 80); cf. Anastassiou and Irmer, eds., *Testimonien,* 464.

117. "evident causes" *(asbāb bādiya):* probably in the sense of "external causes." Nathan ha-Meʾati reads the Arabic as *asbāb bādiʾa* and translates הסבות המתחילות (initial causes).

118. "can be easily repaired" *(sahl al-talāfi):* possibly reading *sahl al-ittilāf;* Deller translates this as "leicht an Verderben."

119. *Pinus pinea.*

120. Galen, *In Hippocratis Epidemiarum* 6.8 (ed. Wenkebach and Pfaff [CMG 5.10.2.2], 504 lines 29–35; Deller translation, 543, no. 112).

121. Galen, *In Hippocratis Epidemiarum* 6.1–8 (ed. Wenkebach and Pfaff [CMG 5.10.2.2], 336 line 20; Deller translation, 540, no. 98).

122. Lit., his whole body is empty because of the evacuation of fluid and pneuma from it.

123. "to weaken and extinguish": lit., to extinguish and weaken. Galen, *De semine* 1.16 (ed. De Lacy, 140 line 5), has διαλύειν.

124. "animal faculty": i.e., vital faculty; cf. aphorism 6.21 in this volume.

125. The quotation actually features in Galen, *De semine* 1.16 (ed. De Lacy, 140 lines 2–6).

126. Galen, *De symptomatum causis* 3.5 (ed. Kühn, 7:238–39).

127. Galen, *De symptomatum causis* 3.5 (ed. Kühn, 7:238).

128. Galen, *In Hippocratis Epidemiarum* 6.5 (ed. Wenkebach and Pfaff [CMG 5.10.2.2], 306 line 32–307 line 3; Deller translation, p. 539, no. 93).

129. This pseudo-Galenic treatise is perhaps identical with *Maqāla fi l-ḥuqan wa-l-qūlanj (De clysteribus et colica)* cited by Ibn Abī Uṣaybiʿa in *ʿUyūn al-anbāʾ,* 1.102 (p. 149); cf. Meyerhof, "Schriften Galens," 543, no. 62; Sezgin, *Medizin-Pharmazie,* 3:128, no. 100.

130. "Pain with numbness": cf. Galen, *In Hippocratis Epidemiarum* 6.1 (ed. Wenkebach and Pfaff [CMG 5.10.2.2], 26 line 23), which has ὀδύνην ναρκώδη. Deller, 532, no. 58, translates this as "Schmerz verbunden mit Kälte" following **L**. Cf. the introduction to this volume.

131. Galen, *In Hippocratis Epidemiarum* 6.1 (ed. Wenkebach and Pfaff [CMG 5.10.2.2], 26 lines 22–25; Deller translation, 532, no. 58.). Cf. the introduction to this volume.

132. "peel and strip": cf. Galen, *De causis morborum* 7 (ed. Kühn, 7:33), which has ῥυπτόμενα.

133. Galen, *De causis morborum* 7 (ed. Kühn, 7:33).

134. "in a row" *(fī ṣanf wāḥid):* lit., of one kind. Cf. Galen, *De symptomatum differentiis* 6 (ed. Kühn, 7:81), which reads οἷον στίχον τινὰ.

135. Galen, *De symptomatum differentiis* 6 (ed. Kühn, 7:81).

136. Galen, *De symptomatum causis* 1.2 (ed. Kühn, 7:95–96).

137. "foods": lit., the thing.

138. "the matter residing in the tongue": i.e., the faculty of taste.

139. Galen, *De symptomatum causis* 1.4 (ed. Kühn, 7:105).

140. Cf. the introduction to this volume and the Arabic translation, entitled *Fī l-ḥarakāt al-muʿtāṣa*, MS Ayasofia 3631, fol. 106a (forthcoming edition and translation by Bos and Nutton): "But laughter occurring through tickling the armpits at the outside and under the footsoles does not fall under this category. I do not see any way at all to find out the reason why these spots, when they are touched, create the same movement as that which occurs when seeing or hearing comical things."

141. "generic form" *(al-ṣūra al-nawʿiyya):* cf. Maimonides, *Dalālat al-ḥāʾirin*, ed. Munk, 1.1; Efros, *Philosophical Terms*, 104, s.v. *zurah minit:* "generic form, i.e., the inner essential characteristics of the whole species."

142. See the introduction to this volume.

143. Galen, *De semine* 2.5 (trans. De Lacy, 194 lines 7–10).

144. "the eyes": lit., vision.

145. "And sometimes nature molds the eyes and sketches them in a hidden way and forms them without completing their strength as with the mole": cf. Galen, *De semine* 2.1, 5 (trans. De Lacy, 193): "If it (i.e., nature) should lack the strength for the final act, it leaves unfinished the thing being made, as is seen, for instance, in the whole race of moles; their eyes were sketched internally but were unable to emerge to the outside, their nature having lost the strength for this, so that it did not complete the work it had proposed to do."

## The Eighth Treatise

1. I.e., less nutrition.

2. Galen, *De acutorum morborum victu et Galeni commentarius* 2.36, 37 (ed. Helmreich, 196 lines 9–10; 197 lines 14–17).

3. Galen, *In Hippocratis Epidemiarum* 1.2 (ed. Wenkebach and Pfaff [CMG 5.10.1], 72 line 33–73 line 3; Deller translation, 522, no. 8).

4. Galen, *In Hippocratis De humoribus commentarius* 1 (ed. Kühn, 16:53); cf. Deichgräber, *De humoribus*, 49–50.

5. "reaching its climax": lit., at the end of its increase. Cf. Galen, *De totius morbi temporibus* 7 (ed. Kühn, 7:459), which has ἐπὶ πλεῖστον ηὔξηται.

6. Galen, *De totius morbi temporibus* 7 (ed. Kühn, 7:459); cf. Maimonides, *Aphorisms: Treatises 1–5*, ed. Bos, 3.101.

7. Galen, *De totius morbi temporibus* 7 (ed. Kühn, 7:459).

8. Galen, *De totius morbi temporibus* 8 (ed. Kühn, 7:460).

9. This quotation does not appear in this text in this form. In 2.19 (ed. Kühn, 17B:490), Galen says that chronic diseases are caused by thick, cold, and viscous humors and cannot be easily cocted.

10. "who is likely to be afflicted for some time": following Galen, *Ad Glauconem de methodo medendi* 1 (ed. Kühn, 11:35–36), which has ἐν χρόνῳ πλείονι ταλαιπωρεῖσθαι μέλλουσαν.

11. Galen, *Ad Glauconem de methodo medendi* 1 (ed. Kühn, 11:35–36).

12. Galen, *De crisibus* 1.13 (ed. Kühn, 11:610; ed. Alexanderson, 107 lines 6–10).

13. "nature": **E, L, B,** and **P** read "strength."

14. Galen, *De methodo medendi* 9.10 (ed. Kühn, 10:639–40).

15. Galen, *De methodo medendi* 12.8 (ed. Kühn, 10:863–64).

16. Galen, *De methodo medendi* 14.7 (ed. Kühn, 10:969).

17. "irritating": cf. Galen, *In Hippocratis Aphorismos commentarius* 4.10 (ed. Kühn, 17B:668), which has ὀργᾶν.

18. "a major organ": Galen, *In Hippocratis Aphorismos commentarius* 4.10 (ed. Kühn, 17B:668), which has κύριόν μόριον (i.e., heart, liver, brain, testes).

19. Galen, *In Hippocratis Aphorismos commentarius* 4.10 (ed. Kühn, 17B:668).

20. Galen, *In Hippocratis Aphorismos commentarius* 1.3 (ed. Kühn, 17B:365–66).

21. Galen, *In Hippocratis Epidemiarum* 1.2 (ed. Wenkebach and Pfaff [CMG 5.10.1], 74 lines 21–27; Deller translation, 522, no. 9).

22. Galen, *In Hippocratis Epidemiarum* 6.2 (ed. Wenkebach and Pfaff [CMG 5.10.2.2], 64 lines 18–26; Deller translation, 533–34, no. 66); cf. Anastassiou and Irmer, eds., *Testimonien*, 309 (ed. Littré 5.476.10).

23. Galen, *In Hippocratis De humoribus commentarius* 1.14 (ed. Kühn, 16:154); cf. Deichgräber, *De humoribus*, 53.

24. Galen, *In Hippocratis De humoribus commentarius* 1.14 (ed. Kühn, 16:154–55); cf. Deichgräber, *De humoribus*, 52–53.

25. Galen, *In Hippocratis De humoribus commentarius* 1.14 (ed. Kühn, 16:255–56); cf. Deichgräber, *De humoribus*, 46.

26. "pains in the joints": i.e., arthritis.

27. Galen, *De victu attenuante* (ed. Kalbfleisch, 433 lines 3–18) and Introduction, XLIX; Galen, *Thinning Diet*, trans. Singer, 305.

28. Galen, *In Hippocratis Epidemiarum* 6.5 (ed. Wenkebach and Pfaff [CMG 5.10.2.2], 254 lines 22, 27ff; Deller translation, 538, no. 86).

29. The original Greek text of this treatise has been lost. For the Arabic version, cf. Galen, *On Examinations* 3 (ed. Iskandar, 54 line 15–56 line 4).

30. Galen, *De consuetudinibus* (ed. Schmutte, 6); German translation from the Arabic by F. Pfaff, ibid., 40–41; Arabic translation, ed. Klein-Franke, *The Arabic Version of Galen's* Περὶ ἐθῶν, 140, English trans., ibid., 128–29.

31. Galen, *De methodo medendi* 7.6 (ed. Kühn, 10:492).

32. Galen, *In Hippocratis De acutorum morborum victu et Galeni commentarius* 1.43 (ed. Helmreich, 156 lines 15–17, 157 lines 4–5).

33. "Barley groats": cf. Galen, *In Hippocratis De acutorum morborum victu et Galeni commentarius* 1.26 (ed. Helmreich, 146 line 20), which has πτισάνη.

34. *Allium porrum.*

35. *Anethum graveolens.*

36. "moderate amount": Nathan ha-Meʾati and Zeraḥyah translate "a small amount."

37. "the nerves": lit., some of the nervous parts. Cf. Galen, *In Hippocratis De acutorum morborum victu et Galeni commentarius* 1.26 (ed. Helmreich, 147 line 8), which reads τὰ νεῦρα.

38. Galen, *In Hippocratis De acutorum morborum victu et Galeni commentarius* 1.26 (ed. Helmreich, 146 lines 20–23; 147 lines 4–9).

39. "barley broth": cf. Galen, *In Hippocratis De acutorum morborum victu et Galeni commentarius* 3.35 (ed. Helmreich, 249 line 14), which has ῥόφημα.

40. "disturbance": cf. Galen, *In Hippocratis De acutorum morborum victu et Galeni commentarius* 3.35 (ed. Helmreich, 249 line 26), which reads ταραχὴ.

41. Galen, *In Hippocratis De acutorum morborum victu et Galeni commentarius* 3.35 (ed. Helmreich, 249, lines 13–15, line 23–250 line 5).

42. See aphorism 7.65 above.

43. "drinks abundantly" *(yashrab sharāban kathīran):* cf. Galen, *In Hippocratis Epidemiarum* 1.3 (ed. Wenkebach and Pfaff [CMG 5.10.1], 133 line 19), which has πίνῃ δὲ δαψιλῶς.

44. Galen, *In Hippocratis Epidemiarum* 1.3 (ed. Wenkebach and Pfaff [CMG 5.10.1], 133 lines 18–25; Deller translation, 523, no. 12).

45. "Similarly": MSS **S, L, B, O,** and **P** have "therefore."

46. "tumor": cf. Pseudo-Galen, *In Hippocratis De humoribus commentarius* 1.17 (ed. Kühn, 16:165), which has ἀπόστημα (abscess).

47. Pseudo-Galen, *In Hippocratis De humoribus commentarius* 1.17 (ed. Kühn, 16:165–66).

48. "[inflamed] tumors": cf. Galen, *In Hippocratis Epidemiarum* 6.4 (ed. Wenkebach and Pfaff [CMG 5.10.2.2], 225 line 5), which has φλεγμονὴ.

49. Galen, *In Hippocratis Epidemiarum* 6.1–8 (ed. Wenkebach and Pfaff [CMG 5.10.2.2], 225 lines 5–7; Deller translation, 537, no. 81).

50. "affections for the soul": see aphorism 7.12 herein.

51. See Pseudo-Galen, *In Hippocratis De humoribus commentarius* 1.18 (ed. Kühn, 16:174–75), which reads ὅπου τοίνυν ἐν τῷ σώματι ψυχροί τε καὶ φλεγματικοὶ χυμοὶ περιττεύουσι, δεῖ μὴ μόνον τῇ τοῦ σώματος κινήσει, ἀλλὰ καὶ τῇ τῆς διανοίας ανεγείρειν καὶ οἷον ἀνάπτειν τὸ ἔμφυτον (wherever cold and phlegmatic humors become abundant in the body, it is necessary to stir up and, so to speak, arouse the innate heat not only by the movement of the body but also by that of the mind). Thus, the work of reducing these cold humors is to be done by the innate heat.

52. "[from the inner parts to the outer parts] of the body": the text reading "to the inner parts of the body" seems to be corrupt; cf. Pseudo-Galen, *In Hippocratis De humoribus commentarius* 1.18 (ed. Kühn, 16:174–75), which has εἰς τὰ ἔξωθεν.

53. Pseudo-Galen, *In Hippocratis De humoribus commentarius* 1.18 (ed. Kühn, 16:165–66).

54. "Joyful thoughts and expectations": lit., to think of joyful things and to expect them.

55. "rejoice": lit., dilate.

56. "distress": lit., contract.

57. Galen, *In Hippocratis De humoribus commentarius* 2.31 (ed. Kühn, 16:329).

58. "belly": "body" in **L**; cf. Arabic translation ed. Nabielek, "Schlaf und Wachsein," 67.10.

59. Nabielek, "Schlaf und Wachsein," 34; cf. aphorism 7.51 above.

60. "feebleness": lit., fainting; cf. Galen, *Ad Glauconem de methodo medendi* 1.15 (ed. Kühn, 11:51), which has ἐκλύσεις.

61. "moistures": lit., things.

62. "illness which causes a derangement of the mind": cf. Galen, *Ad Glauconem de methodo medendi* 1.15 (ed. Kühn, 11:51), which reads παρακρουστικόν τι πάθος.

63. "and": Galen, *Ad Glauconem de methodo medendi* 1.15 (ed. Kühn, 11:51), reads ἐν (in the case of, with).

64. Galen, *Ad Glauconem de methodo medendi* 1.15 (ed. Kühn, 11:51–52).

65. "concentrated grape juice": cf. Fellmann, *Aqrābādhin al-Qalānisī,* 239; Schmucker, *Materia medica,* no. 749.

66. Galen, *Ad Glauconem De methodo medendi* 2.2 (ed. Kühn, 11:81–82).

67. Galen, *De methodo medendi* 7.6 (ed. Kühn, 10:493).

68. "vaporous wind": Galen, *De methodo medendi* 12.8 (ed. Kühn, 10:869), reads πνεῦμα φυσῶδες.

69. "strong heating": lit., with a strong fire.

70. Galen, *De methodo medendi* 7.6 (ed. Kühn, 10:493).

71. "narcotics": lit., drugs that benumb the sensation [of pain].

72. "severe sleeplessness": lit., sleeplessness that causes agitation.

73. The text does not feature in book 8 of *De compositione medicamentorum secundum locos* but is probably an adaptation of book 9 (ed. Kühn, 13:266); cf. Zeraḥyah: בט' המיאמיר בט'.

74. "the remedy named after him": lit., his remedy.

75. Galen, *De compositione medicamentorum secundum locos* 9.4 (ed. Kühn, 13:267).

76. "that symptom": lit., the symptoms.

77. Galen, *De methodo medendi* 12.1 (ed. Kühn, 10:811–12).

78. Galen, *De methodo medendi* 12.1 (ed. Kühn, 10:811–12).

79. Galen, *De methodo medendi* 12.8 (ed. Kühn, 10:861).

80. "by operative treatment" *(bi-ᶜilāj al-ḥadīd):* Galen, *De compositione medicamentorum secundum locos* 14.13 (ed. Kühn, 13:990), has διὰ χειρουργίας; see as well Spink and Lewis, eds., *Albucasis,* 354: "Albucasis also sometimes uses the simple expression *ḥadīd*—iron—as a general term for operative (as opposed to medical or drug) treatment."

81. Galen, *De compositione medicamentorum secundum locos* 14.13 (ed. Kühn, 13:990).

82. "animal": Galen, *De morborum differentiis* 5 (ed. Kühn, 6:854), has ζωτικόν (vital); cf. aphorism 6.21 above.

83. "systems": lit., instruments *(ālāt).* Galen, *De morborum differentiis* 5 (ed. Kühn, 6:854), has ὄργανον; cf. Savage-Smith, "Galen on Nerves," 43.

84. Galen, *De morborum differentiis* 5 (ed. Kühn, 6:854).

85. "of that part": lit., of the homogeneous parts. Corrected after Galen, *De symptomatum differentiis* 5 (ed. Kühn, 7:78) τῶν τοιούτων σωμάτων.

86. Galen, *De symptomatum differentiis* 5 (ed. Kühn, 7:78).

87. Galen, *De curandi ratione per venae sectionem* 6 (ed. Kühn, 11:270); cf. aphorism 6.5 above.

88. Galen, *De methodo medendi* 4.4 (ed. Kühn, 10:260).

89. "although not widespread [in the body]": lit., although its quantity is small.

90. Galen, *De methodo medendi* 4.6 (ed. Kühn, 10:288–89).

91. Galen, *In Hippocratis De natura hominis commentarius* 3.15 (ed. Mewaldt, 101 lines 10–14).

92. "an extremely severe heat [of the urine]": cf. Galen, *In Hippocratis Aphorismos commentarius* 1.24 (ed. Kühn, 17B:448), which has ὑπερβαλλόντος ἐστὶ θερμὰ καὶ πυρρώδη τὰ οὖρα.

93. "inflamed tumor": Galen, *In Hippocratis Aphorismos commentarius* 1.24 (ed. Kühn, 17B:448), has φλεγμονὴ.

94. Galen, *In Hippocratis Aphorismos commentarius* 1.24 (ed. Kühn, 17B:448); cf. Anastassiou and Irmer, eds., *Testimonien*, 76–77 (ed. Littré, 4.472.4–5), 142 (ed. Littré, 4.602.8–9).

95. Galen, *In Hippocratis De acutorum morborum victu et Galeni commentarius* 2.1 (ed. Helmreich, 164 lines 14–19); cf. Maimonides, *Aphorisms: Treatises 1–5*, ed. Bos, 3.106.

96. Galen, *In Hippocratis Epidemiarum* 1.2 (ed. Wenkebach and Pfaff [CMG 5.10.1], 100 lines 7–13; Deller translation, 522, no. 10).

97. Galen, *In Hippocratis Epidemiarum* 2.6 (ed. Wenkebach and Pfaff [CMG 5.10.1], 394 lines 10–19; Deller translation, 527–28, no. 36); cf. Anastassiou and Irmer, eds., *Testimonien*, 227 (ed. Littré, 5.136.19).

98. For this text cf. Deichgräber, *De humoribus*, 50–51. Deichgräber's conclusion that Maimonides' summary of the text is unique for its brevity is no longer valid because that conclusion is based on the corrupt short Latin version, which is similar to **E** and **L**, and not on the correct longer version of **S**, **G**, and **B**. See the introduction to this volume.

99. "Similarly . . . into the whole body": cf. Arabic text, in Nabielek, ed. and trans., "Über Schlaf und Wachsein," 69 line 3ff; English translation, Gerrit Bos: "If someone wants to use his voice, he should train it slowly, especially if there is a superfluity in the stomach that has not descended or if his veins are full. If this is the case you should forbid him to use the movement through the voice for fear that those foods or drinks or [superfluous] matters which are in the veins may descend to [other] parts of the body and harm them."

100. Galen, *De somno et vigilia* (ed. and trans. Nabielek, 31; 69 line 3ff; 83 line 22–84 line 5); see aphorism 7.56 above.

101. Galen, *De arte parva* 34 (ed. Kühn, 1:394; ed. Boudon, 374.2). Boudon does not deal with Maimonides' quotations in her admirable edition.

102. "borax": cf. Maimonides, *Drug Names*, ed. Rosner, no. 51: "natron, impure carbonate of soda."

103. Galen, *Ad Glauconem De methodo medendi* 1.10 (ed. Kühn, 11:33).

104. "*skirros*": Galen, *Ad Glauconem De methodo medendi* 2.6 (ed. Kühn, 11:103), has σκίρρος.

105. Galen, *Ad Glauconem De methodo medendi* 2.6 (ed. Kühn, 11:103–4).

106. Galen, *De sanitate tuenda* 5.3 (ed. Kühn, 6:325; trans. Green, 198).

107. Galen, *De methodo medendi* 7.5 (ed. Kühn, 10:470–71).

108. "the main parts": Galen, *De methodo medendi* 7.5 (ed. Kühn, 10:471), speaks about the very substance of the homoiomerous parts (τῶν ὁμοιομερῶν σωμάτων).

109. Galen, *De methodo medendi* 7.5 (ed. Kühn, 10:470–71).

110. "which is like drizzle": Galen, *De methodo medendi* 7.5 (ed. Kühn, 10:471), reads δροσοειδῶς.

111. "and adapts itself to a [particular] part to provide it with food": cf. Galen, *De methodo medendi* 7.5 (ed. Kühn, 10:471): ταύτην οὖν ἐνθεῖναι τοῖς μορίοις οὐχ οἷον τε χωρὶς τροφῆς (It is not possible to replace this moisture in the body without nutriment).

112. "in those parts of the body that are of a moist, nearly coagulated, and hardened substance—just like fat and flesh—that then liquefies and dissolves"; lit., when they liquefy and dissolve. Cf. Galen, *De methodo medendi* 7.5 (ed. Kühn, 10:471), which has τῶν ἐκ τῆς ὑγροπαγοῦς οὐσίας συνεστώτων ὁποῖόν ἐστι πιμελὴ καὶ σάρξ.

113. Galen, *De methodo medendi* 7.5 (ed. Kühn, 10:471).

114. Galen, *De methodo medendi* 7.5 (ed. Kühn, 10:470).

115. Galen, *De methodo medendi* 11.15 (ed. Kühn, 10:787).

116. "properties": lit., powers.

117. Galen, *De arte parva* 34 (ed. Kühn, 1:399; ed. Boudon, 379–80, 16).

118. Galen, *Ad Glauconem de methodo medendi* 1.5 (ed. Kühn, 11:18).

119. Cf. Galen, *De compositione medicamentorum secundum locos* 8.3 (ed. Kühn, 13:153).

120. Galen, *In Hippocratis De acutorum morborum victu et Galeni commentarius* 2.2 (ed. Helmreich, 165 lines 18–24); cf. Anastassiou and Irmer, eds., *Testimonien,* 282 (ed. Littré, 6.92.10–11).

121. Galen, *De locis affectis* 6.3 (ed. Kühn, 8:394).

122. The medieval term *maghrib* (Islamic West) refers both to the modern Maghreb (Northwest Africa) and to al-Andalus (Muslim Spain), cf. Blau, "At Our Place," 293–95); Maimonides, *On Asthma,* ed. Bos, 4.4.

123. This text and the preceding one dealing with diabetes are quoted by R. Moshe Narboni (c. 1300–1362) in his medical compendium *Sefer Oraḥ Ḥayyim* (MS Munich 276, fol. 36a) in the form of the Hebrew translation by Nathan ha-Meʾati (cf. MS Paris 1173, fol. 31b). For this medical compendium see Bos, "Philosopher and Physician." See as well the introduction.

124. Galen, *In Hippocrates Epidemiarum* 1.2 (ed. Wenkebach and Pfaff [CMG 5.10.1], 161 lines 7–11; 22–25). Deller does not mention Maimonides' quotation.

125. Galen, *In Hippocratis De humoribus commentarius* 3.13 (ed. Kühn, 16:401).

126. "irritated": lit., burdened.

127. Galen, *Ad Glauconem de methodo medendi* 2.4 (ed. Kühn, 11:98–99).

128. Galen, *Ad Glauconem de methodo medendi* 2.5 (ed. Kühn, 11:103).

129. Galen, *De methodo medendi* 7.12 (ed. Kühn, 10:520).

130. "[to expel it]": cf. Bos, ed., *On Asthma,* 13.25, which reads فتكون هي النافية له.

131. Cf. Bos, ed., *On Asthma,* 13.25.

132. For Ibn Zuhr see aphorism 7.8, above.

## The Ninth Treatise

1. Galen, *In Hippocratis Aphorismos commentarius* 2.45 (ed. Kühn, 17B:548–49).

2. "the vein at the inner side of the arm": i.e., cubital; cf. Galen, *De curandi ratione per venae sectionem* 2 (ed. Kühn, 11:285), which has ἐν ἀγκῶνι φλέβα.

3. "on the side opposite to": Galen, *De curandi ratione per venae sectionem* 2 (ed. Kühn, 11:285), has κατ' εὐθύ.

4. "physicians": "ancient physicians" in **E, L, B,** and **P**.

5. Galen, *De curandi ratione per venae sectionem* 2 (ed. Kühn, 11:285).

6. Galen, *In Hippocratis Epidemiarum* 6.1–8 (ed. Wenkebach and Pfaff [CMG 5.10.2.2], 94 lines 24–28; Deller translation, 534, no. 69).

7. "*sawīq*": cf. Maimonides, *Drug Names,* ed. and trans. Rosner, no. 284 (semolina): "It is wheat, barley and other similar roasted cereals, agitated with butter and then ground." Also cf. Galen, *In Hippocratis Epidemiarum* 6.6 (ed. Wenkebach and Pfaff [CMG 5.10.2.2], 342 line 12; 343 line 6), which reads κυκεών.

8. Galen, *In Hippocratis Epidemiarum* 6.6 (ed. Wenkebach and Pfaff [CMG 5.10.2.2], 342 line 5–343 line 12; Deller translation, 540–41, no. 101); cf. Anastassiou and Irmer, eds., *Testimonien,* 326 (ed. Littré, 6.334.7–8).

9. Galen, *In Hippocratis Epidemiarum* 6.7; (ed. Wenkebach and Pfaff [CMG 5.10.2.2], 403 lines 4–9; Deller translation, 542, no. 106); cf. Anastassiou and Irmer, eds., *Testimonien,* 465.

10. Pseudo-Galen, *In Hippocratis De humoribus commentarius* 1.18 (ed. Kühn, 16:170).

11. Pseudo-Galen, *In Hippocratis De humoribus commentarius* 1.18 (ed. Kühn, 16:170–71); cf. Deichgräber, *De humoribus,* 46–47.

12. Pseudo-Galen, *In Hippocratis De humoribus commentarius* 1.17 (ed. Kühn, 16:166) speaks about sparks (μαρμαρυγαὶ) originating from superfluous humors and appearing to one during one's sleep.

13. "bandaging": lit., pressure; cf. Pseudo-Galen, *In Hippocratis De humoribus commentarius* 1.18 (ed. Kühn, 16:175), which has ἐπίδεσις.

14. Pseudo-Galen, *In Hippocratis De humoribus commentarius* 1.18 (ed. Kühn, 16:175).

15. Pseudo-Galen, *In Hippocratis De humoribus commentarius* 1.18 (ed. Kühn, 16:175).

16. "and making him open his eyes when he closes them": lit., "and the closing of his eyes, to force him to open them." Cf. Pseudo-Galen, *In Hippocratis De humoribus commentarius* 3.19 (ed. Kühn, 16:434), which has διοίγειν τέ ποτε εἰ μυήσειεν ἀναγκάζομεν τὰ βλέφαρα (also cf. Deichgräber, *De humoribus,* 44–45).

17. Pseudo-Galen, *In Hippocratis De humoribus commentarius* 3.19 (ed. Kühn, 16:434).

18. Cf. Galen, *Fī al-ḥarakāt,* in the forthcoming edition entitled *On Problematic Movements,* ed. Bos and Nutton, Cambridge University Press: "I have seen a horse doctor, when he wished to pour an oral medicine for horses into the esophagus, grasp firmly the tongue and the lower jaw so that they could

not move. This reminds me of that which is given as an oral medicine to people when they suffer from a stupor. Personally, in the case of a [sore] throat, I also take a narrow vessel, put some moist, fluid foodstuff in it, make it pass over the base of the tongue, and pour its contents into the esophagus." Cf. introduction to this volume and aphorism 7.71 above.

19. "on his back": lit., on his neck; Galen, *De instrumentu odoratus* 6 (ed. Kollesch, 62 line 24), has ὕπτιοι.

20. "torpor": Galen, *De instrumentu odoratus* 6 (ed. Kollesch, 11 line 25), reads κάρος.

21. Galen, *De instrumentu odoratus* 6 (ed. Kollesch, 62 lines 23–25).

22. Galen, *Puero epileptico consilium* 4 (ed. Kühn, 11:370).

23. "a nosebleed": lit., an evacuation.

24. Galen, *Ad Glauconem de methodo medendi* 1.15 ( ed. Kühn, 11:51).

25. "the leading activities": namely, those of the rational soul. Cf. Galen, *De locis affectis* 3.6 (ed. Kühn, 8:163): αἱ μὲν τοῦ λογιστικοῦ τῆς ψυχῆς ἐνέργειαι καλείσθωσαν ἡγεμονικαὶ.

26. Galen, *De locis affectis* 3.6 (ed. Kühn, 8:163–64).

27. "is comparable to the general harm": cf. Galen, *De locis affectis* 3.10 (ed. Kühn, 8:181), which has τῷ κοινῷ λόγῳ τῆς βλάβης. Trans. Siegel, 89, has "according to the general rule of this illness."

28. Galen, *De locis affectis* 3.10 (ed. Kühn, 8:181–82).

29. Galen, *De methodo medendi* 13.21 (ed. Kühn, 10:930).

30. *Papaver somniferum* and var.

31. Galen, *De methodo medendi* 13.21 (ed. Kühn, 10:930–31).

32. Galen, *De methodo medendi* 13.21 (ed. Kühn, 10:931–32).

33. "When the lethargy stops getting worse": cf. Galen, *De methodo medendi* 13.21 (ed. Kühn, 10:931), which reads ἑξῆς ("thereafter," namely, after the application of medications that dissolve the thick humor in the brain).

34. Galen, *De methodo medendi* 13.21 (ed. Kühn, 10:931).

35. *Lactuca sativa* or. *L. serriola*.

36. "has a cooling effect": lit., extinguishes (i.e., the heat).

37. *Brassica oleracea*.

38. *Lens esculenta*.

39. "becomes lax": cf. Galen, *De compositione medicamentorum secundum locos* 2.1 (ed. Kühn, 12:516), which has ἀνατρέπεται (becomes upset).

40. *Punica granatum* and var.

41. *Cydonia oblonga*.

42. Galen, *De compositione medicamentorum secundum locos* 2.1 (ed. Kühn, 12:515–18).

43. *Melilotus officinalis*.

44. *Trigonella foenum graecum*.

45. Galen, *De compositione medicamentorum secundum locos* 4.3 (ed. Kühn, 12:714).

46. "torpor": cf. Galen, *De symptomatum causis* 4.8 (ed. Kühn, 7:144), which has ἀποπληξίαι (apoplexies).

47. Galen, *De symptomatum causis* 4.8 (ed. Kühn, 7:144).

48. "a disturbance": lit., an objectionable occurrence. Cf. Latin translation, ed. Bologna 1487: "Ait. Moyses. Stupor et somnus ad excitandum difficilis est ex perturbatione operationum. Et cum spasmus epilenticus et angustia est ex amissione operationum sicut videtur." It seems that "ex perturbatione operationum" should be exchanged for "ex amissione operationum," whereby "perturbatio" is a translation of *jarayān munkar.*

49. Galen, *De compositione medicamentorum secundum locos* 2.1 (ed. Kühn, 12:499–500).

50. Galen, *De compositione medicamentorum secundum locos* 3.1 (ed. Kühn, 12:601–2).

51. Galen, *De compositione medicamentorum secundum locos* 3.1 (ed. Kühn, 12:603–4).

52. Galen, *De compositione medicamentorum secundum locos* 3.3 (ed. Kühn, 12:690).

53. Galen, *De compositione medicamentorum secundum locos* 5.4 (ed. Kühn, 12:863).

54. The physician al-Tamīmī (tenth century), originally from Jerusalem, served Ya'qūb ibn Killīs, the vizier of the first Fatimid caliph in the city of Cairo. His famous book on foodstuffs, *K. al-murshid fī jawāhir al-aghdhiya wa-quwā l-mufradāt mina l-adwiya* (Guide to the Substances of Foods and the Powers of Simple Drugs) has only been partially preserved and is still in manuscript; see Ullmann, *Medizin im Islam,* 269–70.

55. "Chinese snow": i.e., saltpeter; cf. Dozy, *Dictionnaires arabes,* 1:163; Goltz, *Studien,* 166–71, especially 167 n. 330: "Nach *Lippmann* I (1906), 135 kam die Kenntnis des Salpeters von China her, seine ältesten Namen seien 'Schnee' oder 'Salz von China' gewesen."

56. Golz, *Studien,* 295; Maimonides, *Drug Names,* ed. and trans. Rosner, no. 382.

57. Golz, *Studien,* 130ff; Maimonides, *Drug Names,* ed. and trans. Rosner, no. 342.

58. Maimonides, *Drug Names,* ed. and trans. Rosner, no. 226; Ibn al-Bayṭār, *Traité des simples,* trans. Leclerc, no. 2129: "On lit dans le *Morched* de Temīmy que la *mashaqounyā* est l'écume qui se forme sur la verre en fusion."

59. "glass of Pharaoh": cf. Dozy, *Dictionnaires arabes,* 1:581; Maimonides, *Drug Names,* ed. and trans. Rosner, no. 146: "The antique white glass is the one which one calls 'the glass of Pharaoh.'"

60. "the white opacity of the eye": i.e., leucoma.

61. Cf. **C**: "Says Galen: The inhabitants of the first country (i.e., a hot country) often suffer from ophthalmia, and [when this is the case] they quickly recover from it. But [the case] of those (i.e., the inhabitants of cold countries) is the opposite to these. They do not [often] suffer from ophthalmia, but when it happens to them, their eyes rupture. And ophthalmia is especially so rare amongst them because of the cold of their countries. Similarly, it only happens to a few people during the winter, but if it happens it is severe and painful." See as well the Hebrew translation: Galen, *Airs, Waters, and Places,* ed. Wasserstein, 33, 37 ([217, 221]).

62. *In Hippocratis Epidemiarum* 1.2 (ed. Wenkebach and Pfaff [CMG 5.10.1], 241 lines 37–42; 242 line 8ff; 243 lines 40–41; Deller translation, 524–25, no. 22); cf. Anastassiou and Irmer, eds., *Testimonien*, 426 (ed. Littré, 2.176.2–5) and 428 (ed. Littré, 2.176.7–12).

63. "soups" (*aḥsāʾ*, sing. *ḥasāʾ*): cf. Lane, *Lexicon*, 2:572: "A well-known kind of food, soup; i.e. what is supped, sipped; thin cooked food, that is supped or sipped made of flour and water and oil or grease, and sometimes sweetened."

64. "has the same effect as": lit., replaces.

65. *In Hippocratis Epidemiarum* 1.2 (ed. Wenkebach and Pfaff [CMG 5.10.1], 375 lines 8–15; Deller translation, 526–27, no. 31).

66. Galen, *In Hippocratis De humoribus commentarius* 1.18 (ed. Kühn, 16:175–76).

67. The quotation does not appear in *In Hippocratis De humoribus commentarius* 1.

68. Galen, *De symptomatum causis* 2.5 (ed. Kühn, 7:185–86).

69. Galen remarks that these drugs are necessary to prepare the way for the astringent ones. *De compositione medicamentorum secundum locos* 7.4 (ed. Kühn, 13:74).

70. Galen, *De compositione medicamentorum secundum locos* 7.4 (ed. Kühn, 13:74).

71. Galen, *De compositione medicamentorum secundum locos* 7.4 (ed. Kühn, 13:74), remarks that sometimes very cold drugs are mixed with those for the spitting of blood in order to induce a lethargic sleep.

72. I.e., the sleep.

73. Galen, *De compositione medicamentorum secundum locos* 7.4 (ed. Kühn, 13:74).

74. Galen, *De methodo medendi* 5.14 (ed. Kühn, 10:373–74).

75. Galen, *In Hippocratis Aphorismos commentarius* 6.13 (ed. Kühn, 18A:23); cf. Anastassiou and Irmer, *Testimonien*, 137 (ed. Littré 4.572.8–9).

76. "extremely" (*ʿalā l-istiqsāʾ*): Not reading *ʿalā l-istiqsāʾ* but *ʿalā l-istiqḍāʾ*, Deller (524, no. 19) translates: "gemäss (dem Ergebnis) einer gründlichen Untersuchung." Cf. Nathan: לנמרי and Zeraḥyah: על הקצה.

77. Galen, *In Hippocratis Epidemiarum* 1.3 (ed. Wenkebach and Pfaff [CMG 5.10.1], 199 lines 15–18; Deller translation, 524, no. 19).

78. Galen, *In Hippocratis Epidemiarum* 1.3 (ed. Wenkebach and Pfaff [CMG 5.10.1], 393 lines 5–28; Deller translation, 527, no. 35).

79. Galen, *De locis affectis* 5.6 (ed. Kühn, 8:341–42).

80. Cf. Galen, *De locis affectis* 5.6 (ed. Kühn, 8:342): φυσώδης.

81. Galen, *De locis affectis* 5.6 (ed. Kühn, 8:342).

82. "[hiera] picra": cf. Galen, *De sanitate tuenda* 6.7 (ed. Koch [CMG 5.4.2], 182 line 18), which has τὸ δι᾽ ἀλόης πικρόν (a bitter medicine with aloe as its main component); see Ullmann, *Medizin im Islam*, 296; for its composition see next aphorism.

83. Galen, *De sanitate tuenda* 6.7 (ed. Koch [CMG 5.4.2], 182 lines 9–12, 16–18).

84. Cf. Galen, *De methodo medendi* 7.9 (ed. Kühn, 10:508): μίγνυσθαι δ᾽ αὐτῇ ποτὲ μὲν ὑγρότητα, ποτὲ δὲ ξηρότητα.

85. Galen, *De methodo medendi* 7.9 (ed. Kühn, 10:508).

86. Aloe vera.

87. One *mithqāl* is 4.464 grams; see Hinz, *Islamische Masse*, 4.

88. *Cinnamomum ceylanicum.*

89. *Valeriana jatamansi.*

90. *Crocus sativus* and var.

91. *Asarum europaeum.*

92. *Commiphora opobalsamum.*

93. Galen, *De methodo medendi* 7.11 (ed. Kühn, 10:515–16).

94. *Ruta graveolens* and var.

95. *Cuminum cyminum* and var.

96. *Carum carvi.*

97. *Apium graveolens* and var.

98. Galen, *De methodo medendi* 8.5 (ed. Kühn, 10:576–78).

99. Galen, *De methodo medendi* 8.5 (ed. Kühn, 10:578).

100. "pale or yellowish wine": Galen, *De methodo medendi* 12.4 (ed. Kühn, 10:837), has κιρρός.

101. See Moshe Narboni, *Sefer Oraḥ Ḥayyim* (MS Munich 276, fols. 87b–88a), following the translation by Nathan ha-Meʾati.

102. Galen, *De methodo medendi* 12.4 (ed. Kühn, 10:836–37).

103. Galen, *De compositione medicamentorum secundum locos* 8.2 (ed. Kühn, 13:132).

104. "druglike fluid": cf. Galen, *De compositione medicamentorum secundum locos* 8.3 (ed. Kühn, 13:148), which has φαρμακώδης ἰχώρ.

105. "upset the soul": cf. Galen, *De compositione medicamentorum secundum locos* 8.3 (ed. Kühn, 13:149), which reads τὸν στόμαχον ἀνατρέπειν (upset the stomach); cf. aphorism 9.55 below. How a transposition from stomach to soul came to be made is unclear to me.

106. Galen, *De compositione medicamentorum secundum locos* 8.3 (ed. Kühn, 13:148–49).

107. Galen, *De compositione medicamentorum secundum locos* 8.3 (ed. Kühn, 13:154–55).

108. *Mentha pulegium.*

109. *Mentha piperita.*

110. "prick their chests": cf. Galen, *De compositione medicamentorum secundum locos* 8.4 (ed. Kühn, 13:176), which has τάς τε σιαγόνας νύσσοντας (prick their jaws or cheeks); the Arabic صدورهم (chests) is possibly a corruption of خدودهم (cheeks).

111. Galen, *De compositione medicamentorum secundum locos* 8.4 (ed. Kühn, 13:175–76).

112. Cf. Galen, *De symptomatum causis* 1.7 (ed. Kühn, 7:135): "The kind of bad food and drink one wants to take is analogous to the dominating [kind of] dyscrasia."

113. Galen, *De symptomatum causis* 1.7 (ed. Kühn, 7:134–35).

114. "upsets the soul": cf. Galen, *De sanitate tuenda* 6.10 (ed. Koch, 189 line 14), which has ἀνατρέπει τὸν στόμαχον (upsets the stomach); cf. aphorism 9.51 above.

115. "garum": cf. Schmucker, *Materia medica*, no. 721, s.v. *murrī*: "Das γάρον des Dioscurides, ist Garum: Sauce oder Brühe aus marinierten Fischen." However, in medieval medical texts not derivative from classical sources, it is a cereal-based preparation (see Waines, "Tale of a Condiment").

116. Galen, *De sanitate tuenda* 6.10 (ed. Koch, 189 lines 11–23).

117. Galen, *De methodo medendi* 8.5 (ed. Kühn, 10:573).

118. "salve" *(qīrūṭī):* Galen, *De methodo medendi* 8.5 (ed. Kühn, 10:574), has κηρωτὴ; cf. Ullmann, *Medizin im Islam*, 299; Fellmann, *Aqrābādhīn al-Qalānisī*, 256.

119. Galen, *De methodo medendi* 8.5 (ed. Kühn, 10:574–75).

120. I.e., a bain-marie.

121. This remark about the special preparation of this salve does not feature in Galen and is therefore a personal note by Maimonides; see the introduction.

122. Galen, *De methodo medendi* 8.5 (ed. Kühn, 10:573).

123. "the membrane covering them": i.e., the peritoneum.

124. This text does not appear in the mentioned book; however, cf. Galen, *Introductio sive medicus* 13 (ed. Kühn, 17:746).

125. Cf. Galen, *In Hippocratis De humoribus commentarius* 1.12 (ed. Kühn, 16:111–12); Deichgräber, *De humoribus*, 49.

126. Cf. Galen, *In Hippocratis De humoribus commentarius* 1.12 (ed. Kühn, 16:112); Deichgräber, *De humoribus*, 49.

127. Galen, *In Hippocratis De humoribus commentarius* 2.27 (ed. Kühn, 16:298).

128. [most of them]: cf. Galen, *Ad Glauconem de methodo medendi* 2.7 (ed. Kühn, 11:109), which has οἱ πλεῖστοι.

129. Galen, *Ad Glauconem de methodo medendi* 2.7 (ed. Kühn, 11:109).

130. Galen, *Ad Glauconem de methodo medendi* 2.12 (ed. Kühn, 11:145).

131. Galen, *De symptomatum causis* 3.5 (ed. Kühn, 7:234): διαπήδησις.

132. Galen, *De symptomatum causis* 3.5 (ed. Kühn, 7:234).

133. Galen, *De locis affectis* 5.7 (ed. Kühn, 8:351–54).

134. Galen, *De locis affectis* 5.7 (ed. Kühn, 8:351–54).

135. "a slow digestion": Galen, *De sanitate tuenda* 6.7 (ed. Koch, 182 line 2), has βραδυπεψία.

136. Galen, *De sanitate tuenda* 6.7 (ed. Koch, 181 line 37–182 line 3).

137. *Artemisia absinthium* and var.

138. Galen, *De methodo medendi* 11.16 (ed. Kühn, 10:789–91).

139. Lit., do not approach it.

140. Galen, *De methodo medendi* 13.14 (ed. Kühn, 10:908).

141. *Carthamus tinctorius.*

142. *Urtica pilulifera.*

143. *Polypodium vulgare.*

144. *Helleborus niger.*

145. "mint": The Arabic *fūdhanj* is a generic term for the different species of mint; cf. Galen, *De methodo medendi* 13.15 (ed. Kühn, 10:914), which has ὀρίγανον (origanum).

146. *Citrullus colocynthis.*

147. *Centaurium minus.*

148. Galen, *De methodo medendi* 13.15 (ed. Kühn, 10:913–14).

149. *Pistacia terebinthus.*

150. Galen, *De compositione medicamentorum secundum locos* 8.6 (ed. Kühn, 13:191–92).

151. *Cichorium endivia* and var. or *C. intybus* and var.

152. "they make those serous moistures and other moistures flow and descend [from the body]": cf. Galen, *De compositione medicamentorum secundum locos* 8.8 (ed. Kühn, 13:207), which reads ἐπ' οὖρα προάγει τὴν ὑγρότητα (it leads the [excess] moisture to become urine).

153. Galen, *De compositione medicamentorum secundum locos* 8.8 (ed. Kühn, 13:206–7).

154. Galen, *De compositione medicamentorum secundum locos* 8.8 (ed. Kühn, 13:216).

155. Aspidium filix-mas SW.

156. "taste": cf. Galen, *De compositione medicamentorum secundum locos* 8.8 (ed. Kühn, 13:208), which reads "quality" (ποιότης).

157. Galen, *De compositione medicamentorum secundum locos* 8.8 (ed. Kühn, 13:208).

158. Lit., remedies.

159. Galen, *De compositione medicamentorum secundum locos* 8.1 (ed. Kühn, 13:117).

160. Galen, *De methodo medendi* 13.14 (ed. Kühn, 10:908–9).

161. Galen, *De methodo medendi* 11.16 (ed. Kühn, 10:795).

162. *Capparis spinosa.*

163. Galen, *De methodo medendi* 11.16 (ed. Kühn, 10:796–97).

164. Gum resin of *Ferula communis* var. *gummifera* or *F. tingitana.*

165. Galen, *De methodo medendi* 14.5 (ed. Kühn, 10:959–60).

166. "the soul becomes upset": cf. Galen, *De locis affectis* 6.1 (ed. Kühn, 8:378), which reads τὸ φερόμενον εἰς τὴν γαστέρα ... πολλάκις δ' ἀνατροπήν (frequently the stomach becomes upset); cf. aphorism 9.51.

167. "when the craving is spoiled in another way": cf. Galen, *De locis affectis* 6.1 (ed. Kühn, 8:378), which has ὅταν ἑτέραν τινά ἔχῃ διαφθοράν (trans. Siegel renders this "since [the residues] are corrupted in some other manner").

168. Galen, *De locis affectis* 6.1 (ed. Kühn, 8:378).

169. Galen, *De methodo medendi* 13.17 (ed. Kühn, 10:921).

170. "so that a crisis is not hindered": Galen, *In Hippocratis De acutorum morborum victu et Galeni commentarius* 1.32 (ed. Helmreich, 150 line 18), remarks that if one administers barley groats the patient suffers great harm (μεγάλως βλάψει τὸν κάμνοντα).

171. Galen, *In Hippocratis De acutorum morborum victu et Galeni commentarius* 1.32 (ed. Helmreich, 150 lines 8–18.

172. Galen, *In Hippocratis De acutorum morborum victu et Galeni commentarius* 2.3 (ed. Helmrcich, 166 lines 8–14); cf. Anastassiou and Irmer, eds., *Testimonien*, 11 (ed. Littré, 2.268.10–11).

173. "[inhalation] of the vapor": following Galen, *De acutorum morborum victu et Galeni commentarius* 2.4 (ed. Helmreich, 166 line 27), which reads ἡ τῆς ἀτμίδος εἰσπνοὴ.

174. "pleurisy" *(shawṣa):* for this term and the regular *dhāt al-janb* to indicate this illness, see Dols, *Medieval Islamic Medicine,* 123, esp. n. 18; Ullmann, *Rufus von Ephesos,* 125.

175. Galen, *De acutorum morborum victu et Galeni commentarius* 2.4 (ed. Helmreich, 166 lines 26–28).

176. Cf. Galen, *In Hippocratis De humoribus commentarius* 3.33 (ed. Kühn, 16:481–82).

177. I.e., the symptoms of an inflammation of the nervous part of the diaphragm are the same as those of severe pleuritis; cf. Galen, *De praesagitione ex pulsibus* 4.5 (ed. Kühn, 9:401), which reads ἀνάλογον δὲ τοῖς ἐπὶ τῷ νευρώδει τοῦ διαφράγματος ἔπεται πάντα ταῖς μεγάλαις πλευρίτισιν.

178. Galen, *De praesagitione ex pulsibus* 4.5 (ed. Kühn, 9:401).

179. Cf. Galen, *De methodo medendi* 14.12 (ed. Kühn, 10:986): ἔστι δὲ καὶ ἄλλα πολλὰ μὲν τοιαῦτα.

180. Cf. Galen, *De methodo medendi* 14.12 (ed. Kühn, 10:986): θηριακὴ (theriac), a confection originally given as an antidote to snakebite and occasionally later as a general tonic. In *De theriaca ad Pisonem* and *De theriaca ad Pamphilianum* (ed. Kühn, 14:1–310), we find detailed descriptions of the different theriacs.

181. "and less good are the drugs prepared with water mint" *(Mentha aquatica)*: cf. Galen: τῶν δ᾽ εὐτελῶν ἄριστόν ἐστιν τὸ ἡμέτερον, ὃ διὰ τῆς Κρητικῆς καλαμίνθης σκευάζομεν (of the simple drugs the best one is ours, which we prepare with Cretian mint).

182. Galen, *De methodo medendi* 13.17 (ed. Kühn, 10:921).

183. Galen, *De compositione medicamentorum secundum locos* 7.6 (ed. Kühn, 13:105).

184. This statement is quoted by Moshe Narboni, *Sefer Oraḥ Ḥayyim* (MS Munich 276, fols. 87b–88a), following the translation by Nathan ha-Meʾati.

185. *Adiantum capillus veneris.*

186. *Agrimonia eupatoria.*

187. *Cymbopogon schoenanthus.*

188. *Tamarix gallica.*

189. *Pistacia vera* and var.

190. *Urtica pilulifera* and var.

191. *Commiphora opobalsamum.*

192. *Aristolochia clematis.*

193. I.e., white or blue lily (*Lilium candidum* and *Iris florentina*).

194. *Ecbalium elaterium.*

195. *Rheum palmatum.*

196. *Asphodelus ramosus.*

197. *Cheiranthus cheiri.*

198. *Juniperus sabina.*

199. *Gentiana lutea.*

200. *Athamanta cretensis.*

201. *Cinnamomum ceylanicum.*

202. *Hypericum perforatum.*

203. *Acorus calamus.*

204. *Hyssopus officinalis* and var.

205. *Populus nigra (jūz rūmī = ḥawar rūmī);* cf. Dietrich, trans. and ed., *Dioscorides triumphans,* 1:51.

206. Its identification is impossible; cf. Dietrich, trans. and ed., *Dioscorides triumphans,* 1:2.

207. *Piper cubeba.*

208. *Origanum majorana* and var.

209. *Ammi visnaga.*

210. *Thymus serpillum* and var.

211. *Ruta graveolens* and var.

212. *Cinnamomum cassia.*

213. *Ferula persica.*

214. *"mint" (fūdhanj):* See Maimonides, *Drug Names,* ed. and trans. Rosner, no. 309, where the various species of *fūdhanj* are specified.

215. *Foeniculum vulgare.*

216. *Nigella sativa* and var.

217. *Mesua ferrea;* see Maimonides, *Drug Names,* ed. and trans. Rosner, no. 250.

218. *Elettaria cardamomum.*

219. Cf. Maimonides, *Drug Names,* ed. and trans. Rosner, no. 116.

220. Galen, *In Hippocratis Aphorismos commentarius* 7.37 (ed. Kühn, 18A:140).

221. Galen, *In Hippocratis Aphorismos commentarius* 7.55 (ed. Kühn, 18A:165).

222. "eaten away": cf. Galen, *De usu partium* 5.12 (ed. Helmreich, 1:283 line 24): ἀπεσάπη.

223. Galen, *De usu partium* 5.12 (ed. Helmreich, 1:283 lines 23–25).

224. For this treatise see aphorism 7.65 above.

225. *Panicum miliaceum.*

226. Galen, *De methodo medendi* 12.8 (ed. Kühn, 10:866–67).

227. Cf. Galen, *Introductio sive medicus* 13 (ed. Kühn, 14:755), has ἀσκαριδές (ascarids). Al-Mājūsī, *Kāmil al-ṣināʿa,* 1:370, calls these "worms that originate in vinegar" *(al-dūd al-mutawallid fī l-khall).*

228. Galen, *Introductio sive medicus* 13 (ed. Kühn, 14:755), has κειρίαι (tapeworms).

229. Galen, *Introductio sive medicus* 13 (ed. Kühn, 14:755), has στρογγύλαι (round-worms).

230. Galen, *In Hippocratis Epidemiarum* 1.2 (ed. Wenkebach and Pfaff [CMG 5.10.1], 160, lines 4–9, 24–31; Deller translation, 523, 13.

231. Cf. Galen, *De symptomatum causis* 3.8 (ed. Kühn, 7:251), which reads ἐν ταῖς φλεψί.

232. Galen, *De symptomatum causis* 3.8 (ed. Kühn, 7:251).

233. "abscess": translated after Galen, *De locis affectis* 6.3 (ed. Kühn, 8:391), which reads ἀπόστημα. The Arabic *waram* normally means "tumor."

234. "cicatrization" *(idmāl wa-khatm):* lit., healing and sealing. Cf. Galen, *De locis affectis* 6.3 (ed. Kühn, 8:391), which reads ἐπουλώσις.

235. Galen, *De locis affectis* 6.3 (ed. Kühn, 8:391).

236. Galen, *De symptomatum causis* 3.8 (ed. Kühn, 7:248).

237. "that are not hot when they are washed": cf. Galen, *De compositione medicamentorum secundum locos* 9.6 (ed. Kühn, 13:307): ταῦτα γὰρ πλυνθέντα χωρὶς τοῦ δάκνειν ἐργάζεται τὸ δέον (for when they are washed, they do what is necessary without any biting effect).

238. Galen, *De compositione medicamentorum secundum locos* 9.6 (ed. Kühn, 13:306–7).

239. Cf. Galen, *De tumoribus praeter naturam* 13 (ed. Kühn, 7:727), which has ἐν ταῖς φλεψί.

240. "smell bad": cf. Galen, *De tumoribus praeter naturam* 13 (ed. Kühn, 7:727), which reads δυσώδεις εἰσι.

241. Galen, *De tumoribus praeter naturam* 13 (ed. Kühn, 7:727); cf. Maimonides, *Aphorisms: Treatises 1–5*, ed. Bos, 2.16.

242. "have misled": lit., have caused to stumble.

243. Galen, *In Hippocratis Epidemiarium* 6.1–8 (ed. Wenkebach and Pfaff [CMG 5.10.2.2], 483 lines 11–19; Deller translation, 543, no. 111.)

244. "parching": cf. Galen, *De marcore* 9 (ed. Kühn, 7:701), which has περιφρυγέσιν.

245. "that is accompanied by syncope": lit., which is called "the syncope one"; Galen, *De marcore* 9 (ed. Kühn, 7:701).

246. "barley gruel": cf. Galen, *De marcore* 9 (ed. Kühn, 7:702), which reads πτισάνη.

247. "groats of Roman wheat" *(khandarūs):* cf. Galen, *De marcore* 9 (ed. Kühn, 7:702), which reads χόνδρος; see as well aphorism 6.17 above.

248. Galen, *De marcore* 9 (ed. Kühn, 7:701–2).

249. For this text, which I could not identify, see the introduction.

250. I.e., hydrocele.

251. Galen, *De examinatione medici* 14 (ed. Iskandar, 134 lines 12–19, 136 lines 1–2).

252. "[that patient]": cf. Pseudo-Galen, *"De Theriaca ad Pisonem,"* ed. Richter-Bernburg, Arabic translation, 124b13, which reads *dhālika l-insān*.

253. Galen, *De theriaca ad Pisonem* 15 (ed. Kühn, 14:274–75; ed. Richter-Bernburg, 124b9–125a1 [Arabic translation]).

254. "especially when the affected organ is evidently cold": cf. Galen, *De arte parva* 34 (ed. Kühn, 1:396; ed. Boudon, 377, 9): "especially when the affected spot lies on the surface."

255. "When the organ is markedly cold": cf. Galen, *De arte parva* 34 (ed. Kühn, 1:397; ed. Boudon, 377, 11): "But if the parts on the surface are not affected at all..."

256. Galen, *De arte parva* 34 (ed. Kühn, 1:396–97; ed. Boudon, 377, 9, 11).

257. "The kind of shingles that is associated with corrosion": cf. Galen, *Ad Glauconem de methodo medendi* 2.3 (ed. Kühn, 11:86): οἱ ἀναβιβρωσκόμενοι ἕρπεις.

258. "vine tendrils": cf. Galen, *Ad Glauconem de methodo medendi* 2.3 (ed. Kühn, 11:86): ἕλικας ἀμπέλου.

259. *Rubus fruticosus.*

260. *Plantago major.*

261. "fine" *(fī riqqatihi):* possibly a corruption of *fī waqtihi* (at some time). Cf. Galen, *Ad Glauconem de methodo medendi* 2.3 (ed. Kühn, 11:86): ποτε.

262. *"sawīq* of barley" *(sawīq al-shaʿīr):* for *sawīq,* cf. aphorism 9.4 above; Galen, *Ad Glauconem de methodo medendi* 2.3 (ed. Kühn, 11:86), reads ἄλφιτον (barley groats); cf. Maimonides, *Aphorisms: Treatises 1–5,* ed. Bos, 5.16.

263. Galen, *Ad Glauconem de methodo medendi* 2.3 (ed. Kühn, 11:86); cf. Maimonides, *Aphorisms: Treatises 1–5,* ed. Bos, 25.54.

264. *Polygonum aviculare.*

265. *Lemna.*

266. *Nymphaea.*

267. *Plantago psyllium* and var.

268. *Portulaca oleracea.*

269. *Sempervivum arboreum.*

270. *Solanum nigrum* and var.

271. Galen, *Ad Glauconem de methodo medendi* 2.3 (ed. Kühn, 11:86); cf. Maimonides, *Aphorisms: Treatises 1–5,* ed. Bos, 25.54.

272. Cf. introduction to Maimonides, *On Asthma,* ed. Bos, about the bad air in Alexandria.

273. Galen, *Ad Glauconem de methodo medendi* 2.12 (ed. Kühn, 11:141–42).

274. "which should be consumed in abundance" *(aktharuhā):* cf. Galen, *Ad Glauconem de methodo medendi* 2.12 (ed. Kühn, 11:143): pleonast°on.

275. *Malva silvestris* and var.

276. *Atriplex hortensis.*

277. *Amaranthus blitum.*

278. The generic name *qarʿun* can refer to the following species: *Cucurbita maxima, Cucurbita pepo,* or *Lagenaria vulgaris.*

279. "those that can be sighted amongst the rocks": cf. Galen, *Ad Glauconem de methodo medendi* 2.12 (ed. Kühn, 11:143): ἰχθύων δὲ τοῖς πετραίοις [χρηστέον] (amongst the fish they should use the rockfish); cf. aphorism 8.25 above.

280. *Anethum graveolens.*

281. *Allium porrum* and var.

282. Galen, *Ad Glauconem de methodo medendi* 2.12 (ed. Kühn, 11:143–44).

283. "its sting gets fixed in": cf. Galen, *De locis affectis* 3.11 (ed. Kühn, 8:196): ἐναπερείσηται τὸ κέντρον εἰς.

284. Galen, *De locis affectis* 3.11 (ed. Kühn, 8:196).

285. "evil thoughts": cf. Galen, *De locis affectis* 6.5 (ed. Kühn, 8:418), which reads δυσέλπιδας (despondent).

286. Galen, *De locis affectis* 6.5 (ed. Kühn, 8:418).

287. Galen, *De simplicium medicamentorum temperamentis ac facultatibus* 8 (ed. Kühn, 12:267–68).

288. Galen, *De sanitate tuenda* 3.10 (ed. Koch, 97 lines 13–14, 17–19).

289. Galen, *De locis affectis* 5.2 (ed. Kühn, 8:304–5).

290. Galen, *De methodo medendi* 5.6 (ed. Kühn, 10:313–32).

291. "affliction": cf. Galen, *De methodo medendi* 6.3 (ed. Kühn, 10:408), which reads θλίσις (contusion).

292. *Vicia faba.*
293. Galen, *De methodo medendi* 6.3 (ed. Kühn, 10:407–8).
294. Lit., dissolution.
295. Lit., dissolve.
296. Galen, *De methodo medendi* 12.5 (ed. Kühn, 10:847–48).
297. "the glands swell very rapidly": cf. Galen, *De methodo medendi* 13.5 (ed. Kühn, 10:881–82), which reads τάχιστα μὲν οἱ βουβῶνες ἀνίστανται (swollen glands arise most rapidly). For the Arabic *al-laḥmu al-rakhwu* for "glands," cf. *WKAS* 2.1.358–59; see as well Maimonides, *Aphorisms: Treatises 1–5*, ed. Bos, 1.8, where the term *ghadad* appears for "glands."
298. Galen, *De methodo medendi* 13.5 (ed. Kühn, 10:881–82).
299. Lit., therefore.
300. I.e., to the affected part.
301. "But if one is slow": cf. Galen, *De methodo medendi* 13.5 (ed. Kühn, 10:883): βραδύνοντος.
302. Galen, *De methodo medendi* 13.5 (ed. Kühn, 10:882–84).
303. Lit., "medications."
304. Cf. Galen, *De methodo medendi* 13.6 (ed. Kühn, 10:896), which reads ἡ τοίνυν μέθοδος . . . διττὸν ἔχει τὸν σκοπόν, κένωσίν τε καί ἀλλοίωσιν τοῦ τὴν ὀδύνην ἐργαζομένου (In treating pains caused by animals or noxious drugs, one should aim at two things: to evacuate and to transform that which effects the pain).
305. "hollow horns": cf. Galen, *De methodo medendi* 13.6 (ed. Kühn, 10:896): κοίλα κεράτα.
306. Galen, *De methodo medendi* 13.6 (ed. Kühn, 10:896).
307. Galen, *De methodo medendi* 14.5 (ed. Kühn, 10:959).
308. "cancer": lit., disease.
309. Galen, *De methodo medendi* 14.9 (ed. Kühn, 10:979).
310. "pains in the joints": i.e., arthritis.
311. "detaining and restraining drugs": i.e., those that prevent the fluids from streaming to the hands and feet.
312. "and [this kind of treatment] would increase the overfilling": cf. Galen, *De compositione medicamentorum secundum locos* 10.2 (ed. Kühn, 13:334), which reads συλλαβάνεται τὸ ἐκ τῶν περιεχόντων ἀγγείων αἷμα καὶ μυῶν πρὸς ἐκείνην (because the blood would be gathered to it from the surrounding vessels and muscles).
313. Galen, *De compositione medicamentorum secundum locos* 10.2 (ed. Kühn, 13:334).
314. "by means of food": lit., after the food. Cf. Galen, *De compositione medicamentorum secundum locos* 10.2 (ed. Kühn, 13:335): μετὰ τροφῆς. The Arabic translator has read μετὰ τροφῆν instead of μετὰ τροφῆς.
315. Galen, *De compositione medicamentorum secundum locos* 10.2 (ed. Kühn, 13:335–36).
316. One *mithqāl* is 4.68 grams; see Hinz, *Islamische Masse*, 4.
317. *Juniperus sabina.*
318. The standard *dirham* is 3.125 grams; see Hinz, *Islamische Masse*, 3.

319. *Asphodelus ramosus.* See Maimonides, *Drug Names,* ed. and trans Rosner, no. 935.

320. One ounce is 37.5 grams; see Hinz, *Islamische Masse,* 35.

321. *Myrtus communis.*

322. For al-Tamīmī, see aphorism 9.30 above.

323. Galen, *De methodo medendi* 6.5 (ed. Kühn, 10:439–41).

324. Galen, *De methodo medendi* 13.5 (ed. Kühn, 10:885).

325. Galen, *De methodo medendi* 13.12 (ed. Kühn, 10:905–6).

326. Cf. Aristotle, *Historia Animalium* 9.12 (588a3–6). Galen discusses this matter extensively in his commentary on Hippocrates' *Prognosticon* 3.34 (ed. Kühn, 18B:292–93); the same text is quoted by R. Moshe Narboni in his medical compendium *Sefer Oraḥ Ḥayyim* (MS Munich 276, fols 73a–b) in the form of the Hebrew translation by Nathan ha-Meʾati (cf. MS Paris 1173, fol. 39a); see aphorism 8.69, above, and the introduction.

# Bibliographies

## Translations and Editions of Works by
## or Attributed to Moses Maimonides
(arranged alphabetically by translator or editor)

Bar-Sela, Ariel, Hebbel E. Hoff, and Elias Faris, eds. and trans. *Moses Maimonides' Two Treatises on the Regimen of Health:* Fī tadbīr al-ṣiḥḥa *and* Maqāla fī bayān baʿḍ al-aʿrāḍ wa-al-jawāb ʿanhā. Transactions of the American Philosophical Society, New Series, 54.4. Philadelphia: American Philosophical Society, 1964.

Bos, Gerrit, ed. and trans. *Medical Aphorisms: Treatises 1–5.* Provo, Utah: Brigham Young University Press, 2004.

———, ed. and trans. *On Asthma.* Provo, Utah: Brigham Young University Press, 2002.

Kroner, Hermann, ed. "Der medizinische Schwanengesang des Maimonides: *Fī bajān al-aʿrāḍ* (Über die Erklärung der Zufälle)." *Janus* 32 (1928): 12–116.

———, ed. and trans. "*Fī tadbīr al-ṣiḥḥa:* Gesundheitsanleitung des Maimonides für den Sultan al-Malik al-Afḍal." *Janus* 27 (1923): 101–16, 286–300; 28 (1924): 61–74, 143–52, 199–217, 408–19, 455–72; 29 (1925): 235–58. Reprinted in *Beiträge zur Geschichte der arabisch-islamischen Medizin,* ed. Fuat Sezgin et al. Frankfurt am Main: Institut für Geschichte der arabisch-islamischen Wissenschaften an der Johann Wolfgang Goethe-Universität, 1987.

Leibowitz, Joshua O., and Shlomo Marcus, eds., with the collaboration of M. Beit-Arié, E. D. Goldschmidt, F. Klein-Franke, E. Lieber, and M. Plessner. *On the Causes of Symptoms:* Maqāla fī bayān baʿḍ al-aʿrāḍ wa-al-jawāb ʿanhā, Maʾamar ha-Haḳraʾah, De causis accidentium. Berkeley and Los Angeles: University of California Press, 1974.

Munk, Salomon, ed. *Dalālat al-ḥāʾirīn: Moreh ha-nevukim.* Judeo-Arabic text with variant readings by Issachar Joel. Jerusalem: J. Junovitch, 1930/31.

———, ed. and trans. *Le guide des égarés: Traité de théologie et de philosophie par Moïse ben Maimoun, dit Maïmonide. Traduit pour la première fois sur l'original arabe et accompagné de notes critiques, littéraires et explicatives par S. Munk.* 3 vols. 1856–1866. Reprint, Paris: G.-P. Maisonnueve & Larose, 1970.

Muntner, Süssmann, ed. *Pirke Mosheh bi-refuʾah: be-targumo shel Natan ha-Meʾati.* Jerusalem: Mosad ha-Rav Ḳuḳ, 1959.

Rosner, Fred, trans. *The Medical Aphorisms of Moses Maimonides.* Maimonides' Medical Writings, 3. Haifa: Maimonides Research Institute, 1989.

———, ed. and trans. *Moses Maimonides' Glossary of Drug Names.* Maimonides' Medical Writings 7. Haifa: Maimonides Research Institute, 1995.

Stern, S. M., ed. and trans. "Maimonides' *Treatise to a Prince, Containing Advice on Sexual Matters.*" In *Maimonidis Commentarius in Mischnam ...*, ed. S. M. Stern, 17–21. Corpus codicum Hebraicorum Medii Aevi, 1.3. Copenhagen: Ejnar Munksgaard, 1966.

Zahalon, Jacob. *Shemirat ha-beriʾut leha-Rambam.* Edited by Zohar Amar. Jerusalem: Neveh Tsuf, 2001.

## Editions of Galenic Works

(arranged alphabetically by translator or editor)

Alexanderson, Bengt, ed. *Peri Kriseōn Galenos (De crisibus).* Göteborg: Almquist & Wiksell, 1967.

Boer, Wilko de, ed. *De atra bile.* Corpus Medicorum Graecorum 5.4.1.1. Leipzig: Teubner, 1937.

Boudon, Véronique, ed. *Galien.* Vol. 2, *Exhortation à l'étude de la médecine; Art médical.* Paris: Belles Lettres, 2002.

*De instrumento odoratus.* See Kollesch, Jutta, ed. and trans. *Galen über das Riechorgan.*

De Lacy, Phillip, ed. and trans. *On Semen.* Corpus Medicorum Graecorum 5.3.1. Berlin: Akademie Verlag, 1992.

*De optico medico congnoscendo.* See Iskandar, Albert Z., ed. and trans. *On Examinations by Which the Best Physicians Are Recognized.*

*De somno et vigilia.* See Nabielek, R., ed. and trans. "Die ps.-galenische Schrift 'Über Schlaf und Wachsein.'"

Green, Robert Montraville, trans. *A Translation of Galen's* Hygiene. Introduction by Henry E. Sigerist. Springfield, Ill.: Thomas, 1951. (See also Koch's edition below.)

Helmreich, Georg, ed. *De usu partium corporis humani.* 2 vols. Bibliotheca Scriptorum Graecorum et Romanorum Teubneriana. Leipzig: Teubner, 1907–9. (See also May's translation below.)

———, ed. *In Hippocratis de victu acutorum commentaria.* Corpus Medicorum Graecorum 5.9.1. Leipzig: Teubner, 1914.

Iskandar, Albert Z., ed. and trans. *On Examinations by Which the Best Physicians Are Recognized.* Corpus Medicorum Graecorum, Supplementum Orientale 4. Berlin: Akademie Verlag, 1988.

Kalbfleisch, Karl, ed. *De victu attenuante.* Corpus Medicorum Graecorum 5.4.2. Leipzig: Teubner, 1923.

Klein-Franke, F. "The Arabic Version of Galen's Περὶ ἐθῶν." *Jerusalem Studies in Arabic and Islam* 1 (1979): 125–50.

Koch, Konrad, ed. *De sanitate tuenda.* Corpus Medicorum Graecorum 5.4.2. Leipzig: Teubner, 1923. (See also Green's translation above.)

Kollesch, Jutta, ed. and trans. *Galen über das Riechorgan.* Corpus Medicorum Graecorum, Supplement 5. Berlin: Akademie Verlag, 1964.

Kühn, Karl Gottlob, ed. *Claudii Galeni opera omnia.* 20 vols. 1821–33. Reprint, Hildesheim, Ger.: Olms, 1964–67.

Larrain, Carlos J., ed. and trans. *Galens Kommentar zu Platons Timaios.* Beiträge zur Altertumskunde 29. Stuttgart: Teubner, 1992.

May, Margaret Tallmadge, trans. *Galen on the Usefulness of the Parts of the Body.* 2 vols. Ithaca, NY: Cornell University Press, 1968. (See also Helmreich's edition above.)

Mewaldt, Johannes, ed. *In Hippocratis De natura hominis commentaria tria.* Corpus Medicorum Graecorum 5.9.1. Leipzig: Teubner, 1914.

Nabielek, R., ed. and trans. "Die ps.-galenische Schrift 'Über Schlaf und Wachsein' zum ersten Male herausgegeben, übersetzt und erläutert." Ph.D. diss., Humboldt-Universität zu Berlin, 1977.

Savage-Smith, Emilie, trans. "Galen on Nerves, Veins, and Arteries." Ph.D. diss., University of Wisconsin (Madison), 1969.

Schmutte, Joseph M., ed. *Galeni de consuetudinibus.* With a German translation of Ḥunayn's Arabic version by Franz Pfaff. Corpus Medicorum Graecorum, Supplement 3. Leipzig: Teubner, 1941.

Schröder, Heinrich O., ed. *In Platonis Timæum commentarii fragmenta.* Corpus Medicorum Graecorum, Supplement 1. Leipzig: Teubner, 1934.

Sider, David and Michael McVaugh, trans. "Galen on Tremor, Palpitation, Spasm and Rigor." *Transactions and Studies of the College of Physicians of Philadelphia.* Ser. 5, no. 1 (1979): 183–210.

Siegel, Rudolph E., trans. *Galen on the Affected Parts.* New York: Karger, 1976.

Singer, Peter N. *On the Thinning Diet.* In *Galen: Selected Works.* New York: Oxford University Press, 1997.

Wasserstein, Abraham, ed. and trans. *Galen's Commentary on the Hippocratic Treatise* Airs, Waters, Places: *in the Hebrew Translation of Solomon ha-Meʾati.* Proceedings of the Israel Academy of Sciences and Humanities 6.3. Jerusalem: Israel Academy of Sciences and Humanities, 1983.

Wenkebach, Ernst, ed. *Galeni in Hippocratis Epidemiarum librum III commentaria III.* Corpus Medicorum Graecorum 5.10.2.1. Leipzig: Teubner, 1936.

Wenkebach, Ernst, and Franz Pfaff, eds. *Galeni In Hippocratis Epidemiarum librum I commentaria III; In Hippocratis Epidemiarum librum II commentaria V.* Corpus Medicorum Graecorum 5.10.1. Teubner: Leipzig and Berlin, 1934.

———, eds. *Galeni in Hippocratis Epidemiarum librum VI commentaria I–VIII.* Corpus Medicorum Graecorum 5.10.2.2. Berlin: Academiae Litterarum, 1956.

## General Bibliography

Abū al-Qāsim Khalaf ibn ʿAbbās al-Zahrāwī. *Albucasis on Surgery and Instruments.* Edited and translated by M. S. Spink and G. L. Lewis. Berkeley: University of California Press, 1973.

Anastassiou, Anargyros, and Dieter Irmer, eds. *Testimonien zum Corpus Hippocraticum.* Part 2, *Galen.* Vol. 1, *Hippokrateszitate in den Kommentaren und im Glossar.* Göttingen, Ger.: Vandenhoeck and Ruprecht, 1997.

Aristotle. *Aristotle's* De anima *Translated into Hebrew by Zeraḥyah ben Isaac ben Sheʾaltiel Ḥen: A Critical Edition with an Introduction and Index.* Edited by Gerrit Bos. Leiden: Brill, 1994.

———. *Historia Animalium, History of Animals,* books 7–10. Edited and translated by David M. Balme. Loeb Classical Library 439. Cambridge, Mass.: Harvard University Press, 1991.

Beit-Arié, Malachi, comp., and R. A. May, ed. *Catalogue of the Hebrew Manuscripts in the Bodleian Library: Supplement of Addenda and Corrigenda to Vol. 1 (A. Neubauer's Catalogue).* Oxford: Clarendon, 1994. (See also Neubauer's catalogue below.)

Baron, Salo Wittmeyer. *High Middle Ages, 500–1200: Philosophy and Science.* Vol. 8 of *A Social and Religious History of the Jews.* 2nd ed., rev. and enl. New York: Columbia University Press, 1952–92.

Blau, Joshua. "At Our Place in al-Andalus, At Our Place in the Maghreb." In *Perspectives on Maimonides: Philosophical and Historical Studies,* edited by Joel L. Kraemer. Oxford: Oxford University Press, 1991.

———. *The Emergence and Linguistic Background of Judaeo-Arabic: A Study of the Origins of Middle Arabic.* Script Judaica 5. London: Oxford University Press, 1965.

Bos, Gerrit. "A Recovered Fragment on the Signs of Death from Abū Yūsuf al-Kindī's 'Medical Summaries.'" *Zeitschrift für Geschichte der arabisch-islamischen Wissenschaften* 6 (1990): 189–94.

———. "Maimonides' Medical Works and Their Contribution to His Medical Biography." Forthcoming proceedings of a congress entitled "Moses Maimonides, Talmudist, Philosopher, and Physician" (Yeshiva University and New York University, March 21–23, 2004).

———. "R. Moshe Narboni, Philosopher and Physician: A Critical Analysis of *Sefer Oraḥ Ḥayyim.*" *Medieval Encounters* 1 (1995): 219–51.

Brain, Peter. *Galen on Bloodletting: A Study of the Origins, Development and Validity of His Opinions, with a Translation of the Three Works.* Cambridge, Eng.: Cambridge University Press, 1986.

Brock, Arthur J. *Greek Medicine, Being Extracts Illustrative of Medical Writers from Hippocrates to Galen.* New York: Dutton, 1929.

Cano Ledesma, Aurora. *Indización de los manuscritos árabes de El Escorial.* Madrid: Ediciones Escurialenses, Real Monasterio de El Escorial, 1996.

Davidson, Herbert A. *Moses Maimonides: The Man and His Works.* Oxford: Oxford University Press, 2005.

Deichgräber, Karl, *Hippokrates'* De humoribus *in der Geschichte der griechischen Medizin.* Abhandlungen der Geistes- und sozialwissenschaftlichen Klasse, Jahrgang 1972, Nr. 14. Mainz: Akademie der Wissenschaften und der Literatur.

———. *Medicus gratiosus: Untersuchungen zu einem griechischen Arztbild: Mit dem Anhang* Testamentum Hippocratis *und Rhazes'* De indulgentia medici. Abhandlungen der Geistes- und sozialwissenschaftlichen Klasse, Jahrgang 1970, Nr. 3. Mainz: Akademie der Wissenschaften und der Literatur.

Derenbourg, Hartwig, comp., and Henri Paul Joseph Renaud, ed. *Médecine et histoire naturelle.* Vol. 2, fasc. 2 of *Les manuscrits arabes de l'Escurial.* Publications de l'Ecole nationale des langues orientales vivantes. Paris: LeRoux, 1939.

Deutsche Morgenländische Gessellschaft et al, eds. *Wörterbuch der klassischen arabischen Sprache.* Wiesbaden: Harrassowitz, 1957–.

Dietrich, Albert, trans. and ed. *Dioscurides triumphans: Ein anonymer arabischer Kommentar (Ende 12. Jahrh. n. Chr.) zur* Materia medica. 2 vols. Abhandlungen der Akademie der Wissenschaften in Göttingen, Philologisch-Historische Klasse, Dritte Folge, 172. Göttingen: Vandenhoeck and Ruprecht, 1988.

Dols, Michael W. *Majnūn: The Madman in Medieval Islamic Society.* Edited by Diana E. Immisch. Oxford: Clarendon, 1992.

———. *Medieval Islamic Medicine: Ibn Riḍwān's Treatise* "On the Prevention of Bodily Ills in Egypt." Berkeley: University of California Press, 1984.

Dozy, Rienhart Pieter Anne. *Supplément aux dictionnaires arabes.* 2nd ed. 2 vols. Leiden: Brill, 1927.

Durling, Richard J. *A Dictionary of Medical Terms in Galen.* Leiden: Brill, 1993.

Efros, Israel. *Philosophical Terms in the Moreh Nebukim.* Columbia University Oriental Studies 22. New York: AMS, 1924.

Endress, Gerhard, and Dimitri Gutas, eds. *A Greek and Arabic Lexicon (GALex): Materials for a Dictionary of the Mediaeval Translations from Greek into Arabic.* Fasc. 1ff. Leiden: Brill, 1992–.

Fellmann, Irene. *Das* Aqrābādhīn al-Qalānisī: *Quellenkritische und begriffsanaly-tische Untersuchungen zur arabisch-pharmazeutischen Literatur.* Beirut: Orient-Institut der Deutschen Morgenländischen Gesellschaft, 1986.

Goitein, Shelomoh D. *A Mediterranean Society: The Jewish Communities of the Arab World as Portrayed in the Documents of the Cairo Geniza.* Vol. 2, *The Community.* Berkeley: University of California Press, 1967–1993.

Goltz, Dietlinde. *Studien zur Geschichte der Mineralnamen in Pharmazie, Chemie und Medizin von den Anfängen bis Paracelsus.* Wiesbaden: Steiner, 1972.

Hinz, Walther. *Islamische Masse und Gewichte: Umgerechnet ins metrische System.* Handbuch der Orientalistik 1, Ergänzungs-band 1.1. 1955. Photomecha-nischer Nachdruck mit Zusätzen und Berichtigungen, Leiden: Brill, 1970.

Hippocrates. *Aphorisms.* In *Hippocrates.* Translated by William Henry Samuel Jones. Loeb Classical Library 147–50. 1923–1931. Reprint, Cambridge, Mass.: Harvard University Press, 1979–1984.

———. *Oeuvres complètes d'Hippocrate.* Translated by É. Littré. 10 vols. 1839–1861. Reprint, Amsterdam: Hakkert, 1973–1989.

Hopkins, S., "The Languages of Maimonides." In *The Trias of Maimonides: Jewish, Arabic, and Ancient Culture of Knowledge*, edited by G. Tamer, 85–106. Studia Judaica. Berlin: Walter de Gruyter, 2005.

Ibn Abī Uṣaybiᶜa, ᶜ*Uyūn al-anbāʾ fī ṭabaqāt al-aṭibbāʾ*. Beirut: Dār Maktabat al-Ḥayat, n.d.

Ibn al-Bayṭār. *Traité des simples*. Translated by Lucien Leclerc. 3 vols. 1877–1883. Reprint, Paris: Institut du monde arabe, 1987.

Ibn Isḥāq, Ḥunayn. *Ḥunain ibn Isḥāq über die syrischen und arabischen Galen-Übersetzungen*. Edited by Gotthelf Bergsträsser. Leipzig: Brockhaus, 1925.

———. *Neue Materialien zu Ḥunain ibn Isḥāq's Galen-Bibliographie*. Edited by Gotthelf Bergsträsser. Abhandlungen für die Kunde des Morgenländes 19.2. Leipzig: Deutsche Morgenländische Gesellschaft, 1932.

Ibn Sahl, Sābūr. *Dispensatorium parvum (Al-aqrābādhīn al-ṣaghīr)*. Edited by Oliver Kahl. Islamic Philosophy, Theology, and Science: Texts and Studies 16. Leiden: Brill, 1994.

Kahle, Paul. "Mosis Maimonidis Aphorismorum praefatio et excerpta." In *Galeni in Platonis Timaeum commentarii fragmenta*. Edited by Heinrich Otto Schröder. Corpus Medicorum Graecorum, Supplement 1. Berlin: Teubner, 1934.

Kamal, Hassan. *Encyclopaedia of Islamic Medicine, with a Greco-Roman Background*. Cairo: General Egyptian Book Organization, 1975.

Kaufmann, David. "Le neveu de Maïmonide." *Revue des études juives* 7 (1883): 152–53.

Koningsveld, P. Sj. van. "Andalusian-Arabic Manuscripts from Christian Spain: A Comparative, Intercultural Approach." *Israel Oriental Studies* 12 (1992): 75–110.

Kraemer, Joel L. "Six Unpublished Maimonides Letters from the Cairo Genizah." *Maimonidean Studies* 2, no. 1 (1991): 61–94.

Lane, Edward William. *Arabic-English Lexicon*. London: Williams and Norgate, 1863–1879.

Langermann, Y. Tzvi. "Arabic Writings in Hebrew Manuscripts: A Preliminary Listing." *Arabic Sciences and Philosophy* 6, no. 1 (March 1996): 137–60.

———. "Fūṣūl Mūsā and Maimonides' Method of Composition." Paper presented at "Moses Maimonides, Talmudist, Philosopher, and Physician," a conference held at Yeshiva University and New York University, New York City, March 21–23, 2004.

Larrain, Carlos J. "Galen, *De motibus dubiis:* Die lateinische Übersetzung des Niccolò da Reggio." *Traditio* 49 (1994): 171–233.

Mājūsī, Alī ibn al ᶜAbbās. *Kāmil al-Ṣināᶜa al-ṭibbīya*, 2 vols. Cairo: Būlāq, 1877.

Meyerhof, Max. "The Medical Work of Maimonides." In *Essays on Maimonides: An Octocentennial Volume*, edited by Salo Wittmayer Baron, 265–99. New York: Columbia University Press, 1941.

———. "Über echte und unechte Schriften Galens, nach arabischen Quellen." *Sitzungsberichte der Preussischen Akademie der Wissenschaften: Philosophisch-historische Klasse* 28 (1928): 533–48.

Neubauer, Adolf. *Catalogue of the Hebrew Manuscripts in the Bodleian Library and in the College Libraries of Oxford.* 1886–1906. Reprint, Oxford: Clarendon, 1994. (See also Beit-Arié's supplement above.)

Pertsch, Wilhelm. *Die orientalischen Handschriften der Herzoglichen Bibliothek zu Gotha.* Part 3, *Die arabischen Handschriften.* Vols. 1–5. Vienna: Kais. Kön. Hof- und Staatsdruckerei, 1859–1893.

Ravitzky, Aviezer. "Mishnato shel R. Zeraḥyah ben Isaac ben She²altiel Ḥen." Ph.D. diss., Hebrew University, 1977.

Richter-Bernburg, Lutz, trans. "Eine arabische Version der pseudogalenischen Schrift *De Theriaca ad Pisonem.*" Ph.D. diss., University of Göttingen, 1969.

Rufus of Ephesus. *Krankenjournale.* Edited and translated by Manfred Ullmann. Wiesbaden: Harrassowitz, 1978.

Schacht, Joseph, and Max Meyerhof. "Maimonides against Galen, on Philosophy and Cosmogony." *Bulletin of the Faculty of Arts of the University of Egypt* 5, no. 1 (1937): 53–88 (Arabic section).

Scheyer, Simon B. *Das psychologische System des Maimonides: eine Einleitungschrift zu dessen* More Nebuchim. Frankfurt: Kessler, 1845.

Schmucker, Werner. *Die pflanzliche und mineralische Materia medica im* Firdaus al-Ḥikma *des Ṭabarī.* Bonn: Im Selbstverlag des Orientalischen Seminars der Universität Bonn, 1969.

Sezgin, Fuat. *Geschichte des arabischen Schrifttums.* Vol. 3, *Medizin-Pharmazie-Zoologie-Tierheilkunde bis ca. 430 H.* Leiden: Brill, 1970.

Sirat, Colette. "Une liste de manuscrits du Dalālat al-ḥayryn." *Maimonidean Studies* 4 (2000): 109–33.

Steinschneider, Moritz. "Die griechischen Ärzte in arabischen Übersetzungen." *Virchows Archiv* 124 (1891): 115–36, 268–96, 455–87.

———. *Die Handschriften-Verzeichnisse der Königlichen Bibliothek zu Berlin: Verzeichniss der hebräischen Handschriften.* 2 vols. 1878–1897. Reprint in 1 vol., Hildesheim: Olms, 1980.

———. *Die hebräischen Handschriften der K. Hof- und Staatsbibliothek in München.* 2nd ed., rev. and enl. Munich: Palm'sche Hofbuchhandlung, 1895.

———. *Die hebräischen Übersetzungen des Mittelalters und die Juden als Dolmetscher.* 1893. Reprint, Graz, Austria: Akademische Druck- und Verlagsanstalt, 1956.

Strohmaier, G. "Der syrische und arabische Galen." *Aufstieg und Niedergang der römischen Welt.* Part 2, *Principat,* 37.2. Berlin: de Gruyter, 1994.

Temkin, Owsei. *Galenism: Rise and Decline of a Medical Philosophy.* Ithaca, NY: Cornell University Press, 1973.

Ullmann, Manfred. *Die Medizin im Islam.* Handbuch der Orientalistik 1, Ergänzungsband 6.1. Leiden: Brill, 1970.

———. *Islamic medicine.* Translated by Jean Watt. Edinburgh: Edinburgh University Press, 1978.

Vajda, Georges. *Index général des manuscrits arabes musulmans de la Bibliothèque nationale de Paris.* Publication de l'Institut de recherche et d'histoire des textes 4. Paris: Éditions du Centre national de la recherche scientifique, 1953.

Vogelstein, Hermann, and Paul Rieger. *Geschichte der Juden in Rom.* 2 vols. Berlin: Mayer und Müller, 1895–96.

Voorhoeve, Petrus, comp. *Handlist of Arabic Manuscripts in the Library of the University of Leiden and Other Collections in the Netherlands.* 2nd ed., enl. Boston: Leiden University Press, 1980.

Waines, D., "*Murrī*, the tale of a condiment." *Al-Qantara* 12 (1991): 371–88.

Zotenberg, Hermann, ed. *Manuscrits orientaux: Catalogues des manuscrits hébreux et samaritains de la Bibliothèque impériale.* Paris: Imprimerie impériale, 1866.

# Index of Subjects

*Note: The 0 (zero) refers to the introduction; the numbers before and after the dot refer to the respective chapters and paragraphs.*

superfluity/superfluities, 6.30; 7.24, 32;
    8.13, 17, 47, 49, 63; 9.3, 12, 76, 80
  bilious, 6.35; 8.28
  biting, 7.63
  purely acid, 9.79
  raw uncooked, 8.28
suppository, 9.47, 48
suppuration, 9.118
surgery, 9.102, 124
surmise, 6.93
surplus, 7.14
  of watery moisture, 6.12
swallowing, 9.32
swamps, 8.71
sweat, 6.12
  cold, 6.63
  taste of, 6.65
  that dries up on the face, 6.13
sweating, 6.12
swelling, 9.15, 32, 33, 125
  hard, 6.66
  inflamed, 6.66
  of the uvula, throat, and tonsils, 9.123
  *See also* diaphragm, muscle, testicles
symptom, 6.5; 7.68; 8.40. *See also* phrenitis
symptoms, 6.14, 37, 54, 55, 88, 95; 7.22,
    68; 8.41; 9.91
  bad and malignant, 6.91
  kinds of, 7.8
  very severe, 9.109
syncope, 6.91; 7.9, 11–13, 15, 42; 8.21, 41,
    76; 9.42, 49, 53, 100, 116
  causes of, 7.8, 9, 14
  healing of, 7.8
  quick collapse of the faculties, 7.10
  sudden and rapid, 9.43
systems, 8.44

tamarisk, 9.88
Ṭāmimī, al-, 9.30, 123
tapeworms, 7.31
taste, 6.65
  bitter, 9.73
  faculty of, 7.70
  sense of, 7.73
  *See also* sweat
tear, acid, 6.37
teeth, 7.34; 9.29
temperament, 7.15; 8.25, 63; 9.71
  bad, 6.41, 43, 58; 7.62; 8.44, 45
  balance of the, 7.13
  cold bad, 9.65
  dry bad, 9.66
  hot, 9.104

hot bad, 7.26; 9.46
irregular bad, 9.36
warm, 8.63
warm and moist, 9.97
*See also* esophagus, heart, humors, liver,
    moistures, organs, stomach
temperatures, 6.6
tendons, 9.120
tension, 6.35
testicles, 7.48
  of roosters, 9.116
therapy, 8.7; 9.87, 124
theriac, 9.86. 103
thickness, 7.13, 19, 40; 8.19. *See also*
    humors
thighs, 6.71
things, 8.2; 9.54
  alleviating, 8.6
  astringent, 9.46, 50, 69
  biting, 9.52
  cold, 7.53
  harmful, 8.29
thinking, 7.4
thinness. *See* humors, pneumata, vessels
thirst, 6.9, 41
  lack of, 6.37
  severe, 6.55, 57, 71; 7.57; 8.24
  severity of the, 6.41
thought(s), 6.94
  and considerations, 8.31
  evil, 9.110
  joyful, 8.32
  sad, 8.32
throat
  illness of the, 9.32
  roughness of the, 6.41
  *See also* swelling
throwing up. *See* bile
thyme, 9.88
tickling, 7.71
tissue, 6.82
tongue, 6.24; 7.70; 9.11
  black, 6.51
  colors of the, 6.19
  dry, 6.19
  movement of the, 6.36
  red and black, 6.55
  roughness of the, 6.37
tonsils. *See* swelling
tooth, 7.33
  extraction of a painful, 7.33
  root of the, 7.33
torpor, 9.11, 12, 17, 18, 23, 24, 35, 43
  heavy, 8.27

*About the Editor / Translator*

GERRIT BOS, chair of the Martin Buber Institute for Jewish Studies at the University of Cologne, was born in the Netherlands and educated both there and in Jerusalem. He is proficient in classical and Semitic languages, as well as in Jewish and Islamic studies. He has been research assistant at the Free University in Amsterdam, a research fellow and lecturer at University College in London, a tutor in Jewish studies at Leo Baeck College in London, and a Wellcome Institute research fellow. He currently resides in Germany with his wife and three children.

Professor Bos is widely published in the fields of Jewish studies, Islamic studies, Judaeo-Arabic texts, and medieval Islamic science and medicine, having many books and articles to his credit. In addition to preparing The Medical Works of Moses Maimonides, Professor Bos is also involved with a series of middle Hebrew medical-botanical texts, an edition of Ibn al-Jazzār's *Zād al-musāfir* (Viaticum), and an edition of Averroës' commentary on the zoological works of Aristotle, extant only in Hebrew and Latin translations. He recently received the Maurice Amado award for his work on Maimonides' medical texts.

*A Note on the Type*

The English text of this book was set in BASKERVILLE, a typeface originally designed by John Baskerville (1706–1775), a British stonecutter, letter designer, typefounder, and printer. The Baskerville type is considered to be one of the first "transitional" faces—a deliberate move away from the "old style" of the Continental humanist printer. Its rounded letterforms presented a greater differentiation of thick and thin strokes, the serifs on the lowercase letters were more nearly horizontal, and the stress was nearer the vertical—all of which would later influence the "modern" style undertaken by Bodoni and Didot in the 1790s. Because of its high readability, particularly in long texts, the type was subsequently copied by all major typefoundries. (The original punches and matrices still survive today at Cambridge University Press.) This adaptation, designed by the Compugraphic Corporation in the 1960s, is a notable departure from other versions of the Baskerville typeface by its overall typographic evenness and lightness in color. To enhance its range, supplemental diacritics and ligatures were created in 1997 for the exclusive use of the Middle Eastern Texts Initiative.

TYPOGRAPHY BY JONATHAN SALTZMAN

◆